Principles and Choice of Laser Treatment in Dermatology

Jae Dong Lee • Jong Kook Lee
Min Jin Maya Oh

Principles and Choice of Laser Treatment in Dermatology

With Special Reference to the Asian Population

Springer

Jae Dong Lee
MISODAM Clinic
Daejeon
Republic of Korea

Min Jin Maya Oh
ARA Clinic
Incheon
Republic of Korea

Jong Kook Lee
Research and Development
Cyberlogitec, Inc.
Seoul
Republic of Korea

ISBN 978-981-15-6555-7 ISBN 978-981-15-6556-4 (eBook)
https://doi.org/10.1007/978-981-15-6556-4

This Springer imprint is published by the registered company Springer Nature Singapore Pte Ltd.
The registered company address is: 152 Beach Road, #21-01/04 Gateway East, Singapore 189721, Singapore

Preface

I run a small aesthetic clinic in Korea. During years of skin laser procedures, many questions came to my mind, which I tried to answer by searching for relevant papers or books. Searching for these answers led me to write this book. I would like to clarify that this book is about Korean patients, and from the perspective of a private-practice laser physician. Since Korean skin is similar to Chinese or Japanese, this book may be helpful to private-practice doctors in China or Japan. Also, because the principle of lasers does not change, I believe that by applying the principle of lasers this book may also be of help to private-practice doctors in other countries. Most of all, I am sure that this book will help you answer many of the questions that the laser physician faces daily during skin laser procedures.

It would be ideal to write a medical book based on the papers that the author has personally experimented and published, but in private practice this is quite difficult. This is why I selected and inserted various portions of papers and books that I found relevant and which matched my experience. I also added my personal comments regarding these contents.

From childhood, I found memorizing without understanding very difficult. This led me to love mathematics and physics. Biology and medical studies were rather difficult for me. Fortunately, understanding skin laser required a lot of physics, which made this topic so intriguing for me. However, most papers regarding skin lasers disregarded physics and compared only clinical results, resulting in inconsistent results from paper to paper. Also, it was disappointing to see that most private-practice physicians used only the manufacturer's recommended parameters without thinking about the principle. Fortunately, through the papers and books of world-renowned scholars, I was able to think straight. In particular, I would like to thank and pay tribute and respect to Richard Rox Anderson and Edward Victor Ross Jr.

I would especially like to thank my wife, Mi Ran. Without her support this book would not have been possible. I would also like to thank my two children, my trustworthy and kind firstborn son Jeong Jin and cute and diligent youngest son Yoo Jin. Jeong Jin! You are a son that every father wants. You can do anything! Please remember that your Dad loves you very very much.

Finally, even though it is becoming increasingly difficult for private practices, I hope that my book may be a small beacon for private-practice laser physicians. Let us all shout a Korean cheer!

Aza Aza Fighting!

Daejeon, Republic of Korea Jae Dong Lee
30 April 2020

Contents

About the Authors

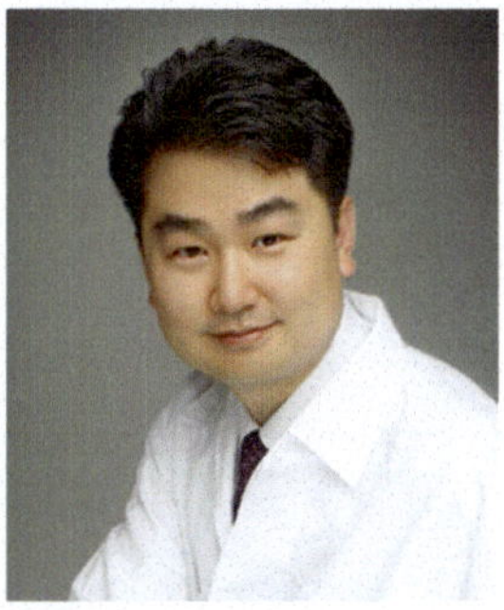

Jae Dong Lee, MD Graduated from Medical College of the Catholic University of Korea

The degree of Master of Medical Science in the Catholic University of Korea

The Chief Academic Officer in Korean Medical Skin Care Society

The Laser Academic Officer in Korean Aesthetic Surgery and Laser Society

The Chairman in Korean Dermatologic Laser Association

Director in MISODAM clinic in Daejeon, Korea

(Writing)

The principles and choice of laser in dermatology (Korean language)

Melasma, diagnosis and treatment of melasma (Korean language)

Laser dermatology: Choice and treatment (Korean language)

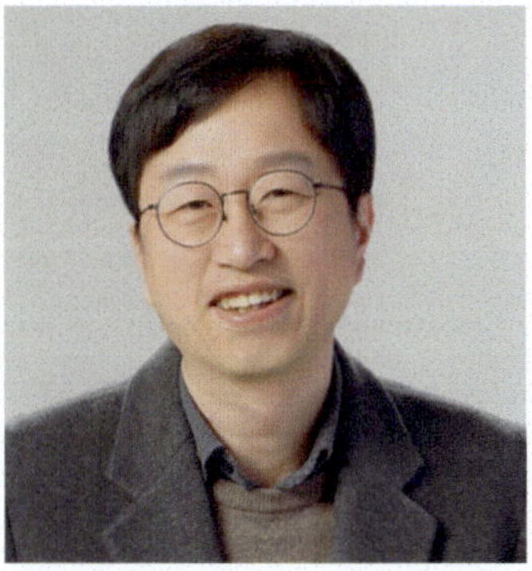

Jong Kook Lee Bachelor of Physics in Korea University

Master of Statistical Physics in Korea University

Ph.D. Candidate of Software Engineering in Soongsil University

Manager of R&D team in Cyberlogitec, Inc.

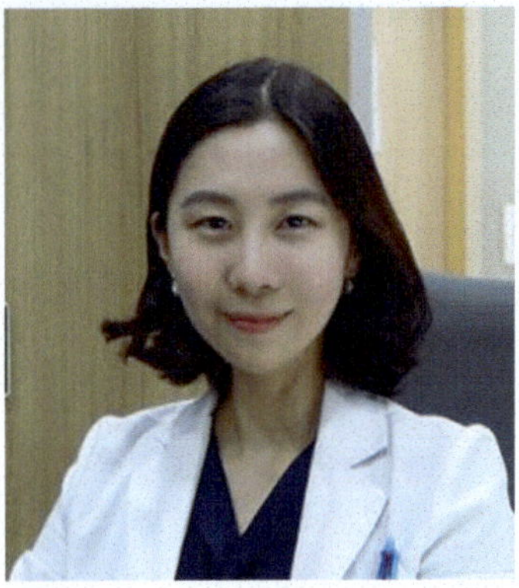

Min Jin Maya Oh, MD Graduated from Medical College of the Catholic University of Korea

The Academic Officer in Korean Academy of Melasma

The Vice-Chairman in Korean Dermatologic Laser Association

Former AsiaPacific Regional Therapeutic Expert for Botox, Allergan

Former Medical reviewer for MFDS (Ministry of Food and Drug Safety)

Director in ARA clinic in Incheon, Korea

Part I

Understanding Lasers and Laser-Tissue Interactions

Principles of Laser

1

1.1 Generation of Laser

The world consists of light and matter. When light and matter meet, they interact with each other and make various physical and chemical changes. For example, if you stand under the clear autumn sky, you can feel your body warming up even in the cool weather (Fig. 1.1). This phenomenon occurs when light is converted into heat in the skin. Conversely, light can be created by applying energy to a material. This phenomenon is used when laser is made.

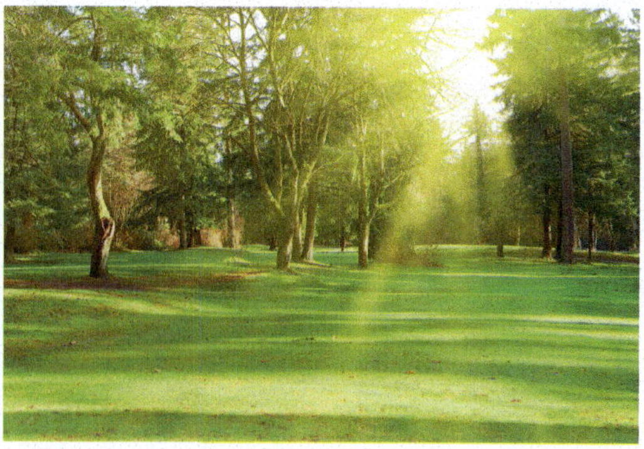

Fig. 1.1 Light and matter

1.1.1 Electromagnetic Radiation

Light refers mainly to the visible range (400–760 nm). But visible light refers to light in the narrow sense, while light in the broad sense refers to electromagnetic radiation (EMR). Electromagnetic waves are all the energy that travels in space in the form of waves by electric and magnetic fields [2]. Electromagnetic waves range from visible rays to short wavelengths of γ-rays and X-rays to the long wavelengths of microwaves and radio waves (Fig. 1.2). Electromagnetic waves have both the properties of waves and energy-bearing particles (photons). This is called wave–particle duality [3]. In the macroscopic world, which is usually visible, it exhibits properties of waves, but in the microscopic world, which can only be seen under a microscope, it exhibits properties of particles.

Each electromagnetic wave has its own wavelength and frequency [4]. Lasers used mainly in the dermatologic field express electromagnetic waves with nanometer (nm), which is a unit of wave. The electromagnetic spectrum used in the dermatological field includes ultraviolet (UV), visible, near-infrared (NIR), mid-infrared (MIR) and far-infrared (FIR) (Table 1.1) [2].

J. D. Lee et al., *Principles and Choice of Laser Treatment in Dermatology*,
https://doi.org/10.1007/978-981-15-6556-4_1

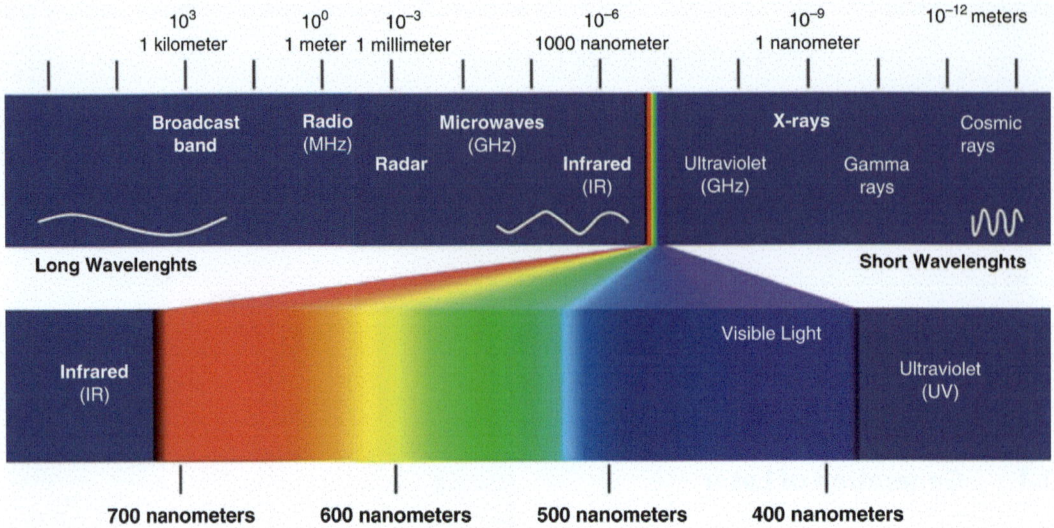

Fig. 1.2 The electromagnetic spectrum. (Reproduced from [1])

Table 1.1 The range and wavelength of electromagnetic waves

Range	Nanometer
Ultraviolet (UV)	200–400
Visual	400–760
Near-infrared (NIR)	760–1400
Mid-infrared (MIR)	1400–3000
Far-infrared (FIR)	>3000

1.1.2 Principles of Laser Generation

The most basic unit of light is photon and the most basic unit of matter is atom. Atoms are composed of a nucleus, containing positively charged protons and neutral neutrons. Negatively charged electrons orbit the nucleus (Fig. 1.3). Electrons orbit in a stable resting state (ground state). This state is the state of lowest energy. When energy comes in from the outside (this is called pumping), the ground state electrons jump to a higher energy level at a position further from the nucleus and will then be in an excited state. But the excited state is a very unstable state and the electron will try to return to the stable ground state. As the excited electrons return to their resting state, they release the energy in the form of photons with the orbit energy difference. This is called spontaneous emission [2].

An Intuitive Explanation about Spontaneous Emission. (Explanation by Physicist Dr. Jong Gook Lee) [5, 6]
To intuitively explain the principle of laser such as spontaneous and stimulated emission, the interaction of atoms and light should be first understood.

First, let's think of light as a particle (photon) and not as wave. Particles are countable (one, two…). Atoms can be excited or unexcited when they receive energy. Atoms are composed of a nucleus and electrons. Light interacts with electrons. When the electron absorbs light, it becomes excited and the energy of the electron increases, and when the electron emits light, the energy of the electron decreases. Now let's suppose that atoms are a staircase on which electrons go up and down. The excited state of atoms means that electrons go up on the staircase. (Atoms and electrons will be distinguished in the following contents. Electrons can be thought of as particles that go up the staircase.)

When we played rock–paper–scissors during our childhood, we went up one

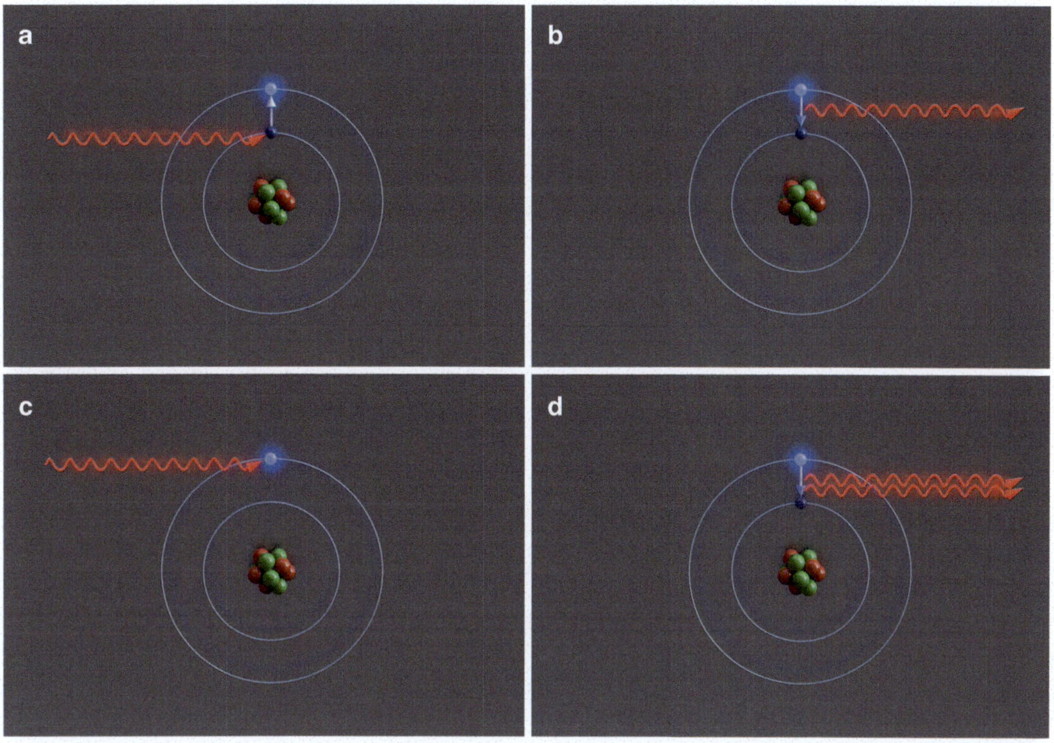

Fig. 1.3 Spontaneous and stimulated emission. The electron is usually located in a low energy orbit (resting state). (**a**) If an electron absorbs energy, it goes up to the excited state. (**b**) As the electron in the unstable and excited state goes back to the low energy state (resting state), it emits photons (spontaneous emission). (**c**) If the already excited electron absorbs yet another photon, (**d**) as the electron return to the resting state, it will emit two photons with the same energy, direction, and frequency (stimulated emission). (Published with kind permission of © Jin Kwon Cho 2019. All rights reserved. Modified from [1])

staircase if we won and went down one staircase if we lost. Similarly, when electron receives a photon, it goes up the staircase and is excited. The bottom of the stairs is the lowest energy state, which is the resting state. The stairs (atoms) on which electrons go up and down are already determined. Let's think about an atom of which the staircase consists only of a resting state and an excited state.

The input light (Fig. 1.4) is considered as a particle (photon) from the atom's point of view. The light enters as a wave but is a particle from the atom's perspective. This concept is called wave–particle duality. The electron in the resting state absorbs photons and goes up the staircase and become excited. The height of the stairs varies from atom to atom, which represents the energy of the photon which can be absorbed by electrons. If a photon with a higher or lower energy than the height of the stairs is thrown at the electron, the electron will not be able to absorb the photon. Electrons have a picky appetite. Electrons can only stay in an excited state for a short period of time and as the excited electrons return to their resting state, they must emit the same number of photons previously absorbed. The emitted photon should have the energy corresponding to the height of the stairs. In conclusion, electrons release the energy previously absorbed (Fig. 1.5).

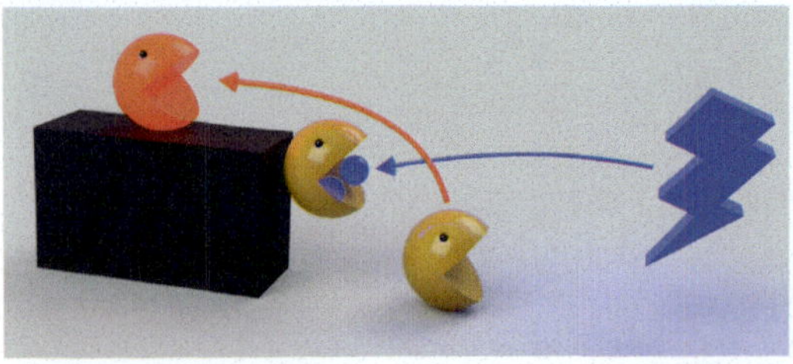

Fig. 1.4 The electron (packman) in the resting state becomes excited when it absorbs light (photon). (Published with kind permission of © Jin Kwon Cho 2019. All rights reserved)

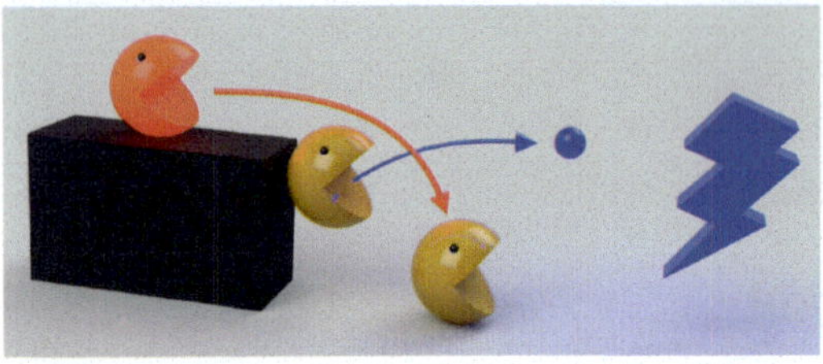

Fig. 1.5 The excited electron (packman) emits light (photon) when returning to the resting state. (Published with kind permission of © Jin Kwon Cho 2019. All rights reserved)

The higher the height of the stairs, the more energy the electron returns. If the height of the stairs is very high, the energy becomes X-rays and γ-rays. If the height of the stairs is very low, the energy becomes infrared light (Energy is inversely proportional to wavelength.)

$$E = \mathrm{h} \cdot v = \frac{\mathrm{h} \cdot c}{\lambda}$$

E: energy of radiation, h: Planck's constant (6.6×10^{-34} Js), *v*: frequency, *c*: constant velocity (299,790 km/s), λ: wave.

Another thing to note is that the excited electrons do not always return to the resting state. However, it is likely that electrons return to the resting state. Also, the electrons in the resting state do not always absorb photons but have a high probability of absorbing photons. Thus, everything in the atomic world is represented by probability.

The above is summarized as follows:

1. Light behaves as particles when entering a microscopic world such as atoms, but they behave as waves in the macroscopic world.
2. Each atom has its own energy staircase.
3. Whether the electron is in the ground state, goes up to the excited state, or comes down from the excited state to the ground state is all decided by probability.
4. Eye for an eye: Electrons return the same amount of energy previously absorbed.
5. The electron only absorbs photons with energy as high as the height of the stairs.

The emitted photons produce the light of a certain wavelength depending on the atoms. In nature, various lights are produced because various atoms are mixed in nature. For example, light from a match is usually red, while light from the stove is mostly blue. This can be easily understood if atoms are thought of as springs. Some springs are strong while others are weak. Regardless of the force applied, the time that spring is stretched and reduced according to its strength is constant. Similarly, atoms have their own frequency (or wavelength) which is called the atom's natural frequency. Atoms emit light as much as it vibrates and the wavelength of the emitted light is inversely proportional to the atom's natural frequency. Thus, if made up of single atoms, only one wavelength of light will be produced. This is the principle of monochromaticity, a characteristic of laser [4].

In some cases, the naturally emitted photons may meet electrons of atoms in excited states. An interesting phenomenon occurs at this time. As the electrons return to the resting state, they emit two photons. This phenomenon is called stimulated emission [2]. The two stimulated emitted photons have the same energy, same shape in time, and space just like twins. This is the principle of coherence, a characteristic of laser [2]. If these two twin photons meet two electrons, then four twin photons are emitted. The four photons emit 8, 16, and 32 photons again, i.e., they increase exponentially. This is the principle of high intensity, a characteristic of laser.

In 1917, Einstein published the theory of stimulated emission of radiation, which is the principle of laser generation [4].

An Intuitive Explanation about Stimulated Emission. (Explanation by Physicist Dr. Jong Kook Lee)

In the above explanation of spontaneous emission, only the irradiation of light to the atoms in resting state was considered. Now let's think about what will happen when light is irradiated to an excited atom. Light with the energy which is equal to the height of stairs should be irradiated; nothing will happen if the energy is larger or smaller. As previously explained, all is decided by probability in the atomic world. Let's think of the electron on top of the stair as a person on top of the mountain. If the wind blows softly, there is little chance that the person will fall from the top but if a typhoon blows, the chances are greater. Likewise, if a photon is thrown at an excited electron, the likelihood that the electron falls to the ground is greatly increased. Throwing photons at excited electrons and making them fall to the resting state is called stimulated emission. The excited light is not absorbed by the electrons, but rather the photons shake electrons, just as the wind shakes the person. However, the electron that falls to the ground must emit photons, so two photons pop out (Fig. 1.6).

Two photons mean that light with twice the energy comes out. In other words, the light coming out is twice as bright as the input light. Matter consists of many atoms. What if all the atoms are excited and they all receive one photon? Because the electron that receives one photon returns two photons and the electrons that receive these photons also return two photons each, ultimately, numerous photons pop out of the matter (Fig. 1.7). These photons have the same energy and become light with the same wavelength, which is laser.

1.1.3 Composition of Laser

The conversion of electrons into the excited state is called "population inversion" [2], and in this state, photons are created exponentially with as many as 10^{20} photons when stimulated emission occurs [4]. Because light travels, if the medium is long enough, it can produce many photons. But because of space constraints, two mirrors are placed at each end of the laser medium and the photons travel between the two mirrors, creating photons exponentially. In this process, the photons that are not reflected vertically to the mirror disappear and only the vertically reflected photons remain (Fig. 1.8). That is the principle of collimation, a characteristic of lasers [2].

One of the two mirrors reflect 100% of light, another mirror passes through the light partially so that some of the stimulated photons go off the two mirrors, past the delivery device, and are col-

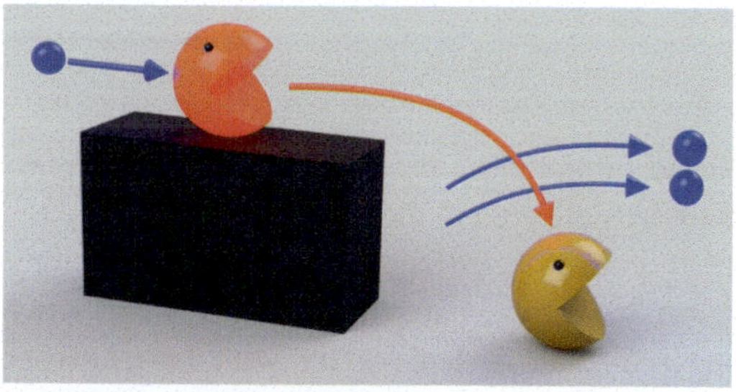

Fig. 1.6 When an excited electron (packman) meets a photon, they fall down to the ground state and two photons pop out. These two photons have the same energy. (Published with kind permission of © Jin Kwon Cho 2019. All rights reserved)

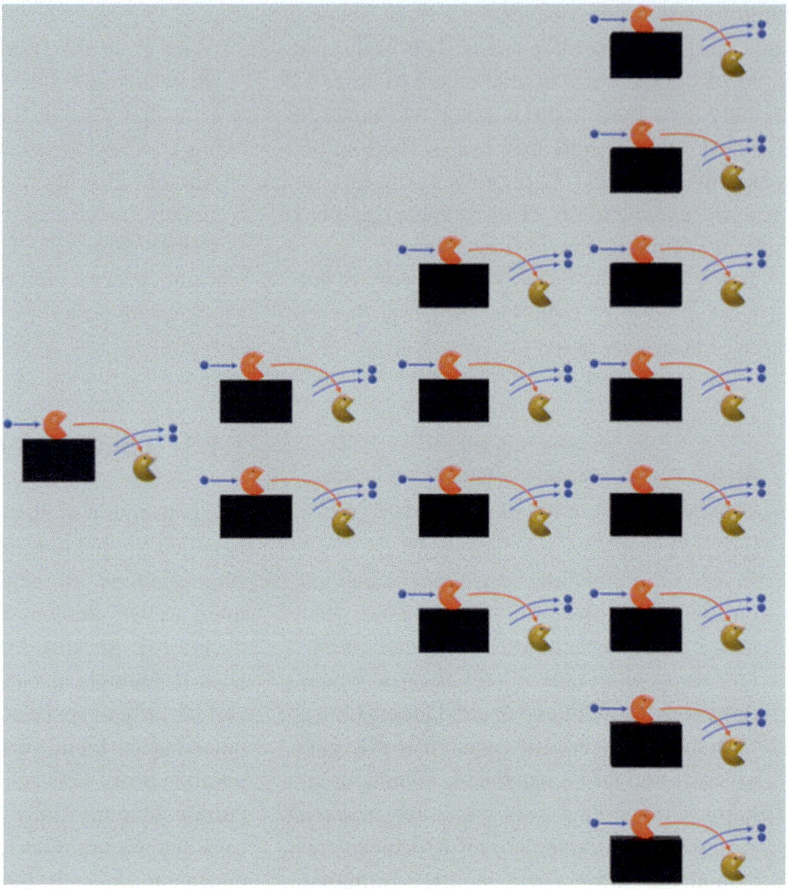

Fig. 1.7. Two photons meet four excited electrons and create four photons. In this way, photon is amplified to produce bright light. (Published with kind permission of © Jin Kwon Cho 2019. All rights reserved)

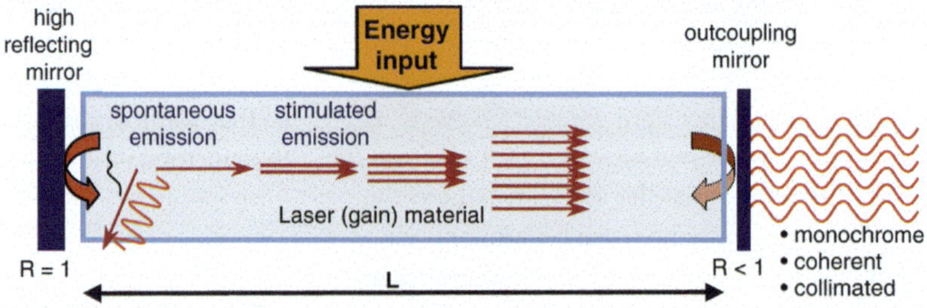

Fig. 1.8 Principle of a laser. (Reproduced from [3])

lected in one place by the lens. Ultimately photons are delivered to the skin (Fig. 1.9).

If you look inside the laser machine, they consist of three parts: pumping system, laser medium, and optical cavity with two mirrors [2]. Additional devices are the cooling device and the delivery system. External energy source serves to supply energy (pumping) and laser medium excites the electrons by the energy received from outside. Electricity or flashlamp is used as an external energy source. The typical laser that uses electricity as external energy source is CO_2 laser and the typical laser that uses flashlamp as external energy source is Q-switched laser.

In laser mediums, there are gas types (CO_2 and argon), liquid types (dye), and solid types (ruby, alexandrite, Nd:YAG, and diode). The wavelength of the laser is determined by the laser medium [2]. For example, CO_2 generates 10,600 nm wavelength, ruby 694 nm wavelength, and alexandrite 755 nm wavelength (Table 1.2).

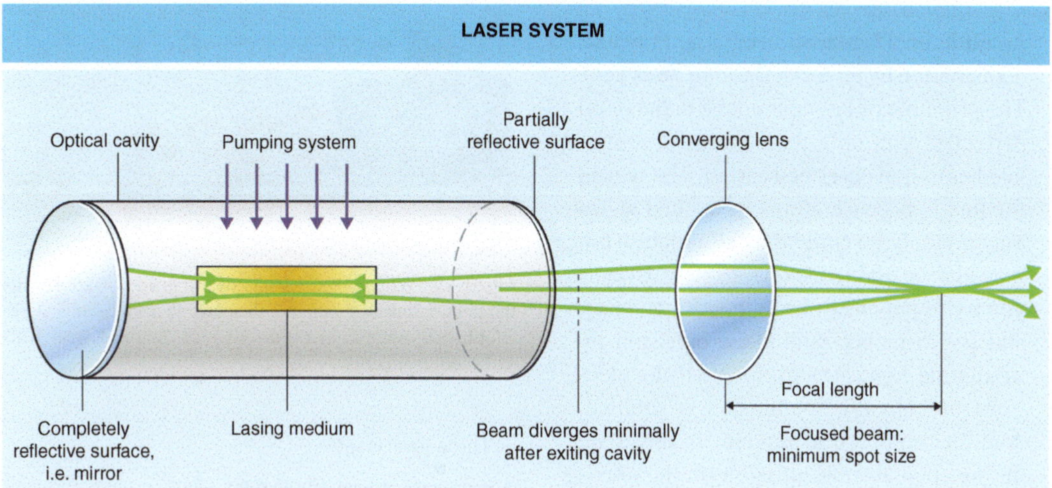

Fig. 1.9 Laser system. Laser consists of lasing medium, pumping system, optical cavity, and delivery system. (Reproduced from [7])

Table 1.2 Laser media and wavelength. (Modified from [2])

Laser type	Lasing media	Wavelength (nm)
Liquid	Dye	585, 595
Gas	CO_2	10,600
	Argon	510
	Excimer	308
Solid	Ruby	694
	Alexandrite	755
	Er:YAG	2940
	Nd:YAG	1064, 1320
	Diode	808, 810, 1450

So, when we talk about the type of laser, when you say ruby laser we know that the wavelength of the laser is 694 nm, and vice versa. Therefore, we must know the wavelength corresponding to the laser medium.

However, Nd:YAG laser can produce 1064, 1320 nm, etc., and diode laser can produce 808, 810, 1450 nm, etc. In other words, some lasers are able to produce multiple wavelengths with one medium. This is why when describing a laser, the wavelength and medium must be described together. For example, "694-nm ruby laser." In addition, because the laser machine itself varies depending on the irradiation time, the irradiation time should also be described. However, I say simply "Q694" or "long1064" in conversation or lectures because of long name.

IPL (intense pulsed light) is different from laser in that it does not have a laser medium and optical cavity. It only has flashlamp as the external energy source [4]. Flashlamps are different from single-wavelength lasers because they emit a variety of lights. Flashlamps are surrounded by water so that wavelength above 1000 nm with high water absorption coefficient is absorbed by the water and disappear, so that only the light below 1000 nm is emitted. If UV wavelength is cut off by the optical cutoff filter, 500–1000 nm wavelength light can be emitted. Various wavelength bands can be selected depending on the optical filter. For example, 640-nm filter emits light in the wavelength range of 640–1000 nm.

1.1.4 Three-Level and Four-Level Lasers

For stimulated emission, the electron in the ground state should move to the excited state. But excited state is unstable so that electrons should move to the ground state before stimulated emission. Therefore, there are no two-level lasers in which only the ground state and the excited state exist. To prevent returning to the ground state, mediums with metastable state—which is a stable state between ground state and excited state—are used in real lasers [8].

An Additional Explanation of Laser Principle (Explanation by Physicist Dr. Jong Kook Lee)

The principle of laser cannot be understood perfectly, with only the concept of stimulated emission described earlier. The reason for this is because atoms in excited states may not only be emitted by stimulation but may also be emitted spontaneously. Even if you try to put electrons in the excited state, and try to induce stimulated emission by irradiating light, it is of no use if the electrons are already spontaneously emitted. And electrons fall at random in any state during spontaneous emission (in the previous figures, ground state was expressed as if it was one, but in fact, there are several ground states) so that miscellaneous kinds of light are emitted and some of the light are absorbed by the electrons again. As a result, light with less energy than the input is emitted. Therefore, it is necessary to have a mechanism that su ppresses spontaneous emission and proceeds only with stimulated emission (Fig. 1.10).

In Fig. 1.10, the concept of metastable state is introduced. Special materials can be used to create metastable states. The rule for changing electron's state is as follows

1. The electrons in the ground state rise up to the excited state by the pumping process.
2. But the excited electron cannot fall to the ground state. It can only fall to the metastable state.

The excited electrons accumulate in a metastable state over time. When a lot of electrons accumulate in the metastable state and light is irradiated, strong light is emitted and the laser we want can be produced.

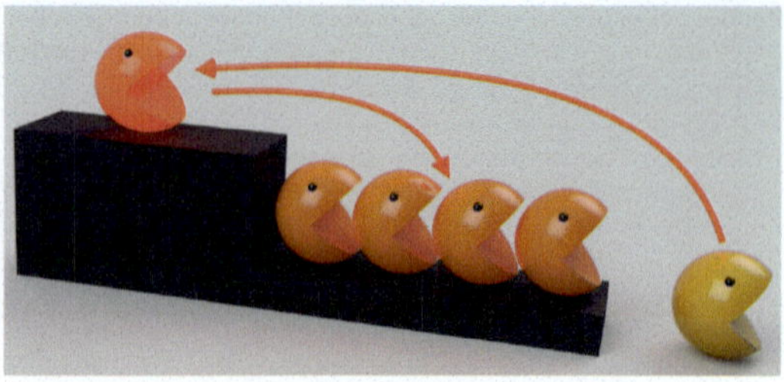

Fig. 1.10 When the electrons in the ground state rise to unstable excited state, it falls back to metastable state. (Published with kind permission of © Jin Kwon Cho 2019. All rights reserved)

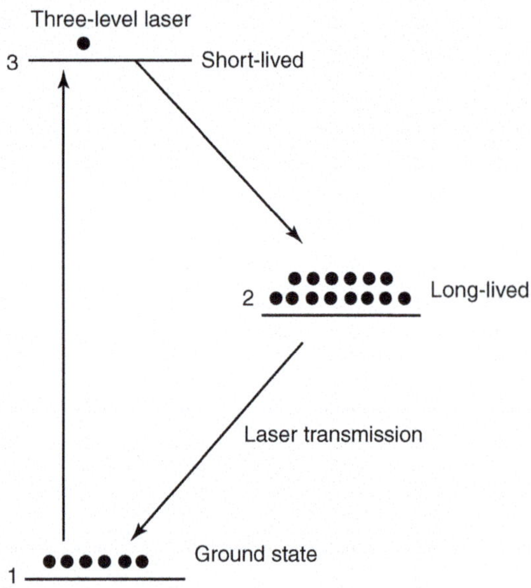

Fig. 1.11 For a three-level laser system, it is possible to achieve a larger population of level 2, as compared to the ground state, by very intense pumping form level 1 to level 2. (Reproduced from [9])

Thus, the laser which has ground, excited, and metastable state is called the three-level laser and the laser that has two metastable state is called the four-level laser. The typical three- and four-level lasers are ruby laser and Nd:YAG laser (Figs. 1.11 and 1.12) [3].

In three-level laser, lower laser level is ground state so that there are many electrons in low energy level. Therefore, high energy is needed for population inversion and a flash lamp with high output is used. Thus three-level lasers are usually pulsed-wave lasers. Because three-level laser needs high output, this makes them expensive but, the laser can produce very high energy (pulse energy 20 J). On the other hand, four-level lasers need low energy for population inversion so that low output flashlamp can be used. Therefore, most continuous-wave lasers use four-level laser [3].

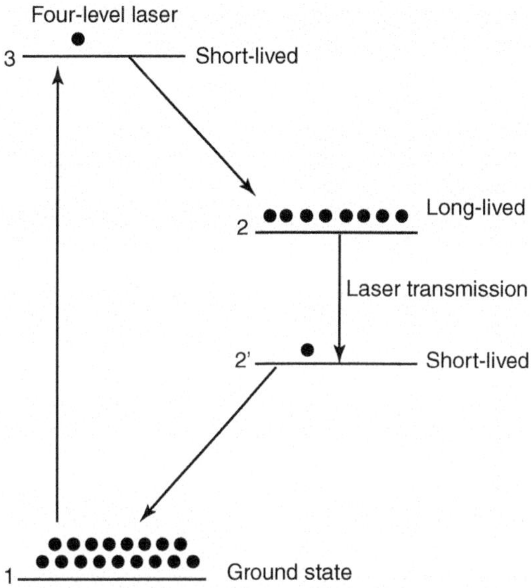

Fig. 1.12 For a four-level laser system, it is possible to achieve, even by weak pumping into the long-lived level 2, a population inversion as compared with the short-lived level 2′, due to its short life, level 2 empties immediately. (Reproduced from [9])

1.2 Characteristics of Laser

Laser is named LASER after the first letter of Light Amplification by Stimulated Emission of Radiation [2]. Currently, lasers can produce from 100 nm to 3 mm wavelength. In dermatology, from 308-nm excimer laser to 10,600-nm CO_2 laser is used. Laser can be divided into continuous wave and pulsed wave by irradiation method; the time of irradiation is from second to femtoseconds (10^{-15} s). Also, laser with a high output density of up to 10^{10} W/cm^2 can be produced [4].

Lasers have four characteristics which are different from light (Fig. 1.13). First, the photons with one wavelength are emitted depending on the laser medium (monochromaticity), and second, the two twin stimulated emitted photons have the same shape in time and space (coherence). Third, the laser goes straight without spreading sideways (collimation). And finally, photons are increased exponentially up to 10^{20} (high intensity). Of the four characteristics, coherence is important for laser manufacturing. Because of coherence, the wavelengths of the photons are overlapped so that the energy of the photons cannot be canceled out and the laser of high intensity can be produced. Therefore, laser can also be called the machine which amplifies low-output light and converts to high-intensity light. However, from the laser physician's point of view, monochromaticity is more important because laser should be selected by target chromophore. Monochromaticity will be discussed later.

> Unit conversion of a second should be understood (Table 1.3). In most laser texts, for example, it is not written as 10^{-3} s, but rather in milliseconds, or simply the abbreviation ms. The novice laser physician may be confused by the unfamiliar second unit. The least you need to know is which units are bigger or smaller. Also, since all the units are shorter than 1 s, you might think that there isn't a big difference between each unit, but you must remember that there's more than 1000 times the difference.

1.2.1 Parameters

Laser has various parameters of energy (Table 1.4). Energy is the number of emitted photons during a single pulse. Because high-quality laser emits a lot of photons during a single pulse, energy is used to represent the power of laser in pulsed wave laser in which irradiation time is fixed. On the other hand, power is the number of emitted photons in unit time. The time concept is included in the power compared with energy. Because power is the number of photons "per hours" in engineering concept, the concept is the output, capacity (force) of a machine. Because "energy = power × time," energy means "the total amount of applied force" or "the amount of work which a machine has done." Power is mainly used to represent the output of continuous-wave laser [10].

Thus, energy and power are all used to express the output of laser. But, for laser physicians, the number of irradiated photons on skin is important, which is why the concept of unit area is needed. Therefore, the parameters of energy density and power density are used. Energy density

Fig. 1.13 Four laser properties. (Modified from [2])

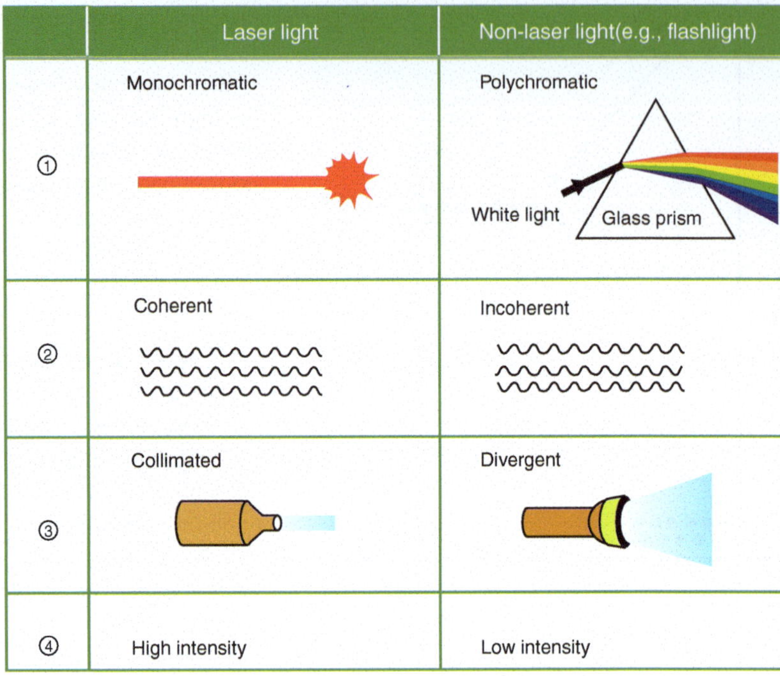

Table 1.3 Unit conversion of a second

Units	Second
Millisecond (ms)	10^{-3}
Microsecond (μs)	10^{-6}
Nanosecond (ns)	10^{-9}
Picosecond (ps)	10^{-12}

Table 1.4 Energy parameters of optical radiation

Parameter	Units	Formula
Energy	Joule (J)	Energy = power × s
Power	Watt (W) = J/s	Power = energy/s
Energy density (fluence)	J/cm²	Energy density = energy/cm²
Power density (irradiation)	W/cm²	Power density = power/cm²

is the number of irradiated photons in a single pulse, in unit area of skin. It is often called fluence. Power density is the number of photons which are irradiated on skin, per unit time and unit area.

So which parameter is more important? Fluence or power density? When laser contacts skin, temperature rises. In other words, light energy is converted into thermal energy. The more the number of photons, the higher the temperature will be. Because the number of photons is included in both fluence and power density, the higher fluence or power, the higher temperature will be. But if the number of photons is the same, which temperature is higher? Ten photons in skin per 1 s or 10 photons per 10 s? Of course, in the former case, the temperature will be higher. For example, in both the former and the latter, fluence is 10 J/cm². But power density is 10 W/cm² in the former case and 1 W/cm² in the latter case. That is, power density is more important than fluence to us. But, you may think that fluence is more important because only fluence appears in the panel of commonly used Q-switched laser and only the fluence can be controlled in Q-switched laser. In even CO_2 laser, the unit of power is not W/cm² but Watt. Therefore, laser physicians should keep power density in mind even if power density is not represented in the laser panel.

Table 1.5 shows the fluence and pulse duration, which is often used clinically for each laser. Corresponding power density was also calculated. The table shows some interesting phenomena. The vertical line of the pulse duration shows that power density increases rapidly as the pulse duration decreases [4]. Even when fluence decreases, power density rises sharply. As mentioned previously, there is a big difference in (1) fluence that is displayed and the (2) real power density.

There is another thing to note in Table 1.5. Power density is somewhat related to the power of the laser because the concept of power is included in power density. The power determines the value of laser machine. Currently, Q-switched laser is much cheaper and there are some IPLs that are expensive, but in the past, Q-switched laser was much more expensive than IPL. Also, according to selective photothermolysis (this will be explained later), smaller targets may be treated by shorter pulse duration. In other words, expensive lasers treat more targets because of the shorter pulse duration, while cheaper laser cannot treat certain targets because it cannot shorten the pulse duration.

The other parameters used for the lasers are shown in Table 1.6.

Table 1.5 My parameters for various lasers

Radiation	Fluence (J/ cm^2 = W/ cm^2 × s)	Pulse duration (ms)	Power density (W/cm^2)
Frequency double Nd:YAG laser (e.g., telangiectases)	18	10	1800
IPL (e.g., freckles)	17, broadband	7	2428
Pulsed dye laser (e.g., port-wine stains)	5.5	0.45	12,222
Q-switched ruby laser (e.g., tattoos)	4	0.00004	1×10^8

Frequency double Nd:YAG laser means 532-nm laser. Because frequency and wavelength are inversely proportional, frequency double Nd:YAG laser means 532 nm, which is half of Nd:YAG's wavelength, 1064 nm

1.2.2 Spatial Mode of Beam

Beam profile is a term that describes the spatial mode of laser beam and represents the spatial distribution of laser intensity. Typical beam profiles are Gaussian mode and flattop (top-hat) mode (Figs. 1.14 and 1.15). There are many other different beam profiles; each beam profile

Table 1.6 Parameters of optical radiation [2]

Parameter	Units
Pulse duration	Seconds, milliseconds, microseconds, nanoseconds
Frequency	Hertz (Hz) = pulses per second
Wavelength	Nanometers (nm)
Spot size	Millimeters (mm)

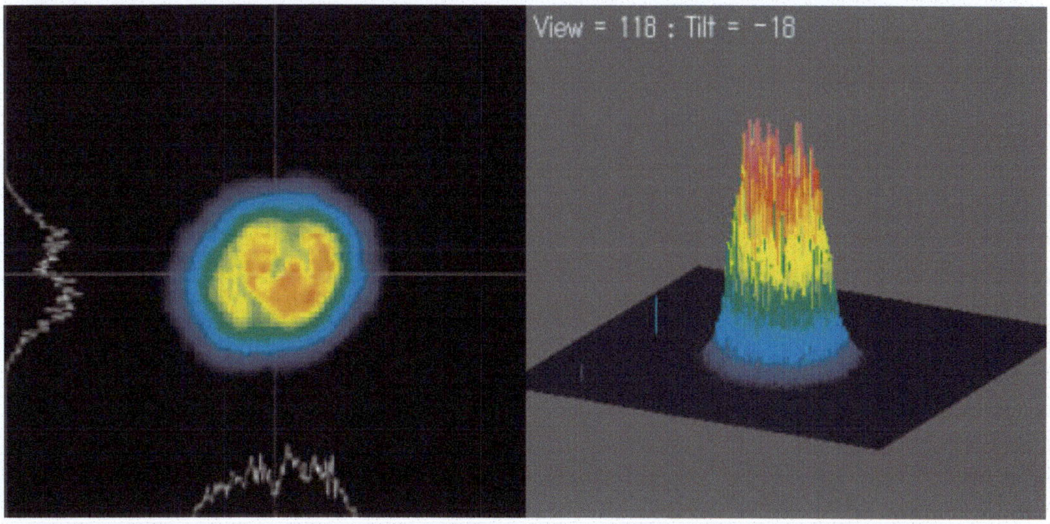

Fig. 1.14 Gaussian mode. 3D-beam profile of the C3 laser (wavelength 1064 nm, spot size 4 mm, energy per pulse 450 mJ/cm^2, pulse duration 8–10 ns, pulse frequency 10 Hz) produced by DataRay v.500 M4 software. This is the typical "Gaussian" profile. (Modified from [11])

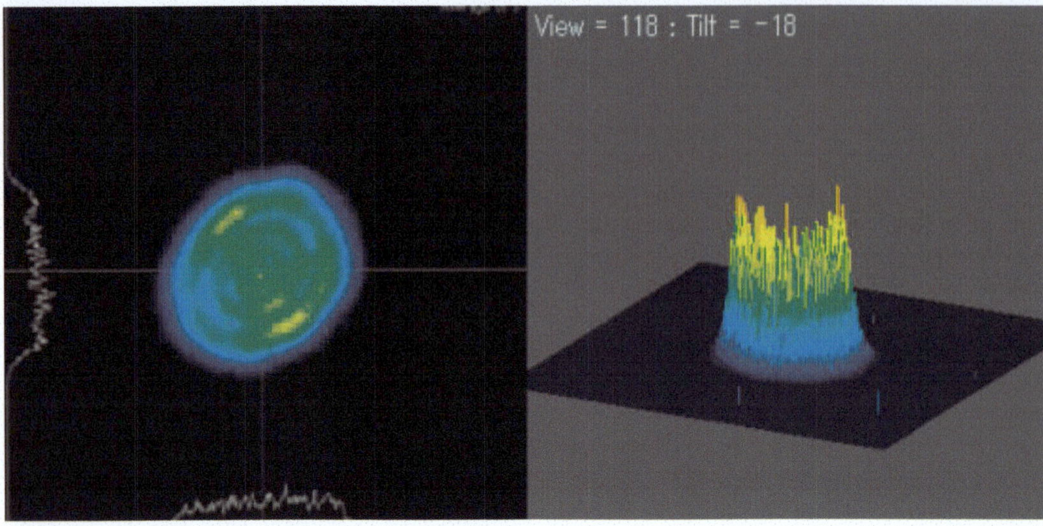

Fig. 1.15 Flat-top mode. 3D-beam profile of the C6 laser (wavelength 1064 nm, spot size 4 mm, energy per pulse 1000 mJ/cm^2, pulse duration 8–10 ns, pulse frequency 10 Hz) produced by DataRay v.500 M4 software. The distribution of the energy density is more homogeneous as compared with C3. The C6 beam has a flat top and most of the area is equal to the average of the energy applied. (Modified from [11])

is represented by the number beside the word of TEM (transverse electromagnetic mode). For example, Gaussian mode is basic mode, called as TEM_{00} and TEM_{10}, TEM_{20} are doughnut-shaped and target-shaped mode [3].

Beam profile is determined by the shape of mirror in optical cavity [3]. Also, beam profile is determined by the delivery system and, in flat-top mode, 80–90% in the center of the cross section has uniform distribution because countless reflections occur in the flexible fiber delivery system of fiberglass [12].

In Gaussian mode, the laser intensity is like Gaussian normal distribution in which the center of the spot is highest in intensity and decreases toward the edge. In Gaussian mode, the point where the laser's intensity drops to 86% is defined as the beam diameter (Fig. 1.16) [2].

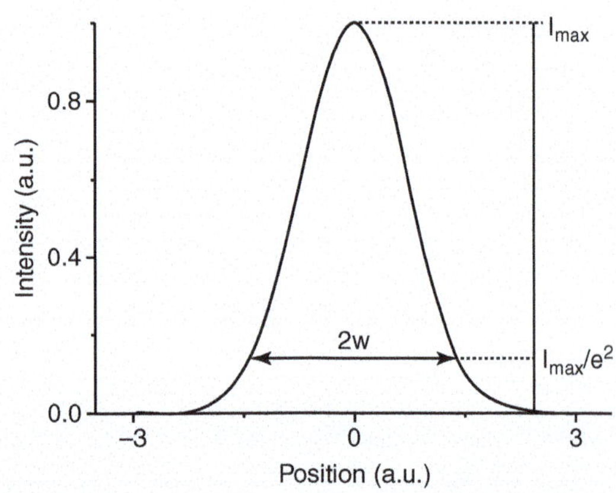

Fig. 1.16 Gaussian output beam distribution; $2w$ shows the spot size diameter measured at a value where the intensity decreases to $1/e^2$ of its maximum. (Reproduced from [13])

Gaussian mode may not be the shape we want. For example, when treating lentigines, the center of the beam may be very strong so that PIH occurs, the middle of the beam may remove lentigines without side effects, while the edge of the beam may not be able to remove lentigines due to very weak energy. Though some degree of overlapping is required to make uniform distribution, it is technically very difficult unless a scanner is attached and mechanically matched correctly. Therefore, flat-top mode is a suitable form to remove lentigines. But it's not right to simply say that flat-top mode is good and Gaussian is bad. It may vary depending on the treatment target which mode should be selected. For example, Gaussian mode is more appropriate than flat-top mode in treating melanocytic nevi.

CO_2 laser can use only joint-delivery system because laser is absorbed and disappear in optical fiber delivery system. Therefore, Gaussian model generated in optical cavity is default in CO_2 laser. Also, in Q-switched laser, only joint-delivery system is possible because optical fiber delivery system may be damaged due to high power. Therefore, though Gaussian mode is default in Q-switched laser, most Q-switched lasers produced recently implement flattop mode by optically uniformly distributing the laser beam within the handpiece.

1.2.3 Temporal Mode of Beam

The temporal mode of laser beam is classified by continuous wave, quasi-continuous wave, and pulsed wave (Fig. 1.17). Continuous wave is used in CO_2 laser, in which irradiation is continuous. In quasi-continuous wave, irradiation is shut off forcibly by using shutters such as propellers in between continuous irradiations [2]. Examples are copper vapor/bromide lasers.

Continuous waves are produced by continuously supplying energy from the external energy source to the laser medium and continuously creating a population inversion. Pulsed waves are produced by supplying energy once, like a flash-lamp on a camera.

Because quasi-continuous waves are based on continuous waves, the power of the quasi-continuous waves is the same as continuous waves. Therefore, quasi-continuous waves are not able to generate high power and the pulse duration is usually from 1 ms to 1 s, which is longer than microsecond or nanosecond. On the other hand, since pulse waves collect photons and emit them all at once in a very short time, the power is much higher than continuous or quasi-continuous waves (Fig. 1.18).

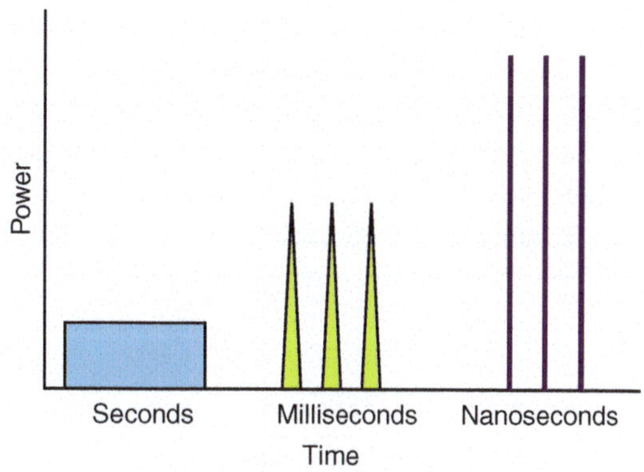

Fig. 1.18 Power of pulsed lasers. (Reproduced from [2])

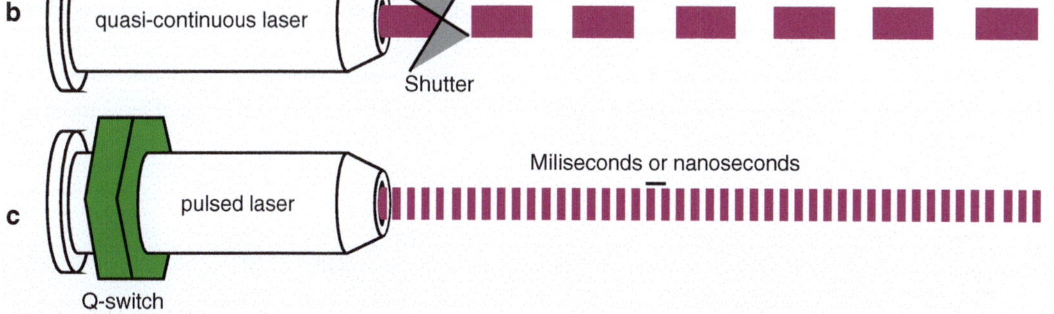

Fig. 1.17 The temporal mode of laser beam. (**a**) continuous wave, (**b**) quasi-continuous wave, and (**c**) pulsed wave. (Modified from [14])

How can pulsed lasers collect photons and emit them all at once? Let's take a look at Q-switched lasers, an example of a pulsed laser.

1.2.4 Q-Switched Laser

Earlier, the optical cavity was described as having two mirrors on each side, one with a 100% reflecting mirror and the other with a partially transmitting mirror, whereby the laser was emitted through some of the transmitting mirrors. On the other hand, both of the mirrors in the Q-switched lasers are 100% reflective, so that the photons move back and forth between the mirrors increasing exponentially. When a certain number of photons are collected, one mirror opens and closes (switching) only for a very short time, emitting photons [4]. Q-switched lasers are lasers that increase the stored energy (Q factor) and emit a large number of photons (high power) when the mirror is momentarily opened (switching).

Q Factor (Quality Factor)

$$Q = 2\pi \times \frac{\text{Peak Energy Stored}}{\text{Energy dissipated per cycle}}$$

Q factor (Quality factor) is the term used in physics and electronic engineering. The term refers to the ratio between stored energy and energy loss in a resonator or oscillator. Therefore, a high *Q* factor means that stored energy is higher than energy loss [15].

For reference, in laser texts, Q-switched lasers usually refer to lasers having a nanosecond pulse duration, and long-pulsed lasers often refer to lasers having a millisecond pulse duration (Table 1.7).

Table 1.7 Pulse durations of Q-switched and long-pulsed lasers

Laser	Pulse duration
Q-switched laser	Nanosecond domain
Long-pulsed laser	Millisecond domain

1.3 Skin Optics

Four phenomena occur when laser contacts skin. These are reflection, transmission, scattering, and absorption (Fig. 1.19) [2]. To increase absorption, which is our goal, we must first reduce reflections and refractions and we must understand scattering.

Transmission, on the other hand, inevitably occurs depending on the wavelength, in which unabsorbed photons pass through the skin and reach deep tissues such as subcutaneous fat tissue. Longer wavelengths reach deeper tissues and result in more transmission. The short wavelength of 300–400 nm is almost scattered in the skin, so little transmission occurs. Transmission is ignored in laser texts as it has little effect on laser–tissue interaction. However, when the IPL or laser is irradiated on the forehead, cheekbone, or mandible, which has less fat than the cheeks, the tissue response is larger and side effects are more likely to occur. I think that this phenomenon may be due to the fact that the photons that penetrate the skin meet the bone, rather than the fat, and is reflected so that it enters the skin again, increasing their absorption, resulting in a stronger tissue response.

1.3.1 Reflection and Refraction

To reduce reflection, the laser should be irradiated 90° perpendicular to skin. However, even if the laser is irradiated 90° perpendicular to skin, 4–6% is reflected from skin [2]. Reflection occurs mainly in the stratum corneum and does not affect the skin. However, the reflected laser can be irradiated to the operator's eye and even to the patient's eye. Therefore, laser operators must wear safety glasses and reflected objects must not be placed in laser rooms and patient's eyes must be covered with safety goggles.

$$\theta = \theta, \frac{\sin\theta}{\sin\theta''} = \frac{n'}{n}$$

The theories applied to refraction are the Law of Snellius and Fresnel equation. Law of Snellius

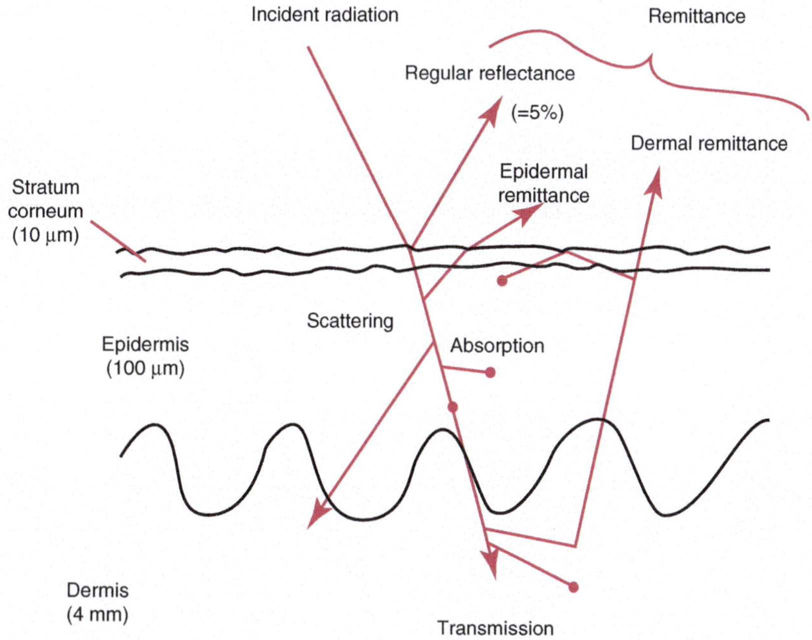

Fig. 1.19 Schematic diagram of optical pathways in skin: Reflection, Transmission, Scattering, Absorption Modified from [16]

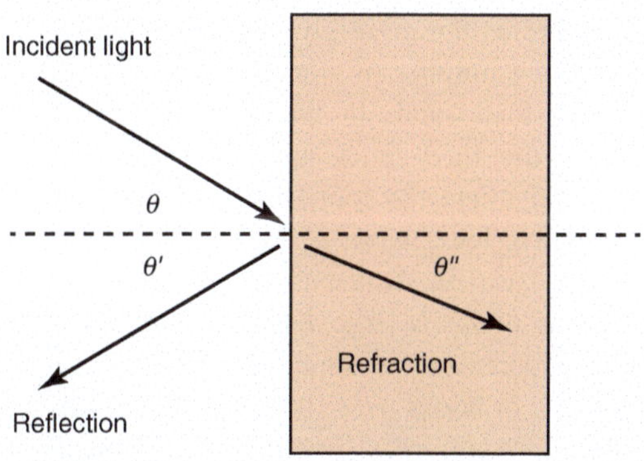

Fig. 1.20 Geometry of specular reflection and refraction. (Reproduced from [17])

is as follows. Incidence angle (θ) and refraction angle (θ″) are related to the ratio of refraction index (*n*) of two matters (Fig. 1.20). We need to minimize the refractive ratio in order to increase absorption in our desired target. Therefore, to minimize the refractive ratio, the ratio of refraction indices of the two media must be small. The reflraction index of air is 1 while the refraction index of the stratum corneum is 1.55, which is larger. To reduce the refractive ratio, alcohol (n = 1.4) or water (n = 1.33) may be applied to the skin. For example, applying water to the skin reduces the refraction ratio of air (n = 1) and water (n = 1.33) and also reduces the refraction ratio of water (n = 1.33) and stratum corneum (n = 1.55) resulting in more laser irradiation to the desired target. For the same reason, ultrasonic gel is applied during IPL procedure.

It is also possible to reduce the refraction ratio by letting the laser arrive at the stratum corneum (n = 1.55) directly through the glass window (n = 1.5) or the sapphire window (n = 1.7) without passing through the air. This is called optical coupling or optical damping [18].

1.3.2 Optical Penetration Depth

Optical penetration depth (OPD) refers to a depth in which the number of photons in the collimated beam is reduced by e^{-1} (37%) [18]. In other words, when ten photons are shot into the skin, the number of photons decreases as they are scattered and absorbed. The depth at which the photons are reduced to 4 is optical penetration depth. Where did Euler' number *e* come from? Changes in the natural world decrease by natural exponential function.

Additional Explanations for Natural Exponential Function and Logarithm and Optical Penetration Depth (OPD) (Explanation by Physicist Dr. Jong Kook Lee) [19, 20]

The rules for determining optical penetration depth follow the Beer–Lambert law. According to the Beer–Lambert law, when light is shot on an object of thickness L, the intensity of light emitted from the object (the amount of light energy per unit area, the number of photons per unit area) decreases rapidly as the thickness increases (Fig. 1.21). In other words, the intensity of the emitted light decreases exponentially with thickness.

Beer–Lambert's law can be easily explained by the previously mentioned rules on spontaneous emission. When light is irradiated on a substance, whether the electrons will absorb or not absorb the light is decided by probability. Assuming a 10% chance of one electron absorbing light, if the material is thinly sliced and always sliced at a constant thickness, the amount absorbed is proportional to the number of electrons, and the number of absorbed electrons is proportional by the volume multiplied by area and thickness. When 100 photons are transmitted, the value is proportional to 10 multiplied by the volume of the material, multiplied by the amount depending on the properties of the material. In conclusion it is absorbed by (constant) × 0.1. For the sake of simplicity, if the constant is 1, 10 are absorbed and 90 passes. That is, 90% of what enters pass by in each step. If it passes by four times, it is as follows.

Step 1: $1 \times 100 \times 0.9$.
Step 2: $1 \times 100 \times 0.9 \times 0.9$.
Step 3: $1 \times 100 \times 0.9 \times 0.9 \times 0.9$.
Step 4: $1 \times 100 \times 0.9 \times 0.9 \times 0.9 \times 0.9$.
Step n: $1 \times 100 \times (0.9)^n$.

The larger the step, i.e., the larger the thickness, the amount of transmitted light decreases exponentially. The above equation can be summarized as follows using the thickness L.

The above equation is an exponential function that decreases rapidly with length. Exponential functions are common in natural phenomena, for two reasons.

1. Because matter is composed of atoms, and the interaction between electrons and light, electrons and energy are expressed as probability. And the number of atoms, including electrons, is enormous, and the number of atoms (the molecule the atoms are bound to, to be precise) in 1 L is 6×10^{23}. If each of these atoms behaves probabilistically, a normal distribution should be used, which is expressed as an exponential function. The normal distribution is used when there is a large number such as an opinion poll.

2. In nature, the size distribution of the same object is represented by an exponential function in many cases. For example, the number of beach rocks and sands is large when the grain is small (sand) and the number rapidly decreases as the grain grows (stone). On the beach, the number of stones is considerably smaller than sand. In the case of English words, the three-letter word is used more frequently than the four-letter word and the use of five-letter word is drastically reduced (Zipf's law). In Amazon, the sales number of cheap books is large, but if the amount of money increases, sales number of books over 50 dollar or books over 100 dollar are sharply reduced. Therefore, selling many cheap books may result in big profit. This is called the Pareto's law, a law of economics which states that, for many events, roughly 80% of the effects come from 20% of the causes.

In Fig. 1.22, 0.9, 0.8, and 0.6 represent the likelihood of the material absorbing light, which is determined by the property of the material. In other words, it is difficult to interpret the graphs due to the graphs varying depending on the nature of the material. Standardization of the shape of the graph is needed. If the probability of being absorbed is 0.9 but we change the exponential function to 0.1.

$$I = I_0 (0.9)^L \cdot I / I_0 = (0.9)^L \left(I_0 : \text{initial input strength}, I : \text{Intensity when passing through thickness } L \right)$$

$$I/I_0 = (0.9)^L = (0.1)^{\alpha L}$$

The same result was obtained when αL was used instead of L and the exponential function was 0.1. At this time, α is 0.9, which is determined by the characteristics of the material and is called the absorption coefficient because it is determined by the probability of light absorption.

The exponent typically uses the value e (natural constant) rather than 0.1. The reason for using natural constants is simply for later computational convenience. This is because using natural constants as exponents simplifies calculations when differentiating or integrating. And since e is greater than 1, $1/e = e^{-1}$.

$$I/I_0 = (0.9)^L = \left(e^{-1}\right)^{\alpha L} = e^{-\alpha L}$$

Now, if you draw the graph in the equation above, you can see figure below (Fig. 1.23).

When αL is 1, the reduction rate of light $I/I_0 = e^{-1}$ is about 0.37. That is, when $\alpha L = 1$, the light is reduced by 37%. Since α is a constant that depends on the material, the amount of light decreases by 37% when light enters the material by depth $L = 1/\alpha$. This penetration depth is defined as optical penetration depth (OPD).

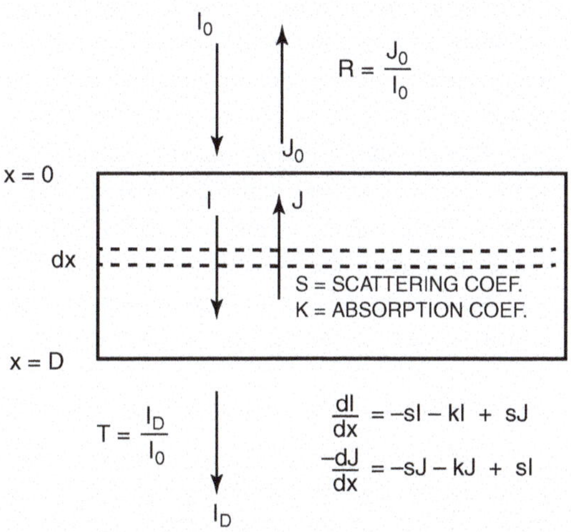

Fig. 1.21 The Kubelka–Munk model for radiation transfer in a turbid, absorbing medium. (Reproduced from [16])

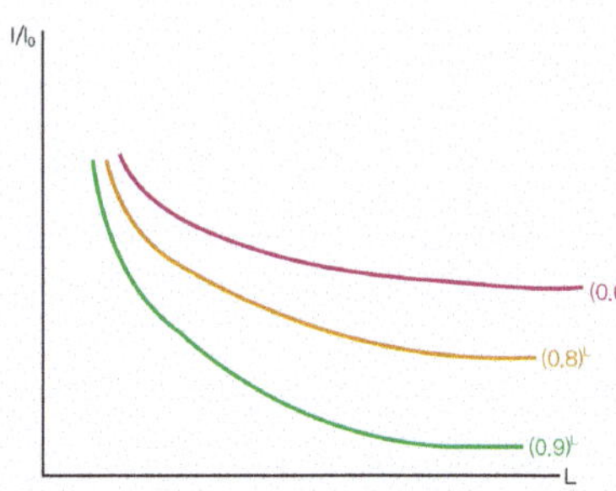

Fig. 1.22 Graph of the rate of light decay, assuming that the material's absorption ratio of light is 0.9, 0.8, 0.6

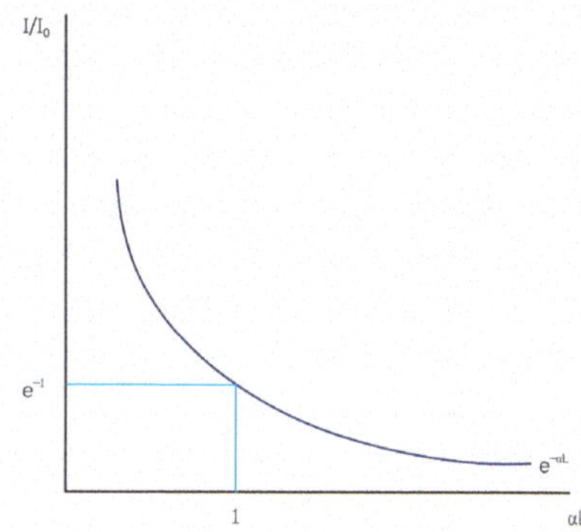

Fig. 1.23 Graph of light decay rate when the absorption coefficient is defined as α using the natural exponential function

When laser contacts the skin, the temperature rises. Changes in the skin occur only if the temperature rises above a certain threshold. The temperature is proportional to the power density. At least four of the ten photons must contact the skin in order to change the skin. The depth at which these changes occur is the OPD. However, as described above, physicists define OPD of the laser when the reduction rate of light is $(I/I_0) = e^{-1}$. Thus, the last remaining photon actually penetrates deeper than the OPD.

1.3.3 Scattering

Absorption occurs when the frequency of the photon and the electrons are same (resonance), resulting in conversion of light energy into thermal energy. In contrast, scattering occurs when the frequencies of photons and electrons do not match [18]. Scattering is the change in the propagation direction of the photon without energy loss.

I like to compare absorption and scattering to billiards. If the cue ball strikes another ball exactly, the cue ball stops and its energy disappears, while the other ball absorbs all the energy and bounces off. This can be compared to absorption. On the other hand, if the cue ball does not strike the other ball exactly, it may bounce off randomly. This may be compared to scattering. (Of course, this is intentional in billiards.)

Scattering is caused by melanin, cell nuclei, type I collagen, etc., but mainly due to collagen in the dermis [21]. At wavelengths below 300 nm, most light is absorbed by chromophores such as epidermal proteins, DNA, and urocanic acid in the epidermal layer, and scattering does not occur. At wavelengths above 1300 nm, the absorption coefficient for water increases and the laser is absorbed directly in the epidermis and scattering does not occur. Therefore, the wavelength at which scattering occurs is mainly at 300–1300 nm.

Scattering occurs better with shorter wavelengths. In other words, scattering is inversely proportional to the wavelength ($\lambda^{3/2}$) [22]. Longer wavelengths are less likely to encounter collagen, resulting in less scattering and deeper penetration (Fig. 1.24). On the contrary, shorter wavelengths have a higher probability of encountering collagen, resulting in more scattering and shallower penetration depth.

According to the definition of optical penetration depth, if there is less scattering, relatively more photons are absorbed. If there are more photons, optical penetration depth increases as the number of photons increases at a same depth. Therefore, as the wavelength increases, scattering decreases and the depth of penetration deepens (Fig. 1.25). Thus, the penetration depth varies depending on the laser.

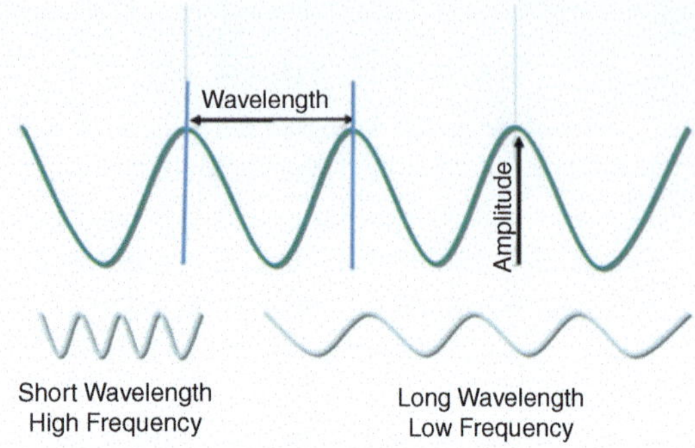

Fig. 1.24 Since light is constant in vacuum, the photon's moving distance per unit time is larger in lights with shorter wavelengths. The more movement per unit time, the more collagen exposure and more scattering [10]. (Reproduced from [1])

But why do Er:YAG lasers and CO_2 lasers have shallower penetration depths than Nd:YAG lasers despite their longer wavelengths? The difference in OPD described so far is due to scattering. The wavelength ranges in which scattering occurs is between 300 and 1300 nm. Er:YAG lasers (2940 nm) and CO_2 lasers (10,600 nm) have wavelengths which are not affected by scattering. Wavelengths above 1300 nm have a high absorption coefficient for water so that the absorption coefficient determines OPD. For example, the Er:YAG laser penetrates shallower because it has a higher water absorption coefficient than the CO_2 laser. In other words, at wavelengths above 1300 nm, where the absorption coefficient for water is high, OPD becomes shallower as the absorption coefficient increases.

1.3.4 Spot Size

When describing scattering, spot size should be considered. The larger the spot size, the deeper the optical penetration depth (OPD) due to scattering. That is, the spot size and OPD are proportional. It is easy to think that as the spot size increases, the number of photons increases, increasing the number of photons absorbed at the same depth, resulting in a deeper OPD. This seems like a simple explanation, but strictly speaking, it is a misconception. Because OPD is a ratio, even if the spot size increases, the depth

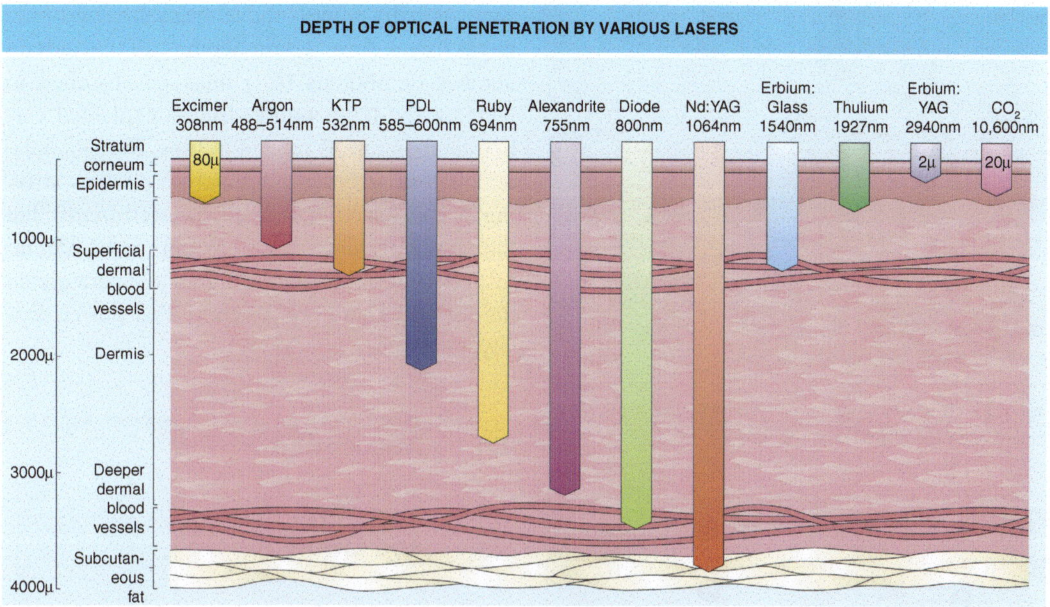

Fig. 1.25 Depth of optical penetration by various lasers. (Reproduced from [7])

will not change as long as the fluence (the unit of fluence is J/cm², i.e., fluence is also a ratio.) is the same. Rather, this can be explained by the spot size effect.

The spot size effect is also called the beam edge effect or the beam dispersion effect [18]. As explained earlier, four phenomena occur when photons contact the skin. Reflection and refraction, absorption, scattering, and transmission. Scattering may seem like a separate phenomenon, and photons may seem to end with scattering, but scattered photons are eventually absorbed or transmitted (Fig. 1.26).

Because scattering and absorption occur probabilistically, the number of photons absorbed increases in the center of the spot and the number of photons absorbed decreases in the outside. Likewise, as photons go deeper into the skin, the number of photons absorbed decreases. The penetration depth of the laser is the depth at which the number of photons per unit area is reduced to e^{-1}. In this depth, four out of ten photons are absorbed. Connecting the points corresponding to this depth form a triangle (Fig. 1.27).

The area outside the triangle is "area outside the OPD," which has less than three out of ten photons. This part will be constant regardless of

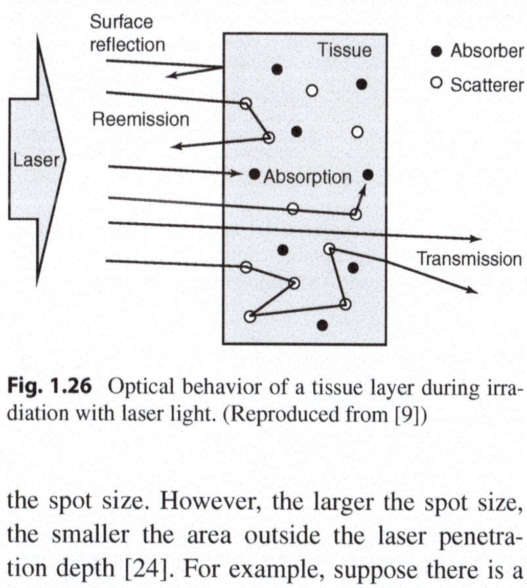

Fig. 1.26 Optical behavior of a tissue layer during irradiation with laser light. (Reproduced from [9])

the spot size. However, the larger the spot size, the smaller the area outside the laser penetration depth [24]. For example, suppose there is a large spot size of 1 cm² and a small spot size of 0.5 cm², ten and five photons were shot respectively, and one photon is in the area outside the OPD. Eight photons will be absorbed by the large spot size and three by the small spot size (Fig. 1.28). Fluence is the number of photons per unit area, so the fluence of the laser is 10 J/cm² in both spot sizes, but inside the skin, the fluence is different (8 J/cm² and 6 J/m², respectively). In other words, the larger the spot size, the higher

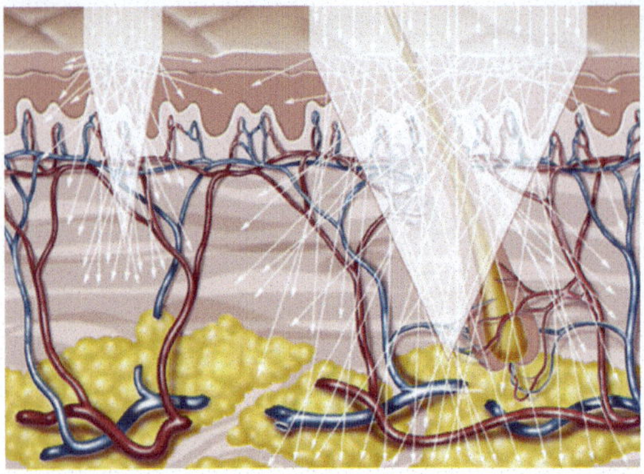

Fig. 1.27 Because of scattering, larger spot sizes penetrate deeper. (Modified from [23])

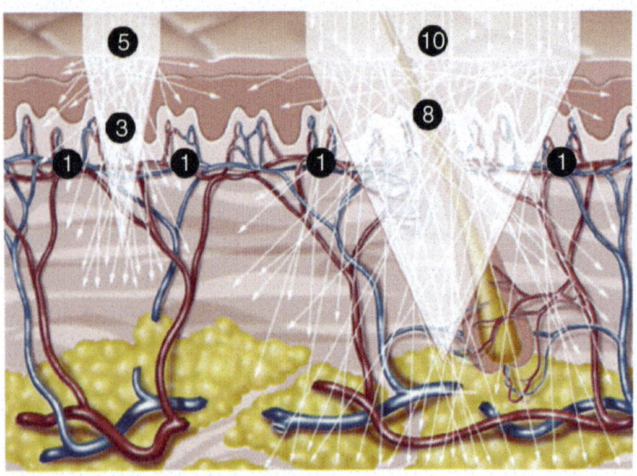

Fig. 1.28 If the spot size is 0.5 and 1 cm^2 and the fluence is both 10 J/cm^2, the number of photons is assumed to be 5 and 10, respectively. (Modified from [23])

Table 1.8 Factors involved in OPD

Optical penetration depth (OPD)
1. Wavelength dependent ↑
2. Spot size dependent ↑
3. Power density dependent ↑

the actual energy in the skin. Assuming that with each depth of 0.1 mm fluence decreases by 1 J/cm^2 due to scattering and absorption, 0.4 mm is the OPD for spot size 1 cm^2 and 0.2 mm is the OPD for spot size 0.5 cm^2. The larger the spot size, the deeper the OPD.

In summary, OPD is decided by three factors (Table 1.8). That is, the longer the wavelength, the larger the spot size, and the larger the power density, the greater the OPD. But in why is power density related to OPD and not fluence? What we eventually want is the temperature rise of the target tissue. At a certain depth (OPD), a certain number of photons (e^{-1}) must be absorbed to increase the temperature. But as explained earlier, temperature is related to time. For example, ten photons arriving at 1 s and ten photons arriving at 10 s have the same fluence (10 J/cm^2), but the power densities are 10 W/cm^2 and 1 W/cm^2 respectively, resulting in higher temperature in the former. Therefore, I believe that power density, not fluence affects OPD.

1.4 Absorption

1.4.1 Monochromaticity and Chromophore

As described earlier, of the four characteristics of the laser, I think monochromaticity is the most important. Lasers produce one particular wavelength depending on the laser medium. In other words, laser is monochromatic. Monochromaticity is important because of the absorption coefficient. Absorption coefficient depends on chromophore and wavelength.

Before we look at absorption coefficients, let's first examine chromophores. Chromophores are "components of the skin that absorb certain light" [2]. The three major chromophores of the skin are melanin, hemoglobin (Hb), and water. In addition, tattoo ink is also considered as a chromophore.

Note that the epidermis contains only melanin and water, while the dermis contains only hemoglobin and water. Of course, in dermal pigmentation disorders such as ABNOM (acquired bilateral nevus of Ota-like macules), nevus of Ota, and tattoos, the dermis may have melanin or tattoo ink, but, basically, the epidermis lacks hemoglobin as a chromophore and the dermis lacks melanin as a chromophore (Table 1.9).

Table 1.9 Chromophores of the epidermis and the dermis

Skin	Chromophore
Epidermis	Melanin, water
Dermis	Hemoglobin, water, (melanin, tattoo ink)

Chromophores and corresponding wavelengths are as follows: The chromophore of ultraviolet light is mainly DNA, proteins, and water, and the chromophore of visible light is melanin, hemoglobin, oxyhemoglobin, hemosiderin, bilirubin, carotenoid, and cytochrome. The chromophore of near-infrared light is melanin, hemoglobin, oxyhemoglobin, and cytochrome while the chromophore of mid-infrared light is water and lipid and the chromophore of far-infrared light is water [2].

1.4.2 Absorption Coefficient

Certain chromophores have a characteristic light absorption rate. This characteristic light absorption rate is the absorption coefficient. For example, melanin, hemoglobin, and water all have different absorption rates for light. This will be explained in detail in "Chap. 3". In addition, the absorption coefficient not only depends on the chromophore but also depends on the wavelength [24].

The absorption coefficient depends on the wavelength and the chromophore (Fig. 1.29) For example, when a 694-nm ruby laser irradiates 1000 photons, 90 photons are absorbed in the chromophore melanin and one photons are absorbed in the chromophore hemoglobin. There is a chromophore that absorbs better depending on the wavelength. On the contrary, there is a wavelength that absorbs better depending on the chromophore [24].

Since the wavelength is determined when purchasing the laser machine, we should purchase a laser for the chromophore we want. For example, for vascular therapy, lasers with a wavelength of 500–600 nm with a high absorption coefficient for hemoglobin are needed. For pigmented lesions and laser hair removal, ruby laser or alexandrite laser with a high absorption coefficient for melanin is needed.

1.5 Laser–Tissue Interactions

What happens after laser is irradiated and absorbed into the skin? Heat is generated. In other words, light energy is converted into heat energy. When converted to heat, the temperature of the chromophore rises. What happens to the skin when the temperature of the chromophore rises?

As the temperature rises in the skin, various phenomena take place. In order from low to high temperature: Denaturation of protein, evaporation of water, carbonization, evaporation, etc.,

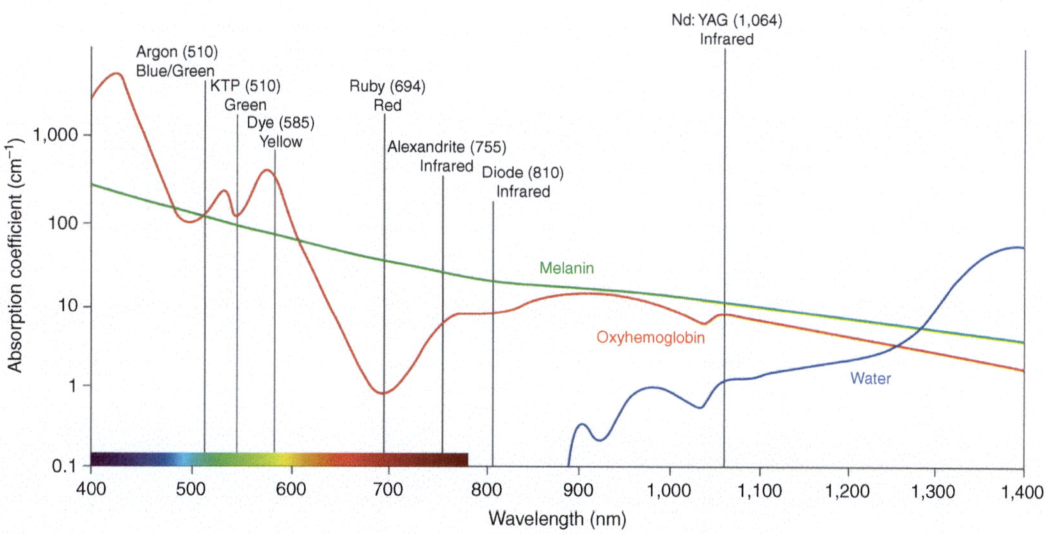

Fig. 1.29 Absorption curves for various wavelengths and chromophores. (Reproduced from [2])

take place [8]. Optical changes are blanching, increased tissue scattering, blackening, increased tissue absorption, and smoke and gas generation. Mechanical changes are drying, damage, and ablation.

The laser–tissue interactions (effects) can be classified into three types: Photothermal effects, photomechanical effects, and photochemical effects.

The photothermal effect refers to laser–tissue interactions by the phenomena of coagulation, vaporization, carbonization, melting [25]. For example, coagulation and formation of scabs when treating lentigines with long-pulsed laser or IPL, or vaporization with a CO_2 laser is considered as a photothermal effect.

Photomechanical effects exhibit laser–tissue interactions by the phenomena of plasma formation, shock wave, cavitation, jet formation [25]. For example, bursting of blood vessels resulting in purpura by 585-nm PDL laser and the breakdown of melanosomes and the damage of melanocytes by Q-switched laser and tattoos removal procedures laser are considered as a photomechanical effect.

Photochemical effects include low-level laser therapy (LLLT) using light-emitting diodes (LEDs) or He–Ne lasers, photodynamic therapy (PDT) using photosensitizers, and excimer lasers for vitiligo.

Previously, we classified laser–tissue interactions into three types, but strictly it can be divided into five types (Table 1.10). Depending on the laser text, the plasma-induced ablation effect and photodisruptive effect are sometimes considered the same as the photomechanical effect while biostimulation is seen as a separate effect, but in other laser texts, it is considered as a part of photochemical effect.

Under what conditions will these three effects occur? Different effects occur depending on the pulse duration and power density (Fig. 1.30). When the pulse duration is in seconds and the power density is low, photochemical effect takes place. When the pulse duration is in milliseconds and the power density is about 1–10^3 W/cm^2,

Table 1.10 Types of laser–tissue interaction

Laser-tissue interaction
1. Plasma-induced ablation effect
2. Photodisruption effect
3. Photoablation effect
4. Photothermal effect
5. Photochemical effect (biostimulation)

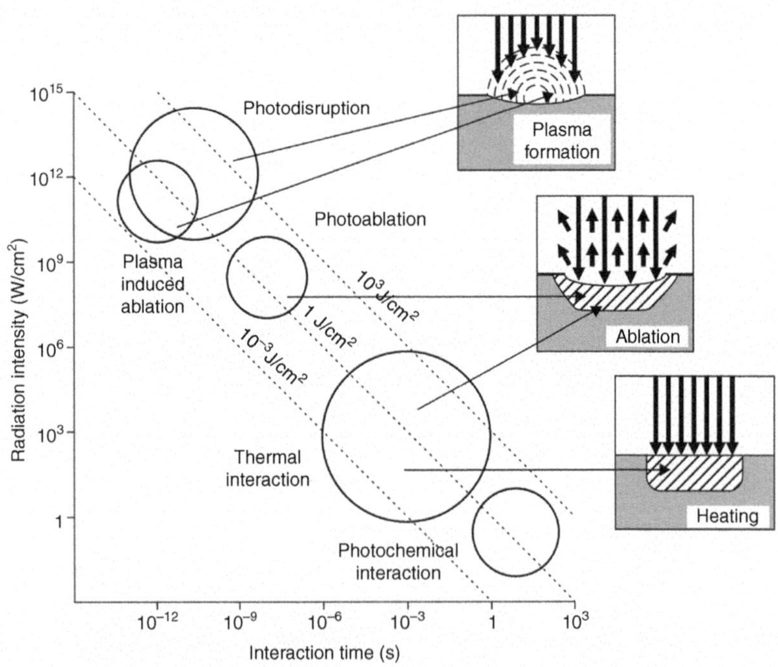

Fig. 1.30 Laser–tissue interactions. Circles indicate laser parameters for each interaction. (Reproduced from [13])

photothermal effect takes place. When the pulse duration is in nanoseconds and the power density is more than 10^{11} W/cm^2, photomechanical effect takes place. This is called "the rule of one microsecond" because the photomechanical and photothermal effects are divided based on 1 μs, usually 10^{-6} s [2].

In other words, laser–tissue interaction depends on the correlation between pulse duration and power density. Even if the pulse duration is short as 10^{-6} s but the power density is as low as 10^{-3} W/cm^2, there will be no effect. Even if the pulse duration is as high as 10^3 s but the power density is as high as 10^6 W/cm^2, only side effects such as burn will occur. In both cases, the desired effect cannot be achieved.

It is also important to note that fluence is not important in Fig. 1.30. Diagonally dotted lines show the same 1 J/cm^2 but depending on the pulse duration and the power density, photochemical, photothermal, and photomechanical effects can occur [25]. Therefore, simply increasing fluence does not give the photomechanical effect for a laser that exhibits a photothermal effect. Details will be explained in "Chap. 2".

1.6 Theory of Selective Photothermolysis

In 1983, Richard R. Anderson and John A. Parrish published the theory of selective photothermolysis in Science [26]. The ultimate goal of the skin laser procedure is to give the laser energy exactly to a specific chromophore (or target tissue) of the skin without damaging the surrounding tissue [21]. As we saw in absorption coefficients earlier, we thought in the past that we could achieve this ultimate goal by selecting a wavelength with a higher absorption coefficient in the target tissue than in the surrounding tissue. But in reality, this did not happen.

In the 1960s, 510-nm argon lasers were used to treat port-wine stains (PWS). Argon lasers were thought to be suitable for vascular therapy because of their high absorption coefficient for hemoglobin, but in fact they affected the surrounding tissues and burned them. Argon lasers are continuous waves that have a high absorption coefficient for hemoglobin, which selectively raises the temperature in blood vessels, but as heat spreads, the temperature of surrounding tissues rises, resulting in burn [28]. On the other hand, a short irradiation with a pulsed wave showed that only the blood vessels were damaged and the damage of surrounding tissues was minimized (Fig. 1.31) [14]. In other words, "heat diffusion" was a problem. To explain this phenomenon, Richard R. Anderson presented the theory of selective photothermolysis. Let's take a closer look at the theory of selective photothermolysis.

During laser irradiation, the light energy absorbed by the target is converted into thermal energy. The target tissue transfers heat to the surrounding tissue (heat diffusion, thermal relaxation), reducing the temperature of the target tissue (Fig. 1.32). This process takes time and the heat is confined to the target tissue during the

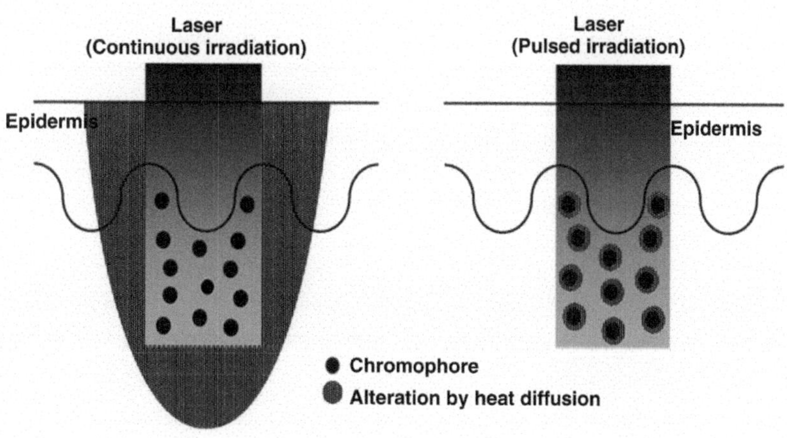

Fig. 1.31 A schema showing the difference between conventional laser therapies using continuous irradiation and selective photothemolysis using pulse irradiation. (Reproduced from [27])

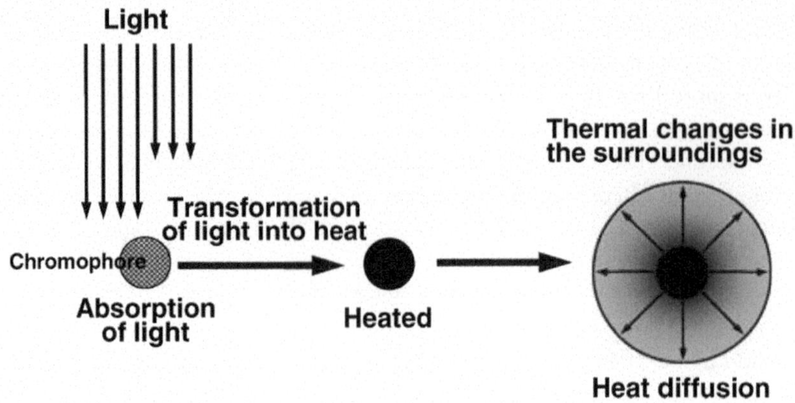

Fig. 1.32 A schema showing the changes of a chromophore after light irradiation that can be absorbed by the chromophores. (Reproduced from [27])

laser irradiation. The theory of selective photothermolysis is simply, "when a small amount of light energy is irradiated for a short time, the light energy received by the target tissue is used only to raise the temperature of the target tissue and does not transfer heat to surrounding tissues." Is this realistically possible?

Richard R. Anderson measured the temperature of target tissue and surrounding tissue during laser procedure (Fig. 1.33) [26]; 75 °C is the target temperature at which the protein denatures to produce the desired effect. There is no change in tissue below the target temperature. T_0 is a temperature before laser irradiation. T_1, T_2 is a temperature during laser irradiation, and T_3, T_4, T_5, T_6 is a temperature after laser irradiation.

The temperature of the target tissue exceeded the target temperature (75 °C) as time passes T_1 and T_2. During laser irradiation, heat is confined to the target tissue, so there is no temperature change in the surrounding tissues. After laser irradiation, T_3, the temperature of the target tissue drops and the target tissue transfers heat to the surrounding tissue, elevating the temperature of the surrounding tissue. As time passes T_4, T_5, and T_6, the temperature of the target tissue gradually decreases while the temperature of surrounding tissue gradually increases, but the surrounding tissue never reaches the target temperature (75 °C). In conclusion, only the target tissue exceeds the target temperature (75 °C), and the surrounding tissue does not reach the target temperature (75 °C).

1.6.1 Thermal Relaxation Time

When is this short time (T_2)? What is it related to? Considering physics theory, this short time (T_2) is related to the thermal conduction time or the thermal diffusion time of the target tissue. This short time (T_2) is defined as the thermal relaxation time (TRT). This will be explained later in Sect. 3.4.1 in "Chap. 3".

Thermal relaxation time (TRT) also decreases exponentially. Thus, the definition of TRT may also be defined as the time it takes for the core temperature to drop to 63% ($e^{-1} = 0.37$). Also, some laser texts define TRT as the time it takes for the core temperature to drop to 50% by a logarithmic function, not 63%.

Physics studies show that TRT is related to the following variables:

$$T_r = d^2 / gk$$

T_r: thermal relaxation time, d: thickness or diameter of the target, g: geometric factor, k: thermal diffusivity.

g is a geometric factor known to be 24–27 if the target tissue is a sphere, 16 for a cylinder [26], and 8 for a plane [26, 29]. In other words, temperatures cool slowly in spherical, cylindrical, and planar order. For example, planes like the epidermal layers cool more slowly than spheres like melanosomes or cylinders like blood vessels.

The important thing to note is that TRT is proportional to the square of the tissue diameter (d^2). In other words, the larger the tissue,

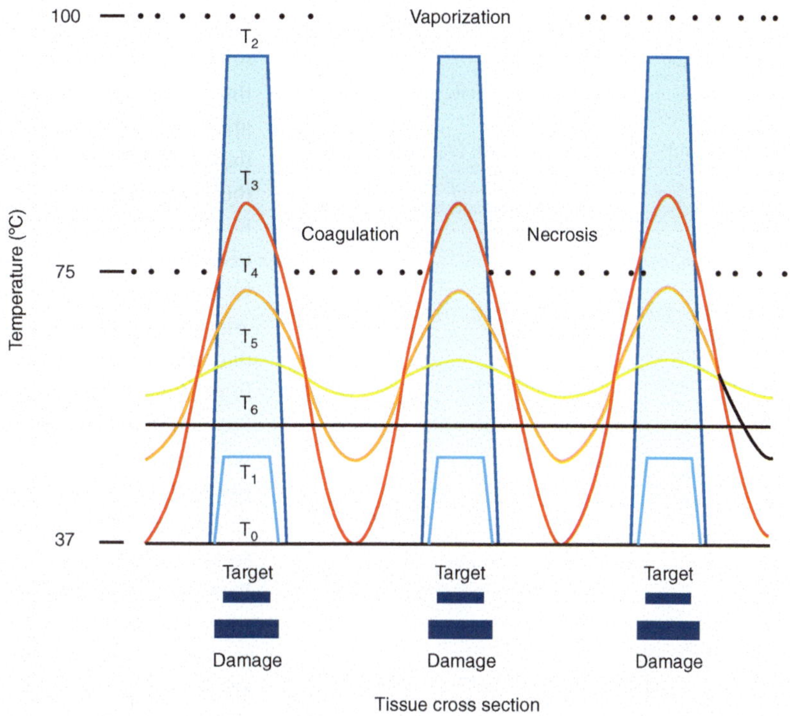

Fig. 1.33 Schematic temperature profiles during selective photothermolysis: T_0, before laser exposure (uniform body temperature); T_1, during laser exposure (selective rapid target heating); T_2, at the end of laser exposure (targets irreversibly damaged); T_3, one thermal relaxation time after laser pulse (targets cooling, surrounding tissue warming); T_4, two thermal relaxation times after laser pulse; T_5, five thermal Target relaxation times after laser pulse; and T_6, tissue slowly returning to ambient thermal equilibrium. (Reproduced from [26])

the larger the TRT and the slower the temperature drop. Conversely, the smaller the tissue, the smaller the TRT and the faster the temperature drop [30]. This phenomenon is easily observed in everyday life. For example, the kimchi stew in the pot slowly cools because it is large, but if you spoon the kimchi stew, it will cool down quickly because it is small.

TRT can be calculated according to the diameter of various sizes (Table 1.11). An interesting phenomenon is seen. For example, the TRT in tissues with a diameter of 0.1–1.0 μm corresponds to nanoseconds of 10^{-7} to 10^{-9} s and skin components corresponding to this diameter are subcellular organelles such as melanosome. TRTs in tissues with a diameter of 10 μm correspond to microseconds at 10^{-5} s and skin components corresponding to this diameter are cells such as RBCs. TRTs in tissues with diameters of 100–1000 μm correspond to milliseconds at 10^{-1} to 10^{-3} s and skin components corresponding to this diameter are skin structures such as the blood vessel or the epidermal layer [26].

Table 1.11 TRT and skin components by tissue size

Spherical targets (diameters) (μm)	TRT (s)	Time domain and skin components
0.1	3×10^{-9}	Nanosecond domain or shorter pulses on the subcellular organelle scale (e.g., Melanosome)
1.0	3×10^{-7}	
10	3×10^{-5}	Microsecond-domain or shorter pulses on the cell-specific scale (e.g., RBC)
100	3×10^{-3}	Millisecond-domain or shorter pulses for noncapillary vessels and other small structures (e.g., epidermis)
1000	3×10^{-1}	

In summary, the treatment of constituents in cells such as melanosomes requires lasers capable of irradiating in nanoseconds, for treatment of cells such as RBCs requires microseconds and treatment of structures such as epidermal layers require milliseconds [26]. In other words,

Table 1.12 Skin components by pulse duration

Time domain	Skin component
Nanosecond (ns)	Subcellular organelle scale (e.g., Melanosome)
Microsecond (μs)	Cell-specific scale (e.g., RBC)
Millisecond (ms)	Noncapillary vessels and other small structure (e.g., epidermis)

Table 1.13 TRT to remember [2, 8, 10, 18, 31]

TRT to remember	
Melanosome	<1 μs (250–1000 ns)
Tattoo pigment	20 ns–3 ms
Melanocyte	1–30 μs
Basal layer	0.4 ms
Epidermis	2 ms (1–10 ms)
Capillaries	4.5 ms (100 : 100 μm corresponds to the size of the smallest visible blood vessel)
Hair follicle	40 ms (10–100 ms)
Water	<1 ms in CO_2 laser, 1 μs in Er:YAG

lasers with different pulse durations should be used depending on the size of the target tissue (Table 1.12).

Thermal Relaxation Time (TRT) to Remember

The TRT to remember when performing skin laser treatment is shown above (Table 1.13).

One thing to note is the epidermal TRT. The TRTs of the epidermis, blood vessels, and hair follicles are all in milliseconds, so when treating the dermis (vascular treatment and laser hair removal) the epidermis may be damaged. Therefore, epidermal cooling is essential.

1.6.2 Pulse Duration Versus TRT

Until now, we reviewed TRT. But in reality, what we actually adjust is not the TRT, but the pulse duration (PD). What is the relationship between PD and TRT, and how do we adjust it? PD can be divided into three based on TRT.

First, PD is longer than the TRT (TRT < PD, middle figure in Fig. 1.34). This is the case when the temperature of T_3 does not go down and is above T_2. In this case, there is a possibility that the surrounding temperature may rise above the target temperature (75 °C). That is, it can not only damage the target tissue but also damage the surrounding tissue. It is a side effect that we do not want. Similarly, irradiating with high energy, irrespective of pulse duration may cause damage to surrounding tissue as the T_2 itself rises high. Another problem is that the temperature of the target tissue may exceed the temperature at which side effects occur (e.g., 100 °C). This temperature alone may cause side effects [21].

Second, PD is shorter than the TRT (TRT > PD, right figure in Fig. 1.34). This is the case when laser irradiation is completed at T_1. Because the temperature of T_1 is low, the surrounding temperature will not reach the target temperature (75 °C), but the target tissue will not reach the target temperature (75 °C) either. That is, neither the target tissue nor the surrounding tissues are damaged. There will be no side effects, but no effects either [21]. However, photomechanical effects can be used with Q-switched lasers. Because Q-switched lasers have very short pulse durations (nanoseconds), they cannot treat keratinocytes or melanocytes with very long TRTs (TRT 1–30 μs) directly. However, melanosomes (TRT 250–1000 ns) can be exploded to indirectly destroy keratinocytes or melanocytes to induce necrosis.

Third, PD and TRT are the same (TRT = PD, left figure in Fig. 1.34). Only the target tissue is damaged without damaging the surrounding tissues. This is the ideal situation. However, this situation is difficult to create. This is because first, the size of the target tissue is not constant, i.e., TRT is not constant. Second, the TRT-derived formula is based on the general heat equation, where the temperature is not an absolute temperature. So, the short time we want (T_2) and TRT are not exactly the same. Therefore, it would be safe to shorten the PD so that it is similar or slightly shorter than TRT. In this case, the photothermal effect is applied.

In summary, a similar or shorter PD should be used when using the photothermal effect to

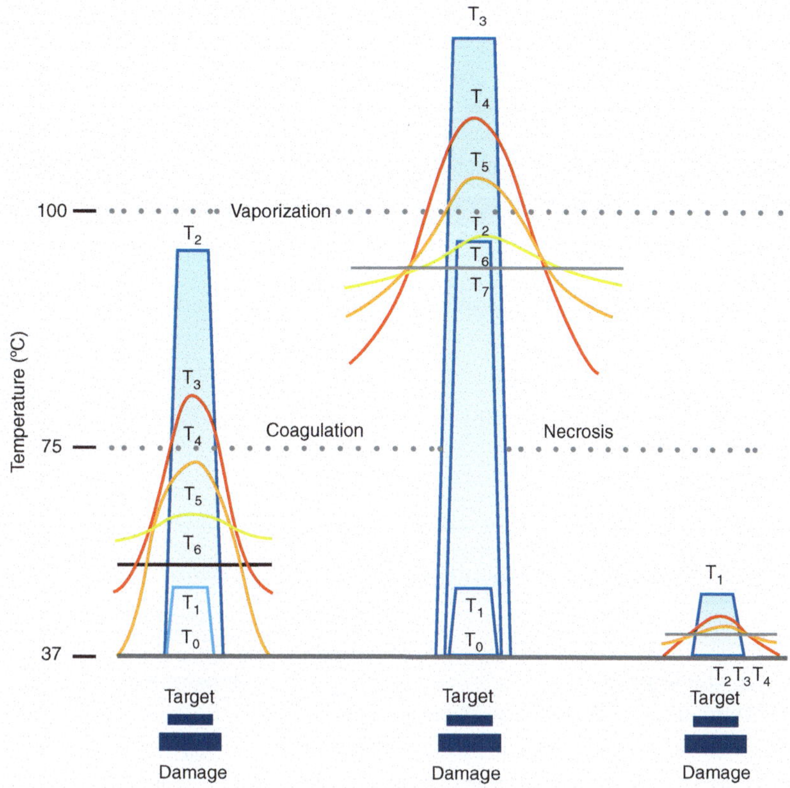

Fig. 1.34 Temperature changes by pulse duration. (Left) PD and TRT are the same (TRT = PD). (Middle) PD is longer than the TRT (TRT < PD) or the energy is high. (Right) PD is shorter than TRT (TRT > PD). (Modified from [26])

Table 1.14 The relationship between PD and TRT according to laser–tissue interaction

Laser–tissue interactions	The relationship of PD and TRT
Photothermal effect	TRT ≥ PD
Photomechanical effect	TRT >> PD
∴ TRT ≥ PD	

selectively treat only the target tissue. When using the photomechanical effect, treatment is possible even with a much shorter PD than TRT (Table 1.14). In conclusion, the same or shorter PD compared to TRT should be used (TRD ≥ PD).

When using photothermal effect, compared to TRT, how short should PD be to be effective? This is not mentioned in the laser texts, but in papers about vascular treatment, effectiveness is seen even if PD about 1/10 of the TRT [21]. This is why I think it would be ineffective if PD is shorter than 1/10 of TRT.

1.6.3 Three Parameters in the Theory of Selective Photothermolysis

The theory of selective photothermolysis is as follows: First, you should choose a wavelength with a higher absorption coefficient of the target tissue (chromophore) than the surrounding tissue. Second, PD should be equal to or shorter than the TRT of the target tissue. Third, as briefly mentioned above, there must be adequate energy (or fluence) to damage the target tissue while preserving the surrounding tissue [21].

Specific examples in which the theory of selective photothermolysis is applied to the skin are as follows. (1) Since blood vessels with a size of 10–100 μm have a TRT of 1–3 ms, a 585-nm pulsed dye laser (PDL) with a high absorption coefficient is used, with the PD set to 450 μs. (2) Melanosomes are 0.5–1 μm in size, and the corresponding TRT is 250–1000 ns. Therefore, a Q-switched ruby laser or a Q-switched alexan-

Table 1.15 The meanings of parameters

Parameters	Meanings
Wavelength	Kind and depth of chromophore
Pulse duration	Size of chromophore
Spot size	Location of chromophore
Fluence	Clinical end point
Frequency (Hz)	Tissue degeneration process
Surface cooling	Epidermal sparing (e.g., vascular lesions, hair removal)

drite laser with a high absorption to melanin is used. The PD of each laser is set to 40 ns and <1 μs, respectively [21].

1.7 Definition of Parameters

The meanings of the parameters are summarized above (Table 1.15).

There are a total of six laser parameters that we must determine. So far, we reviewed the meanings of wavelength, pulse duration, and spot size. "Tissue degeneration process," meaning frequency, will be explained in "Chaps. 3 and 7".

Next, we will review fluence and surface cooling.

1.8 Clinical End Points

Fluence can be determined by the following formula [32], but the calculation is difficult and is not calculated in real practice.

$$\Delta T = \frac{F_Z \mu_a}{\rho c}\left(\frac{\tau_r}{\tau_r + \tau_p}\right)^{g/2}$$

ΔT: temperature increase of a desired target.
μ_a: absorption coefficient,
F_z: local subsurface fluence.
ρ: density,
c: specific heat,
g: geometric factor (1 for planes, 2 for cylinders, and 3 for spheres),
τ_p: laser pulse duration,
τ_r: thermal relaxation time of the target (TRT).

Table 1.16 Clinical end points and corresponding causes

Laser	Clinical end point
Lasers for vascular lesions	Purpura—Vessel rupture Darkening or disappearance—Blood or vessel coagualtion Gray and white discoloration—a sign of necrosis
Lasers for pigmented lesions	Darkening and perilesional erythema—Denaturation of proteins, microvacuole Immediate whitening—Microbubble, Mie scattering Petechial—Vessel rupture
Laser for hair removal	Perifollicular erythema, edema—Peribulbar damage Pop out Gray or white discolorization—a sign of necrosis
Nonablative laser	Erythema?
Ablative laser	Gray—Coagulation Darkening—Carbonization Disappearance—Vaporization
Fractional photothermolysis	No clinical end point

Observation of skin changes during or after laser irradiation usually determines the appropriate fluence. This is called the clinical end point [33]. In your head, you should imagine the phenomena taking place inside the skin, for each clinical end point. Clinical end points and my thoughts about the possible causes of each clinical end point are described above (Table 1.16).

Darkening or disappearance - Blood or vessel coagualtion, a 585-nm PDL with 450 μs uses photomechanical effect to treat blood vessels. The clinical end point is purpura (vessel rupture). On the other hand, a 595-nm PDL with millisecond uses photothermal effect to treat blood vessels. Darkening may be observed (clot formation) or the blood vessel may disappear (vessel coagulation). Too much energy may result in gray or white discoloration (necrosis) (Figs. 1.35–1.39).

After the laser procedure, we are only able to see the clinical end point. This is why we need to think about the cause, conversely. We should carefully observe the changes in the skin after the laser procedure, think about why these changes occurred, and determine whether these changes are appropriate and adjust the fluence.

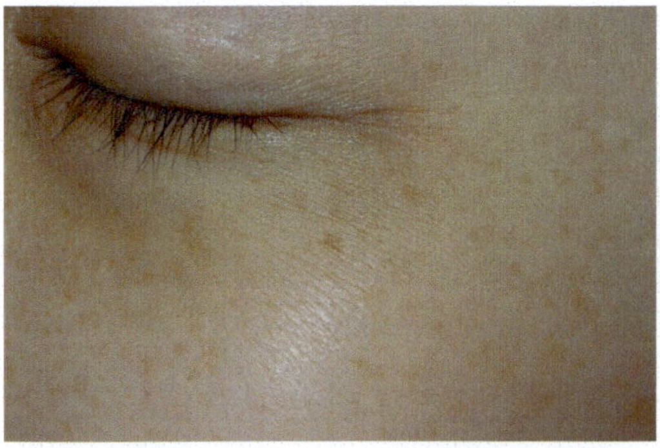

Fig. 1.35 Lentigo before laser treatment

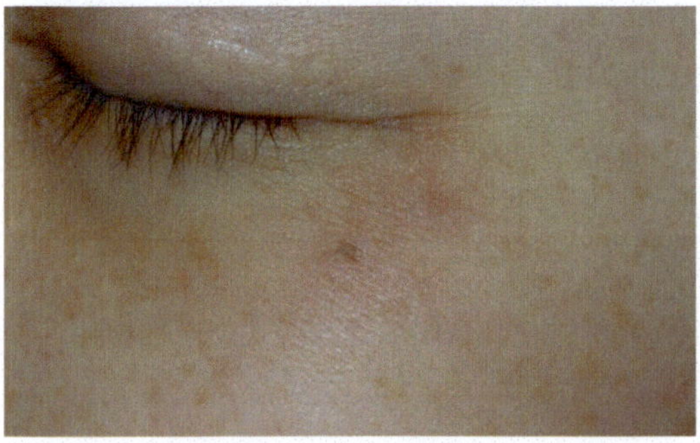

Fig. 1.36 Gray discolorization and perilesional erythema of lentigo immediately after repeat pulse method by 532-nm Q-switched Nd: YAG laser

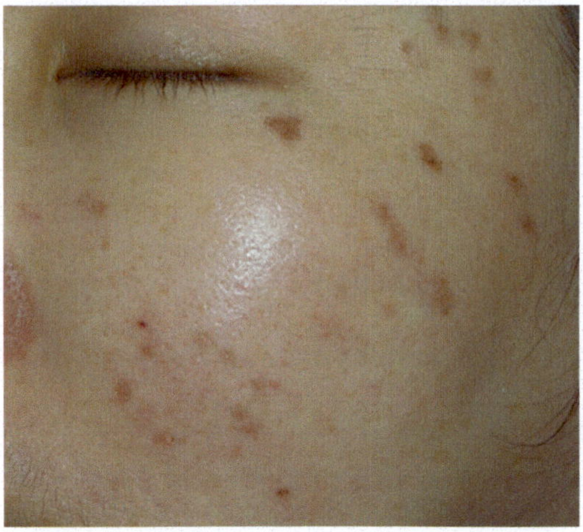

Fig. 1.37 Eschar change of lentigo 24 h after repeat pulse method by 532-nm Q-switched Nd:YAG laser

1.9 Surface Cooling

The main purpose of surface cooling is to protect the epidermis (epidermal sparing) during the

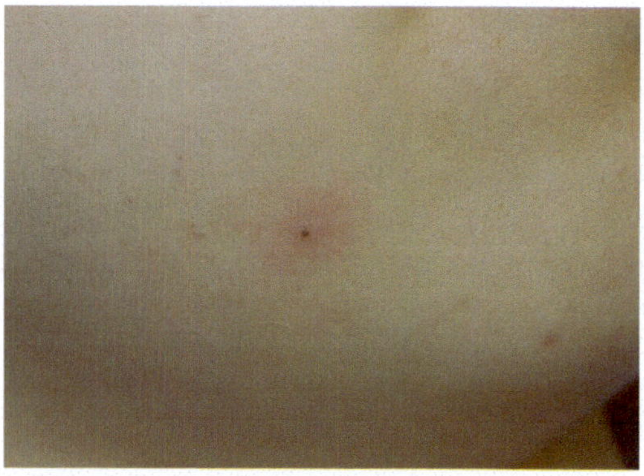

Fig. 1.38 Darkening and perilesional erythema in junctional nevus after 755 nm long-pulsed alexandrite laser

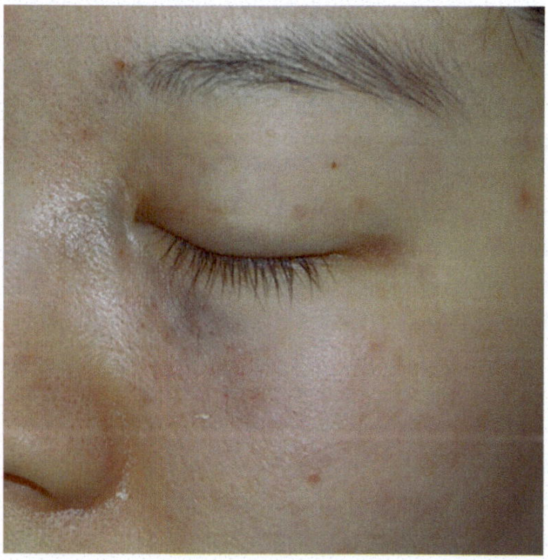

Fig. 1.39 Fine petechia after treatment of nevus of Ota with 1064-nm Q-switched Nd:YAG laser

treatment of the dermis such as vascular therapy, laser hair removal, and nonablative lasers. Photons travel from outside of the skin into the epidermis and then the dermis, i.e., the photons first reach the epidermis and then the dermis. During treatment of the dermis, epidermal photon absorption may cause no effect in the dermis or may cause side effects by elevating epidermal temperatures too high. Epidermal cooling is done to prevent this. It may also be used to reduce pain or edema.

Surface cooling can be divided into precooling, parallel cooling, and postcooling based on the time of laser irradiation [2]. Precooling mainly uses cryogen spray cooling (CSC or dynamic

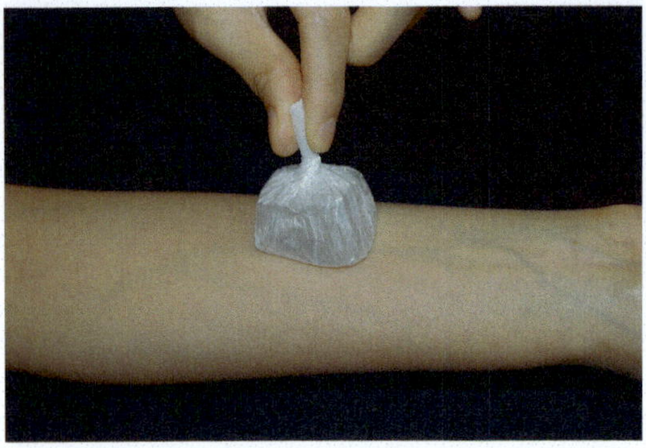

Fig. 1.40 Skin cooling by ice cube

cooling). An example of parallel cooling is the sapphire tip, which circulates water to cool the handpiece tip. This is mainly the preferred cooling for long-pulsed lasers. Postcooling is used to reduce pain and edema rather than affect the effect of the laser [24].

The ice cube can be used as a simple method for epidermal cooling. If an ice cube is in contact with the skin for 10 s, the skin temperature is known to drop to 10 °C (Fig. 1.40) [4].

Surface cooling can also be divided into conductive cooling, evaporative cooling, and convective cooling depending on the principle of cooling [8]. Conductive cooling is also referred to as contact cooling, such as a sapphire tip which cools by direct contact. Evaporative cooling reduces the temperature of the skin as the refrigerant evaporates by CSC (Fig. 1.41). Convective cooling uses cold air to cool the skin.

The pros and cons of each are as follows. Conductive cooling is economical because there are no maintenance costs but is not suitable for procedures requiring high temperatures due to its low cooling effect. Evaporative cooling has a strong cooling effect, but there are maintenance costs. And because spraying time is very short, it is not suitable when pulse duration is long. Convective cooling is effective and inexpensive when treating large areas such as arm and leg laser hair removal, but it is difficult to apply to the face because the patients have difficulty breathing when it is used near the patient's nose.

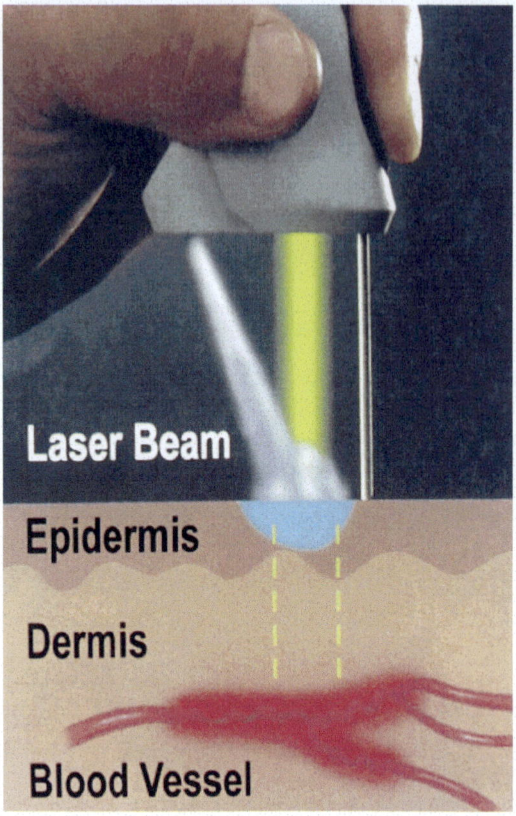

Fig. 1.41 The dynamic cooling device emits bursts of cryogen several milliseconds before the laser pulse. (Reproduced from [34])

1.10 Conclusion

1.10.1 Principles of Laser Therapy

Kim Bumsoo, the creator of Kakao Talk, said, "The essence of a smartphone is communication." Likewise, it is important to understand the "essence" of an object or phenomenon. To grasp the essence, one should be able to define it in one simple sentence so that even children can understand.

Now we will summarize what we reviewed about lasers in a sentence.

The principle of laser treatment is:

1. use a laser, which is a single wavelength of light,
2. select the wavelength, pulse duration, and spot size corresponding to each chromophore,
3. without affecting surrounding tissues,
4. selectively increase the temperature of the chromophore,
5. to induce changes in the chromophore, such as protein denaturation, vaporization, carbonization, etc.

Selective/Photo/Thermo/Lysis

Then what is the essence of laser treatment? What are the keywords? I think "selective" is the keyword. In other words, there are other ways to selectively increase the temperature. This is the theoretical basis for the use of radiofrequency (RF), needle RF, and ultrasound in skin treatment. The strategy of selectively raising the temperature will be discussed in "Chap. 3".

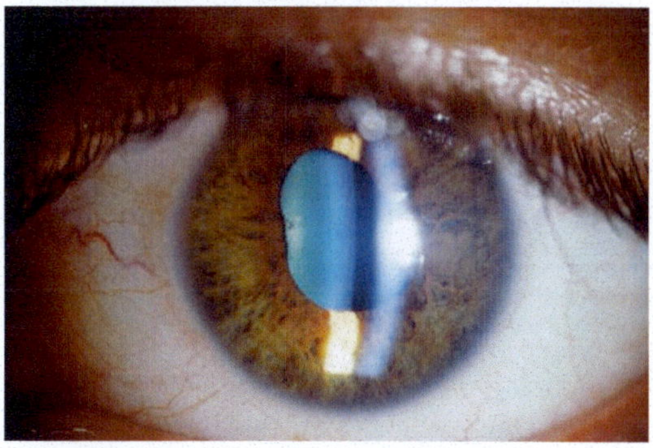

Fig. 1.42 Pupil damage in the left eye after diode laser epilation of eyebrow. (Modified from [35])

1.10.2 Comments by Author

So far, we have reviewed the principles of lasers for laser therapy. But more important than treatment is to prevent side effects and complications. Although this book does not cover the contents regarding "side effects and complications of lasers," studying this part is essential.

One important complication I would like to mention is the eyes, especially blindness (Fig. 1.42). No matter how serious the side effects and complications are from laser treatment, they are not related to the patient's life. However, blindness causes severe and irreversible pain for the patient. Therefore, the patient's eyes should not be irradiated and goggles must be used when treating lesions around the eyelids (Fig. 1.43). The laser physician should also wear safety glasses (Fig. 1.44).

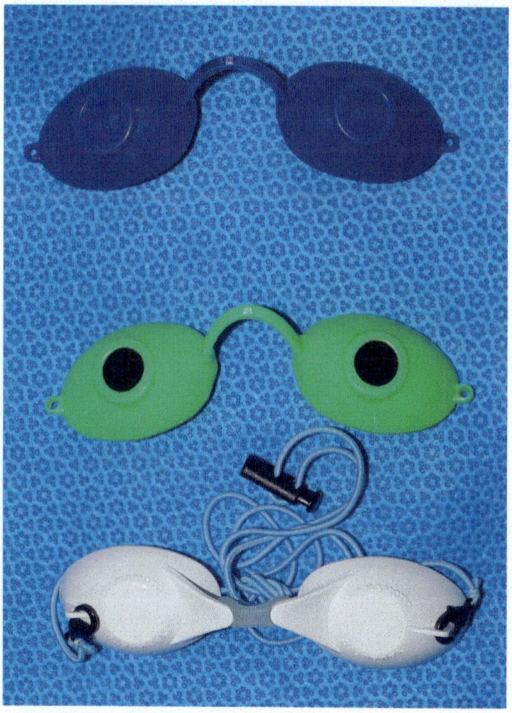

Fig. 1.43 Various eye goggles for patients

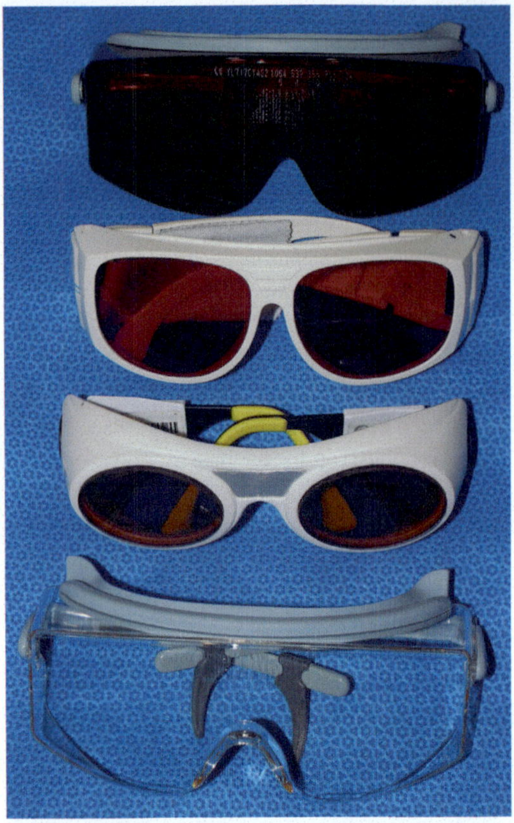

Fig. 1.44 Various laser safety glasses for laser physicians. Nd:YAG, alexandrite, PDL, and Excimer lasers (From top to bottom)

References

1. Issa MCA, Tamura B (2018) Lasers, lights and other technologies. Springer
2. Allemann IB, Goldberg DJ (2011) Basics in dermatological laser applications. Karger Medical and Scientific Publishers
3. Raulin C, Karsai S (2011) Laser and IPL technology in dermatology and aesthetic medicine. Heidelberg: New York
4. Goldsmith LA, Katz SI, Gilchrest BA, Paller AS, Leffell DJ, Wolff K et al (2012) Fitzpatrick's dermatology in general medicine. McGraw-Hill Professional, New York
5. Song SD (1999) Basic principles and applications of lasers (Korean). CheungMookGak, Seoul
6. Lee CW (2011) Optics and lasers (Korean). Gongju University Press, Gongju
7. Bolognia J, Schaffer JV, Cerroni L (2018) Dermatology. Elsevier
8. Kauvar A, Hruza G (2005) Principles and practices in cutaneous laser surgery. CRC Press
9. Berlien H-P (2003) Applied laser medicine. Springer Science & Business Media
10. Lee W (2008) Principles of IPL and its uses (Korean). MD World, Seoul
11. Karsai S, Pfirrmann G, Hammes S, Raulin C (2008) Treatment of resistant tattoos using a new generation Q-switched Nd: YAG laser: influence of beam profile and spot size on clearance success. Lasers Surg Med 40(2):139–145
12. Park SH, Yeo WC, Koh WS, Park JW, Noh NK, Yoon CS (2014) Laser dermatology plastic surgery, 2nd edn (Korean). Koonja, Seoul
13. Jelínková H (2013) Lasers for medical applications: diagnostics, therapy and surgery. Elsevier
14. Franck P, Henderson PW, Rothaus KO (2016) Basics of lasers: history, physics, and clinical applications. Clin Plast Surg 43(3):505–513
15. Jeong JY (2010) Clinical skin care (Korean). MD World, Seoul
16. Anderson RR, Parrish JA (1981) The optics of human skin. J Investig Dermatol 77(1):13–19
17. Niemz M (2019) Laser-tissue interactions. Springer International Publishing
18. Goldman MP (2006) Cutaneous and cosmetic laser surgery. Mosby Elsevier, Philadelphia, PA
19. Zipf's law: Wikipedia; [cited 2020 1 March]. Available from: https://en.wikipedia.org/wiki/Zipf%27s_law
20. Maxwell-Boltzmann distribution: Wikipedia; [cited 2020 1 March]. Available from: https://en.wikipedia.org/wiki/Maxwell%E2%80%93Boltzmann_distribution
21. Stratigos A, Dover JS (2000) Overview of lasers and their properties. Dermatol Ther 13(1):2–16
22. Nouri K (2018) Lasers in dermatology and medicine: dermatologic applications. Springer International Publishing
23. Gold MH (2007) Lasers and light sources for the removal of unwanted hair. Clin Dermatol 25(5):443–453
24. Carroll L, Humphreys TR (2006) LASER-tissue interactions. Clin Dermatol 24(1):2–7
25. Niemz MH (2007) Laser-tissue interactions. Springer, New York
26. Anderson RR, Parrish JA (1983) Selective photothermolysis: precise microsurgery by selective absorption of pulsed radiation. Science 220(4596):524–527
27. Watanabe S (2008) Basics of laser application to dermatology. Arch Dermatol Res 300(1):21–30
28. Parrish JA, Anderson RR, Harrist T, Paul B, Murphy GF (1983) Selective thermal effects with pulsed irradiation from lasers: from organ to organelle. J Invest Dermatol 80(Suppl):75s–80s

29. Altshuler GB, Anderson RR, Manstein D, Zenzie HH, Smirnov MZ (2001) Extended theory of selective photothermolysis. Lasers Surg Med 29(5):416–432
30. Brazzini B, Hautmann G, Ghersetich I, Hercogova J, Lotti T (2001) Laser tissue interaction in epidermal pigmented lesions. J Eur Acad Dermatol Venereol 15(5):388–391
31. Kang WH (2013) Treatment strategies for pigmentation disorders in skin (Korean). Hansol Medical, Seoul
32. Keyvan N (2012) Lasers in dermatology and medicine. Springer-Verlag, London
33. Wanner M, Sakamoto FH, Avram MM, Chan HH, Alam M, Tannous Z et al (2016) Immediate skin responses to laser and light treatments: therapeutic endpoints: how to obtain efficacy. J Am Acad Dermatol 74(5):821–833. quiz 34, 33
34. Alora MBT, Anderson RR (2000) Recent developments in cutaneous lasers. Lasers Surg Med 26(2):108–118
35. Shulman S, Bichler I (2009) Ocular complications of laser-assisted eyebrow epilation. Eye 23(4):982–983

Laser-Induced Tissue Reactions

2

2.1 Intersection of Physics and Dermatology

During Apple's iPad2 launch presentation, Steve Jobs said, "The reason that Apple is able to create products like the iPad is because we've always tried to be at the intersection of technology and the liberal arts... And it's the combination of these two things that I think has let us make the kind of creative products like the iPad." Similarly, we are at the intersection of physics and dermatology. Doctors who treat skin are too ignorant of physics, while physicists and laser-manufacturing companies do not know what is important for skin treatment because they have no experience in dermatology.

In this "Chapter," we will review the physical phenomena caused by lasers and how they impact the skin.

2.2 Laser–Tissue Interactions

First, let's clarify our ultimate goal for laser treatment. The ultimate goal of cutaneous laser surgery is to precisely direct the laser energy at a specific chromophore (or target tissue) of the skin without causing damage to the adjacent tissues [1]. In this sentence, we can see two goals for laser treatment. The first goal is to precisely direct the laser energy at a specific chromophore. The second goal is not to cause damage to the adjacent tissues. When considering safety first, we should focus on the second goal. Taking these into mind, let's review laser-induced tissue reactions.

Before reviewing laser-induced tissue reactions, we should keep in mind that physical phenomena due to temperature change occur first before tissue reactions (effects, interactions) occur. For example, plasma formation, shock wave formation, cavitation, and jet formation are physical phenomena that cause photomechanical reactions (effects) while coagulation, vaporization, carbonization, and melting are physical phenomena that cause photothermal reactions (effects).

In the Sect. 1.5 of "Chap. 1," we reviewed that laser–tissue interactions (laser-induced tissue reactions) can be divided into five reactions (Table 2.1). These five reactions occur depending on pulse duration and power density (Fig. 2.1). Interesting facts are shown in Fig. 2.1; The difference in the power density is large (from 10^{-3} to

Table 2.1 Classification of laser-tissue interactions

Laser-tissue interactions
1. Plasma-induced ablation effect
2. Photodisruption effect
3. Photoablation effect
4. Photothermal effect
5. Photochemical effect (biostimulation)

J. D. Lee et al., *Principles and Choice of Laser Treatment in Dermatology*,
https://doi.org/10.1007/978-981-15-6556-4_2

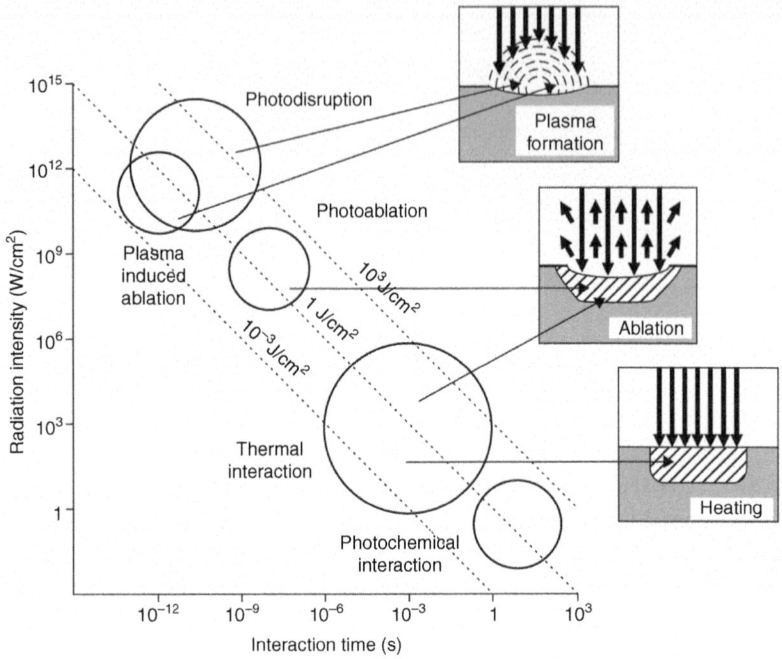

Fig. 2.1 Physical processes occurring during laser radiation interaction with the tissue. (Reproduced from [2])

10^{15} W/cm²), while the difference in the fluence (energy density) is comparatively small (from 10^{-3} to 1000 J/cm²) [3]. Also, the most important parameter in classifying the five reactions is pulse duration [4]. For example, above 1 s, photochemical interactions occur. From 1 μs to 1-min, thermal interactions occur. From 1 ns to 1 μs, photoablation occurs. Below 1 ns, reactions such as plasma-induced ablation and photodisruption occur. In conclusion, various reactions appear depending on power density and pulse duration, but the fluence of these reactions is relatively constant. Pulse duration is the main parameter that can be used to divide the various reactions.

Among the five reactions, water absorption coefficient is important for photothermal effect. The higher the absorption coefficient, the lower the optical penetration depth, and the lower the optical penetration depth, the lower the TRT. Therefore, TRT for water is smallest at 3000 nm which has the highest absorption coefficient for water (Fig. 2.2). The TRT for water at 3000 nm is 1 μs. Therefore, in pulse durations below 1 μs, thermal damage does not occur. For example, heat diffusion in nanosecond or picosecond lasers is negligible. Mechanical effect is the main effect in these lasers. On the other hand, in pulse durations over 1 μs, thermal diffusion is the main effect and thermal damage may take place. Therefore, photomechanical effect is dominant in less than 1 μs, while photothermal effect is dominant in more than 1 μs. This is called the "rule of one microsecond" [4].

In Fig. 2.1, the five laser–tissue interactions can be thought of as separate reactions, but they are not completely independent [2]. Adjacent reactions overlap one another. For example, we assume that there is no temperature change in photochemical effects, but in reality, temperature plays an important role. There are overlapping parts in plasma-induced ablation and photodisruption. Also, temperature elevation is observed when rapidly repeating 10–20 Hz of picosecond laser or femtosecond lasers, which are thought to have no thermal effect due to having a pulse duration of less than 100 ps. For example, water (liquid) must be converted to water vapor (gas) at 100 °C or higher, but water vapor (gas) is also present in indoor air below 100 °C. The overlapping of laser–tissue interactions is partially caused by physical phenomena but they are mostly caused by inhomogeneity of skin tissue [3]. Various reactions occur simultaneously with one laser irradiation.

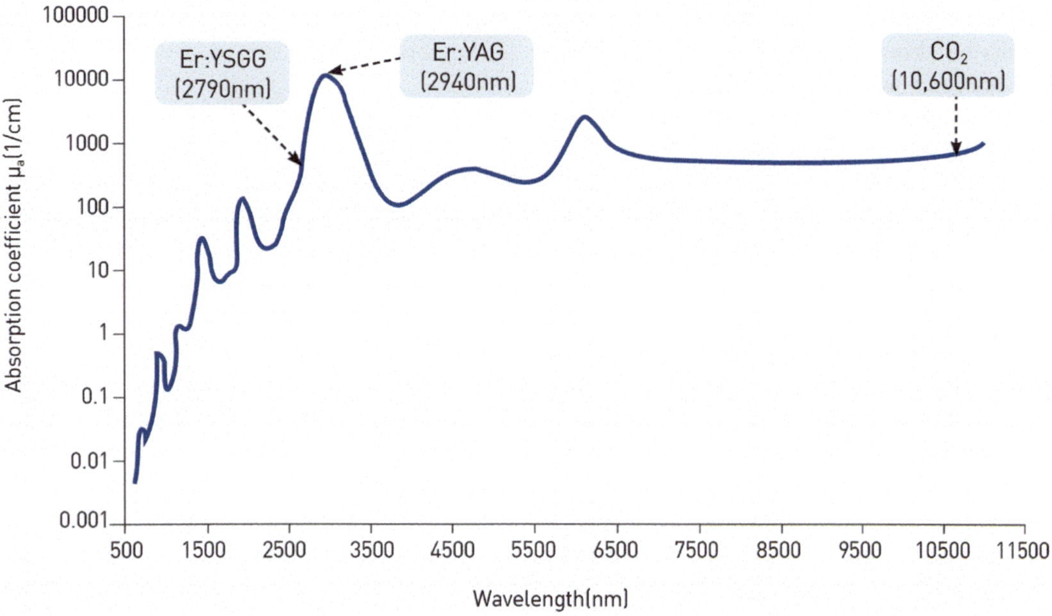

Fig. 2.2 Absorption coefficient of pure water. (Modified from [5])

2.3 Plasma

2.3.1 Generation of Plasma

Now let's look into an unfamiliar physical phenomenon called plasma. Plasma is defined as a gas–state matter which is separated into negative-charged electron and positive-charged ion in ultrahigh temperature. In general, the phase of matter is divided into three: solid, liquid, and gas. Plasma is "the fourth phase of matter" [6]. When energy is applied to solid, it is changed into liquid or gas, and when high energy is applied to the gas phase, it is then separated into electron and atomic nucleus resulting in the plasma phase.

Plasma may seem like an unfamiliar phenomenon, but in the entire universe, plasma is the most common phase. Ninety-nine percent of the universe is presumed to be in the plasma phase. We can see natural plasma in lightning, aurora in the North Pole, and ionosphere in the atmosphere. Artificial plasma commonly observed in everyday life are fluorescent light, mercury lamp, neon signs, and PDP (plasma display panel).

In dermatology, the generation of plasma is usually divided into three methods [6]. First, plasma can be generated by using a very high-power density with a picosecond laser. Second, plasma can be generated with a Q-switched laser. Figure 2.3 shows plasma generation by increasing the power density by focusing on one spot by 1064 nm Q-switched Nd:YAG using a zoom handpiece. Also, when treating tattoos, flash of light is occasionally seen. This is also plasma.

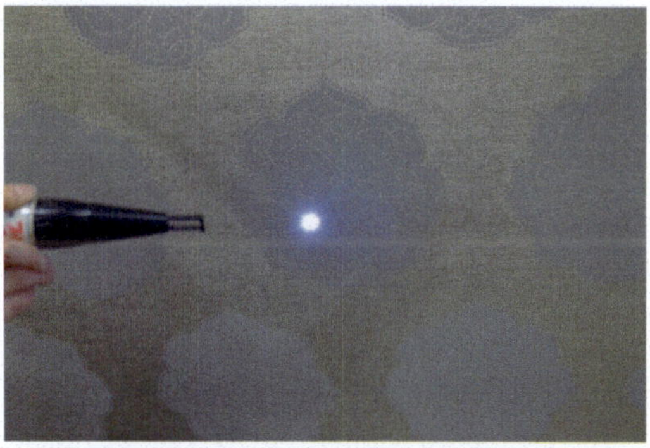

Fig. 2.3 Plasma is generated with 1064 nm Q-switched Nd:YAG laser, using a zoom handpiece

Finally, there is a method of generating plasma using RF (radiofrequency)-excited nitrogen gas. In the past, plasma skin resurfacing was performed using a device called a Portrait PSR system (Rhytec, Inc., Waltham, MA) to create plasma for skin resurfacing [7]. Currently, there is a device called Legato II (Alma Lasers, Inc., Buffalo, Grove, IL, USA) that generates microplasma for fractional skin resurfacing.

2.3.2 Laser-Induced Optical Breakdown

Plasma formation may be referred to as dielectric breakdown because it is a phenomenon in which matter is divided into a positive charge and a negative charge. However, the term optical breakdown is mainly used to emphasize the phenomenon in which ultraviolet rays, visible rays, infrared rays, etc. are absorbed by plasma (inverse Bremsstrahlung) [3]. Therefore, optimal breakdown and plasma formation may be considered as the same expression. In this case, plasma generation by laser can be referred to as laser-induced optical breakdown (LIOB). Therefore, LIOB is "plasma produced by picosecond lasers or femtosecond lasers" and "plasma produced by Q-switched lasers." However, due to the emphasis of picoseconds in private practice and congresses, there is a misconception that LIOB can be made only by picosecond lasers. LIOB only refers to plasma made by lasers and can be created not only with picosecond lasers but also with femtosecond and Q-switched lasers.

As mentioned earlier, LIOB can be made with two lasers. First, it can be made with a Q-switched laser with a nanosecond pulse duration. Q-switched lasers can be used to raise the temperature to emit electrons. This is called thermal ionization and electron emission by thermal ionization is called thermionic emission. Second, mode-locked lasers with pulse durations in picosecond or femtosecond create high electric field intensities, overcoming Coulomb's force, and produce large amounts of electrons. This is called multiphoton ionization. In other words, light energy can separate atoms into positive and negative charges [3].

Electrical force between positive and negative charge is called electric field strength (*I*). The relationship between electric field strength and power density of the photon is known as the following formula [3].

$$I(r,z,t) = \frac{1}{2}\varepsilon_0 c E^2$$

I—local power density, ε_0—dielectric constant, *c*—speed of light, *E*—electric field strength.

It is known that the power density that can produce optical breakdown with picosecond lasers is typically 10^{11} W/cm^2. Substituting this in the above formula, the electric field strength is 10^7 V/cm^2, which is known as the average Coulomb's force between positive and negative charges. Multiphoton ionization typically requires picosecond lasers or femtosecond lasers because multiple coherent photons are required.

Because Q-switched lasers require high energy to produce plasma, plasma is produced at high temperatures. There are also other side effects (shock wave formation, cavitation, and jet formation) other than ionization. Picosecond lasers, on the other hand, produce plasma at low energy, so there are fewer side effects. This will be explained in the following sections.

By these two lasers, few "lucky" electrons induce a lot of free electrons and ions, similar to an avalanche in which few snowballs collapse all the snow on the mountain. This is called the electron avalanche (Fig. 2.4). Specifically, when some free electrons encounter photons, they move faster and collide with surrounding atoms to ionize them into electrons and nuclei. Thus, two free elections are generated. Due to decreased kinetic energy, these two free electrons are slower than before, but when these electrons meet photons and accelerate and meet two nearby atoms, they create four free electrons. This creates exponential ionization and free electrons. This process of absorbing photons and accelerating electrons in the presence of atoms is called inverse Bremsstrahlung [3]. Inverse Bremsstrahlung results in plasma shield effect or multiple plasma generation (described later).

Therefore, plasma generation process is as follows: First, free election is generated by Q-switched laser or mode-locked laser (starting phase). Second, electron is accelerated by photons generating many free elections (electron

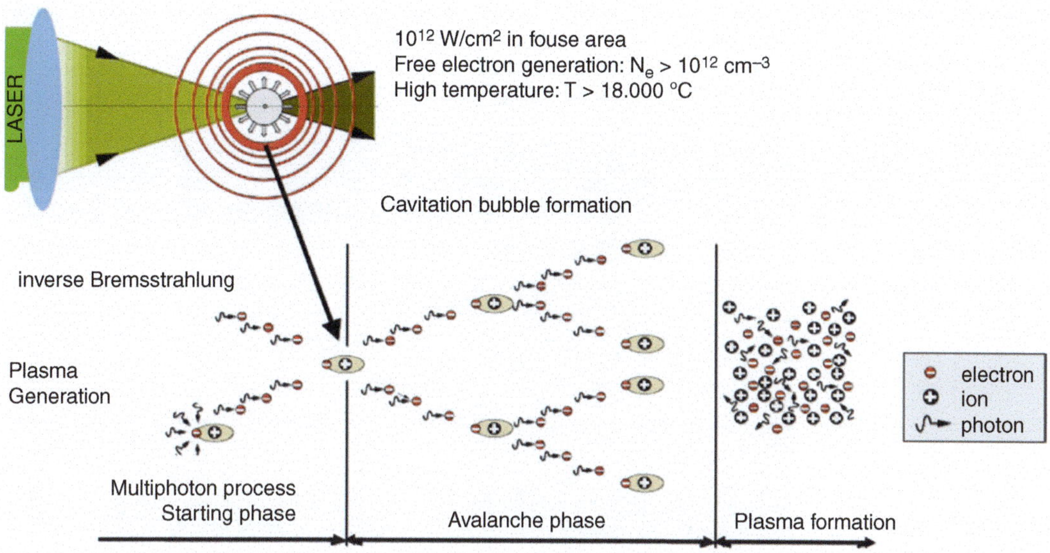

Fig. 2.4 Schematic presentation of the processes responsible for the optical breakdown generated by ultrashort laser pulses. (Reproduced from [8])

avalanche stage). Third, plasma is formed by the separation of many electrons and atomic nuclei (plasma formation stage).

The plasma thus produced can be observed by intense white flashes and acoustic signals. The temperature rises to 15,000–20,000 °C and the pressure rises to 20–60 bar [8]. After plasma generation, cavitation occurs due to pressure and volume expansion, and the size of the cavity varies depending on the energy and pulse duration. In particular, the shorter the pulse duration, less energy is required to make the plasma resulting in smaller size of cavities and reduced side effects. Therefore, Q-switched lasers produce large cavities with many side effects and picosecond lasers produce small cavities with fewer side effects.

Next, we will discuss two reactions that occur on the skin by plasma: plasma-induced ablation and photodisruption.

2.4 Plasma-Induced Ablation

Plasma-induced ablation refers to a reaction in which tissue is ablated by the generation of plasma. One laser text describes this as "very clean and well-defined reaction without evidence of thermal or mechanical damage [4]" (Fig. 2.5). This may be an ideal method in eliminating only the target tissue without damaging the surrounding tissues.

Plasma-induced ablation is used for caries therapy in dental clinic, for corneal surgery in ophthalmic clinic, but is not yet used in dermatology. Plasma-induced ablation requires a very high-power density, which requires more than 10^{11} W/cm^2 for solids and fluids and 10^{14} W/cm^2 in air [3]. It is known to occur only in picosecond lasers, not in nanosecond Q-switched lasers.

2.5 Photodisruption

When plasma is generated, a shock wave is generated due to volume expansion and pressure due to phase change (phase explosion). Due to shock wave, cavitation occurs in soft tissues or fluids, and when a solid is located on one side, the pressure is directed against the solid, creating jet formation in which the pressure is doubled.

The reaction by these phenomena is called photodisruption, using the expression "disruption" derived from the Latin word "ruptus" which means "ruptured" [3]. In other words, photodis-

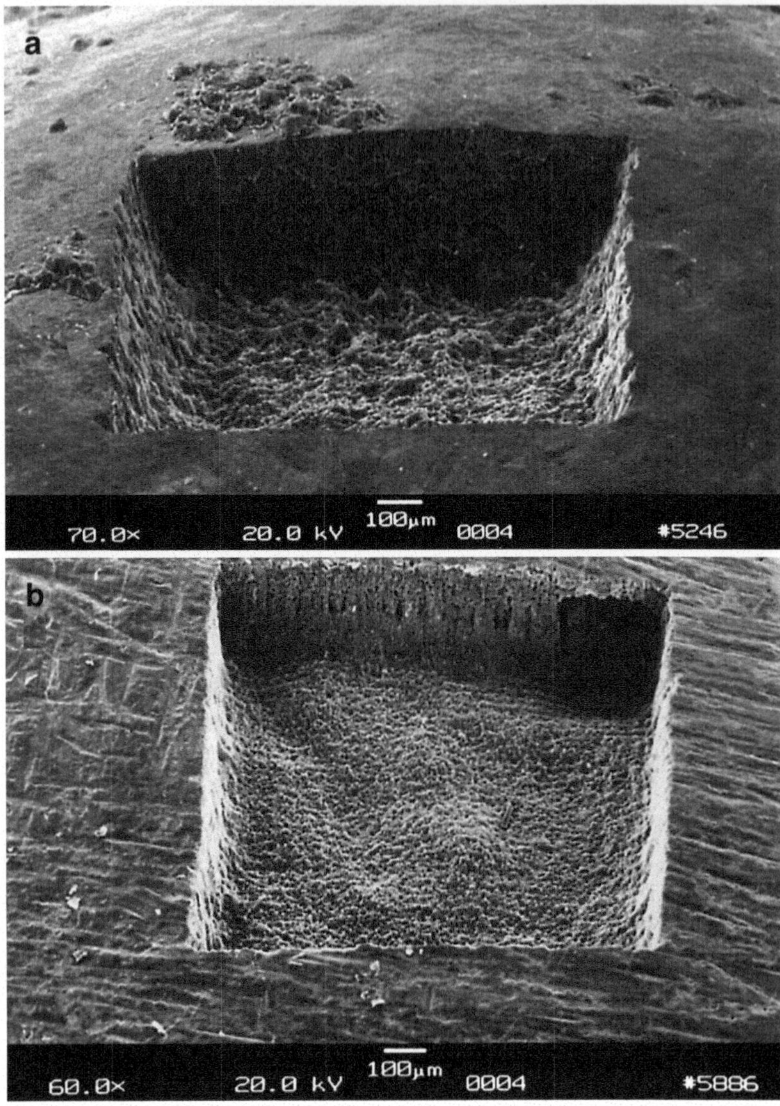

Fig. 2.5 (**a**) Cavity in healthy enamel achieved with 160,000 pulses from an Nd:YLF laser (pulse duration: 30 ps, pulse energy: 1 mJ). (**b**) Cavity in carious enamel achieved with 16,000 pulses from an Nd:YLF laser (pulse duration: 30 ps, pulse energy: 1 mJ). (Reproduced from [9])

ruption is a reaction in which phenomena such as plasma formation, shock wave generation, cavitation, and jet formation all occur.

Figure 2.6 shows immediately after picosecond laser irradiation on glass. In Fig. 2.6 a, the outer rim is thought to be caused by shock wave and cavitation and the cracked portion in the middle is thought to be caused by plasma and jet formation. The higher the energy, the stronger the plasma formation, shock wave generation, cavitation, and jet formation. Thus, overall tissue damage is linearly proportional to energy. On the other hand, plasma-induced ablation is bounded to the area in which plasma is generated, so the shock wave generation or cavitation only has a limited effect on the surrounding tissue [3].

After the plasma generation by laser, shock wave generation, cavitation, and jet formation do not occur sequentially. In more detail, after shock wave is generated by plasma, cavity is generated later by the shock wave. The cavity is reduced in volume due to the pressure of the surrounding tissue, and the reduced volume generates more pressure resulting in a second shock wave, and again due to the second shock wave, second cavitation occurs. The cavity is a phenomenon that

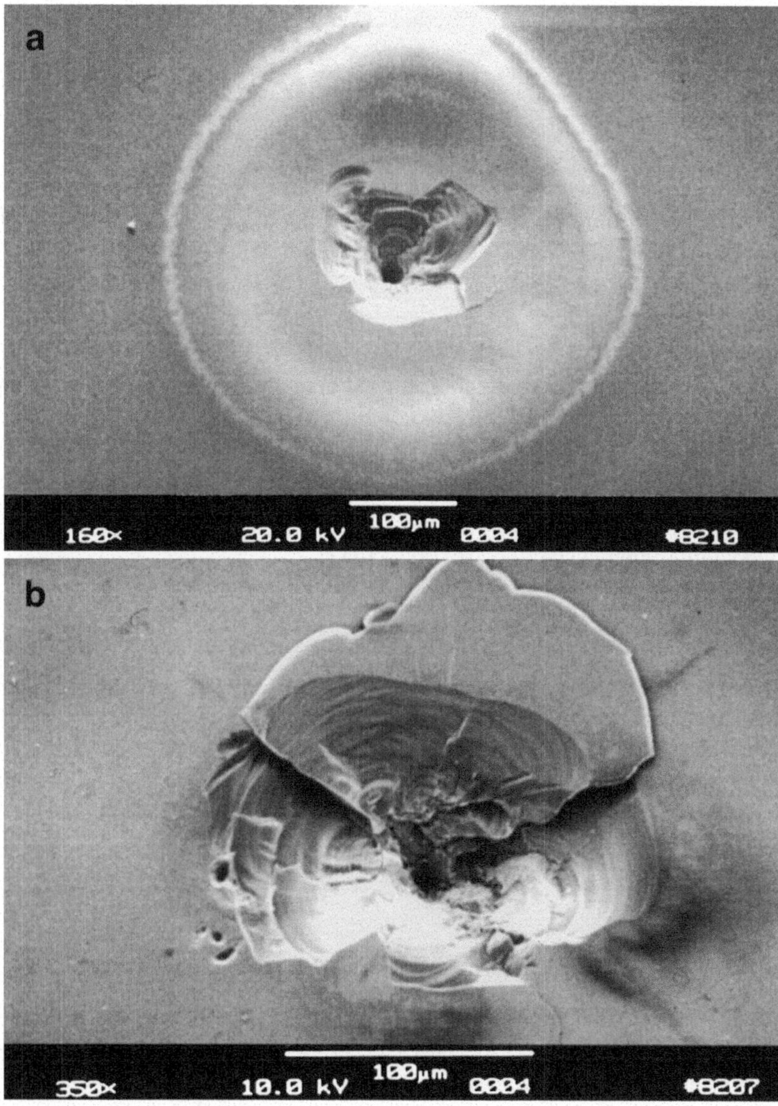

Fig. 2.6 (**a**) Anterior surface of a 90 µm thick glass plate exposed to ten pulses from an Nd:YLF laser (pulse duration: 30 ps, pulse energy: 1 mJ, focal spot size: 30 µm). (**b**) Posterior surface of a glass plate after a similar experiment. (Reproduced from [9])

occurs only in soft tissues and fluids, and if there is a solid nearby, jet formation occurs, and similarly, second jet formation occurs [3].

Next, let's take a closer look at plasma formation, shock wave generation, cavitation, and jet formation [4].

Shock wave is a phenomenon that occurs after plasma. Due to phase changes, volume expansion may occur (phase explosion or expansion). It may also occur secondary after cavitation. Shock waves occur at supersonic speeds and change to normal acoustic waves after 30–50 ns. Shock waves produce mechanical effects such as ablation and fracturing. These mechanical effects are proportional to the energy absorbed. The range of impact of the shock wave is known to be spatially up to 0.2 mm^2. In terms of radius it affects up to 0.252 mm and in terms of depth it affects up to 252 µm. Since the epidermal layer is 60–100 µm thick and the dermal layer is 1000 µm thick, shock waves can affect the entire epidermal layer and part of the dermal layer.

Cavitation is a phenomenon that occurs 50–150 ns after laser irradiation and occurs only in soft tissues and fluids. When the pressure is lowered due to volume expansion, the water around the target vaporizes, and cavitation occurs. This is why cavitation occurs 50–150 ns after laser irradiation, rather than immediately after laser irradiation. The inside of cavitation bubbles made by cavitation consists of gaseous vapor of which water vapor and carbon oxides are the main components. Within one millisecond, the bubble is compressed due to external pressure, causing a secondary cavity to be created again by the compression pressure. Several bubbles occur over several microseconds, resulting in multiple cavities and shock waves. Once the bubble is formed and contracted, about 84% of the energy is lost, mainly by sound. Since the size of the cavitation bubble grows to several millimeters, it can be observed with the naked eye unlike other phenomena (macroscopic effect).

Jet formation is a secondary phenomenon that occurs in fluids when there is a hard solid at the peripheral boundary as the cavity bubbles are compressed. Very high pressures occur as the pressure to be generated inside the solid is added to the opposite side of the solid boundary. Therefore, the skin damage caused by jet formation is more severe than the skin damage caused by cavitation alone.

2.5.1 Three Effects Generated by the Plasma of Photodisruption

In the previous section, we mentioned that plasma can be generated by plasma-induced ablation or by photodisruption. However, plasma by photodisruption requires 100 times more energy than plasma by plasma-induced ablation. Therefore, the density of free election and plasma temperature is higher than plasma by plasma-induced ablation. As a result, plasma only occurs in plasma-induced ablations, but in photodisruption plasma, shock wave, cavitation, and jet formation occur. And another three effects occur in photodisruption and may be more important (Table 2.2) [3].

First, plasma shielding effect occurs. The succeeding laser photons that arrive after the plasma is generated are absorbed as they meet the plasma and cannot pass through the plasma. Therefore, plasma protects the tissue under the plasma by blocking photons like a shield, so it is called the plasma shielding effect. The plasma shielding effect occurs because of inverse Bremsstrahlung. Free electrons mainly absorb the photons in plasma. Higher fluence leads to more free electrons and higher density of free elections. As the density of free electrons increases, they absorb more photons that arrive. Thus, the number of photons passing through the plasma is reduced.

Table 2.2 Three effects generated by the plasma of photodisruption

1. Plasma shielding effect
2. Brillouin scattering
3. Multiple plasma generation

In physical terms, the higher the fluence, the higher the absorption coefficient of the plasma. The absorption coefficient of plasma is 0.1 cm^{-1} in the very low fluence below 10 J/cm^2 but increasing the fluence to 23 J/cm^2 increases the absorption coefficient to 100 cm^{-1} which is 1000 times. When irradiated with fluence twice as high as the threshold of plasma generation, the absorption coefficient increases from 100 to 1000 times. Therefore, the higher the fluence, the better the plasma shielding effect.

I believe that due to the plasma shielding effect, the following result occurs when using picolaser. Figure 2.7 shows the biopsy of 755 nm alexandrite picolaser with different fluences on the skin.

A change occurs in the epidermis because the chromophore of 755 nm picolaser is melanin. It can be observed that if the fluence is higher, the vacuoles, including cellular debris, generate closer to the skin surface. On the other hand, if the fluence is lower, the size of the vacuole becomes smaller and is generated deeper in the epidermis.

The concentration of melanosomes increases as it goes down to the deep basal layer. In long-pulsed lasers or Q-switched lasers, photons pass from the epidermis to the dermis and the highest temperature rises in the basal layer due to highest melanin concentration leading to initial

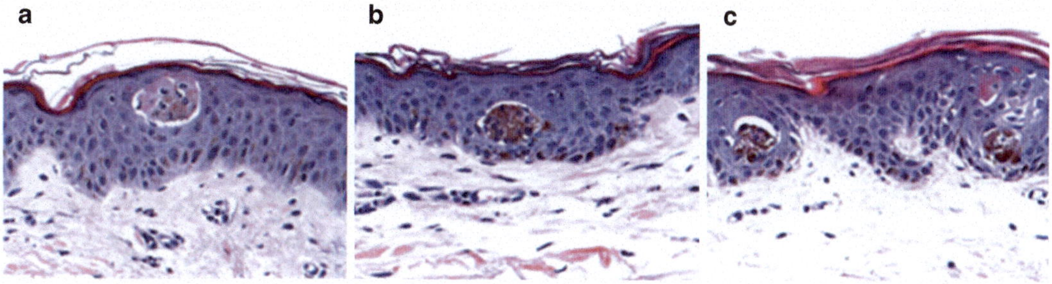

Fig. 2.7 Histology from a skin biopsy at 24 h posttreatment of skin type IV. MI = 31 demonstrating intraepidermal vacuoles created with F = (**a**) 0.71 J/cm^2, (**b**) 0.4 J/cm^2, and (**c**) 0.25 J/cm^2. The vacuoles contain cellular debris and the size and depth of the vacuole appear to diminish and increase, respectively, as the energy per micro-spot decreases. As we decrease the energy the vacuole diameter becomes smaller and the depth becomes deeper probably due to increase in melanin density deeper in the epidermis (200×). (Reproduced from [10])

changes. But in picosecond lasers, because of plasma shielding effect, the higher energy, the more likely plasma is generated in the surface of epidermis layer rather than in the basal layer. Once the plasma is generated, photons cannot pass through so that vacuole occurs only on the epidermis layer and because of the high fluence, the sizes of vacuoles are large.

In view of this result, when treating epidermal pigmentations with 755 nm alexandrite picolasers, treatment with low fluence may brighten the skin tone, but the pigmentations are not completely removed due to small vacuoles. Also, it may affect basement membranes causing side effects. On the other hand, if the fluence is high, it may be safer because the surface is treated first, but it must be repeated several times over several sessions to completely remove the pigmentations of the epidermis.

Of course, the region of pigmentation treatment with 755 nm alexandrite picolaser is not the photodisruption region of plasma generation but photoacoustic effect region. However, I think that plasma shielding effect also appears in photoacoustic effect region as well as photodisruption region (This will be explained later in Sect. 2.6.1).

Second, Brillouin scattering occurs. Brillouin scattering is a phenomenon in which subsequent photons are scattered by thermally amplified acoustic waves after the plasma is generated. In the scattering, we know only the direction of the photon is changed by collagen, not the energy or wavelength, but in Brillouin scattering, the photon changes to a frequency corresponding to the material's inherent phonon frequency. The phenomenon is called as scattering because photons disperse and are not absorbed with frequency changing. In Brillouin scattering, like the plasma shielding effect, photons disappear when encountering plasma and cannot pass through the plasma.

Third, multiple plasma generation occurs. One plasma is generated around ablation threshold; however, multiple plasmas are generated in higher energy. For example, in the focusing beam, one plasma is generated only at the focus. Then, especially in the case of a mode-locked laser, fluence increases during pulse duration and subsequent photons generate new plasma before reaching the focus. Therefore, multiple plasmas are generated from the focus to the laser direction (Fig. 2.8).

2.5.2 Reactions of Q-Switched Lasers and Picolasers

What reactions are produced by Q-switch lasers and picolasers currently released?

I think Q-switched laser does not produce reactions such as by plasma-induced ablation or photodisruption. As shown in Fig. 2.3, plasma is generated only when Q-switched lasers focus on the one point with a zoom handpiece to produce high energy. In practice, flash (plasma) is rarely

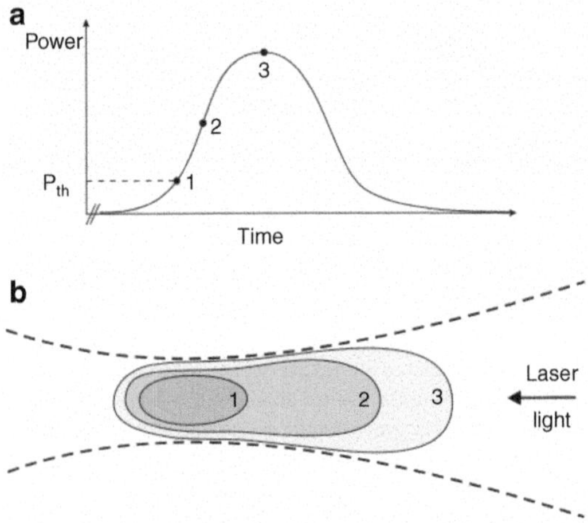

Fig. 2.8 Temporal evolution of the laser power (**a**) and the plasma contours (**b**) during the optical breakdown process at pulse energies above threshold ("moving breakdown"). (1) When the laser power exceeds the optical breakdown threshold, *P*th, a plasma is formed in the focal volume. (2) As the laser power increases during the pulse, the threshold irradiance is exceeded further upstream of the focal volume. (3) The maximum plasma extension is reached when the laser power reaches its maximum. While upstream of the focal volume the plasma contours at times (1)–(3) correspond to iso-irradiance lines, this does not hold for the region "downstream" of the focal volume because of light absorption by the plasma ("plasma shielding"). (Reproduced from [11])

detected during the use of Q-switched lasers for pigmentation and tattoo treatment. Therefore, I think that only shock wave generation, cavitation, and jet formation occur in Q-switched lasers. During tattoo treatment, shock wave is generated by the Q-switched laser and a popping sound is generated by cavitation. Therefore, in one laser text, breaking tattoo particles with shock wave generation and cavitation is called the photoacoustic effect [4]. Therefore, I think that Q-switched laser mainly generates photoacoustic effects.

What kind of laser shows photodisruption, such as plasma shielding effect, Brillouin scattering, and the multiple plasma generation? They appear only when currently released picolaser (strictly speaking, subnanosecond laser) focuses with zoom handpiece.

To call the laser as true picosecond laser, pulse duration must be below tens of picosecond. It is right to call the currently released picolaser as

Table 2.3 Lasers and its effects and reactions

Lasers	Effects	Reactions
Q-switched laser Subnanosecond laser	Photoacoustic effect	Shock wave, cavitation, jet formation
Subnanosecond laser (zoom handpiece)	Photodisruption	Plasma, shock wave, cavitation, jet formation Plasma shielding effect, Brillouin scattering, multiple plasma generation
True picosecond laser Femtosecond laser	Plasma-induced ablation	Plasma

subnanosecond laser because they are hundreds of picoseconds [12–14]. (In the previous chapter, I described subnanosecond laser as picolaser to distinguish it from a true picosecond laser.) In other words, the currently released subnanosecond laser (picolaser) mainly generates shock wave, cavitation, and jet formation. When the laser focuses with a zoom handpiece, photodisruption effect appears such as the plasma shielding effect, Brillouin scattering, multiple plasmas appear together with plasma formation, shock wave generation, cavitation, and jet formation.

If true picosecond laser or femtosecond laser is released, only plasma-induced ablation effect will occur (Table 2.3). Reactions such as plasma shielding effect, Brillouin scattering, multiple plasma generation, shock wave generation, cavitation, and jet formation will not occur.

2.6 Plasma-Induced Ablation Versus Photodisruption

So far, we reviewed the effects of plasma-induced ablation and photodisruption. Which is the optimal response for our purpose? What laser should we buy?

As reviewed above, shock wave generation, cavitation, and jet formation influence the surrounding tissue. Therefore, true picosecond lasers and femtosecond lasers are the safest and the most adequate laser for our purpose. Let's take a closer look at this concept.

The threshold fluence at which plasma is generated depends on the pulse duration. High temperature per hour is required to generate plasma and the parameter related to the phase or reaction change is power density. Therefore, the longer pulse duration, the higher the fluence. On the other hand, the parameter related to volume change and pressure is fluence (the curve in Fig. 2.9 shows the threshold at which the plasma occurs). Therefore, nanosecond laser needs higher fluence than picosecond laser to make plasma. Due to high fluence, large volume changes and high pressures can cause damage to surrounding tissues due to phenomena such as shock waves. In fact, nanosecond lasers are known to generate shock waves even at the threshold at which plasma is generated. Thus, pure plasma-induced ablation does not occur in nanosecond lasers. On the other hand, picosecond and femtosecond lasers produce plasma at low fluence due to the short pulse duration. Due to the low fluence, the volume change is small and no phenomena such as shock waves occur. Therefore, the damages are confined spatially and the predictability increases in picosecond and femtosecond lasers. In conclusion, for our purposes of avoiding damage to surrounding tissues, picosecond or femtosecond lasers that produce plasma-induced ablation are the best lasers.

Let's summarize what we have reviewed. Figure 2.9 shows the areas of plasma-induced ablation and photodisruption that occur by pulse duration and fluence. So, what happens to the lower right area of the curve? Area 1 is the area of the Q-switched laser that we use. That is, in this area, plasma is not generated and phenomena such as shock wave generation, cavitation, and jet formation occur. Area 2 is the area where flash (plasma) is made by using a zoom handpiece with a Q-switched laser. Currently released subnanosecond lasers fall in area 3. This is because no flash (plasma) occurs during pigmentation or tattoo treatment with a subnanosecond laser. Nowadays, subnanosecond lasers are used to treat scars and wrinkles using zoom handpieces (area 4). There is no laser for areas 5 and 6 yet.

What happens if lasers for area 5 and 6 laser are released? In order to make the laser for area 5, the power of the laser must be ten times higher than the subnanosecond laser in area 3. The power determines the cost of the laser machine. Thus, the cost should be about ten times as high. And the area we want is not area 5 but actually area 6. To make a laser for area 6, zoom handpiece is needed and because the zoom handpiece has a small treatment range, many shots should be irradiated. Therefore, a laser about ten times more expensive than the current subnanosecond

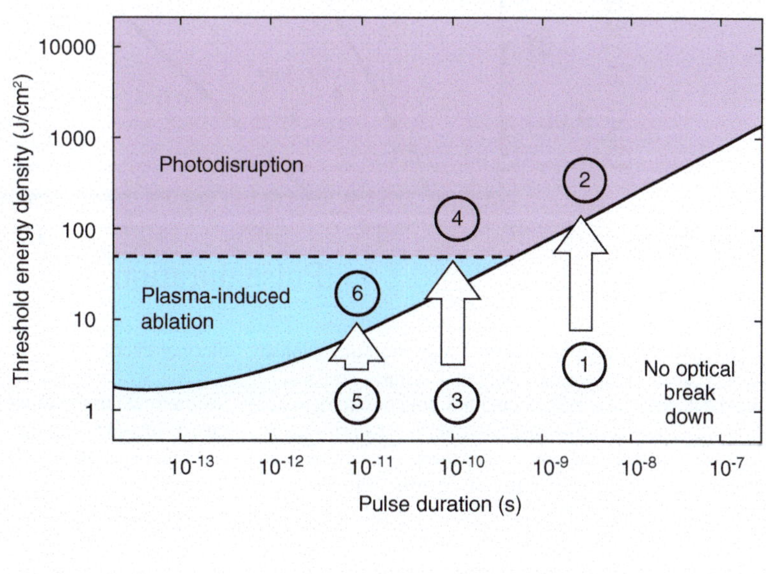

Fig. 2.9 Distinction of plasma-induced ablation and photodisruption according to applied energy density. (Modified from [9])

laser should be released for area 6. Since the cost-effectiveness of treating pigmentations with such expensive lasers is still low, I believe that lasers using pure plasma-induced ablation will not be available for a while.

2.6.1 Stress Confinement Time

Q-switched laser and currently released subnanosecond lasers are in the region of photoacoustic effect, which does not produce plasma. Then what is the difference between Q-switched and subnanosecond lasers?

The keyword in selective photothermolysis is thermal relaxation time (TRT). In other words, the idea is that "if a little light energy is irradiated for a short time, the light energy received by the target tissue is used only to raise the temperature of the target tissue and does not transmit heat to surrounding tissues." In other words, heat is confined in the target tissue (thermal confinement). Similarly, stress confinement can be thought of stress confined in the target tissue [6]. In other words, "if a little light energy is irradiated for a short time, the light energy received by the target tissue is used only to give stress and damage the target tissue and does not transmit stress to surrounding tissues."

Figure 2.10 shows the zone of thermal confinement and stress confinement and the corresponding laser. The zone corresponding to the theory of selective photothermolysis is the thermal confinement zone in Fig. 2.10. On the other hand, there is a stress confinement zone which is affected by shock waves affects and the corresponding lasers are 1064 nm Q-switched Nd:YAG lasers and subnanosecond lasers. To put it simply 1064 nm Q-switched Nd:YAG lasers and subnanosecond lasers are lasers that break target tissue. These zones are not clearly divided. For example, Q-switched Nd:YAG lasers not only have only a mechanical effect but also thermal effects. But the main effect is mechanical.

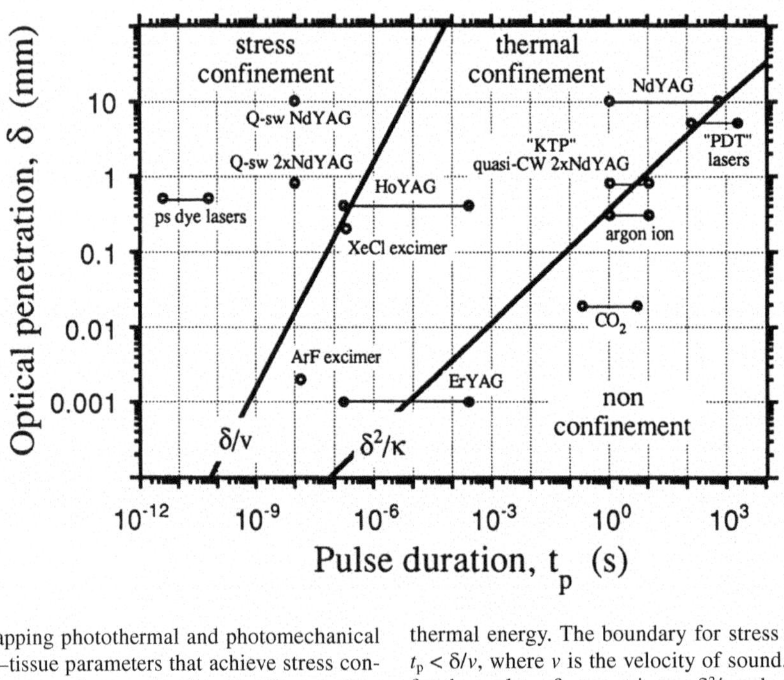

Fig. 2.10 Mapping photothermal and photomechanical effects. Laser–tissue parameters that achieve stress confinement, thermal confinement, and nonconfinement are mapped in terms of the optical zone, δ, of laser energy deposition and the laser pulse duration, t_p. Shallow penetration requires shorter pulses to confine the stress or thermal energy. The boundary for stress confinement is $t_p < \delta/v$, where v is the velocity of sound. The boundary for thermal confinement is $t_p < \delta^2/\kappa$, where κ is the thermal diffusivity. Example lasers are shown in terms of t_p and approximate δ for typical tissues. (Reproduced from [15])

Similar to the thermal relaxation time (TRT), stress relaxation time (SRT) or stress confinement time can be considered in the stress confinement zone. The formula of SRT is as follows [16]:

$$\tau_S = \frac{\Delta}{c_S}$$

τ_s: stress confinement time,
c_S: sonic velocity inside the tattoo, $c_s \fallingdotseq 4 \times 10^5$ cm/s,
Δ: characteristic length in the tattoo material.

SRT is a concept to mainly use in tattoo treatment so that Δ depicts the size of tattoo particles. Let's look at SRT in tattoo treatment. The size of tattoo particles varies from text to text, but it is known that the size usually is from 0.5 to 5 μm and as small as 25 μm (Fig. 2.11). Calculated SRT is from 125 ps to 1.25 ns and as small as 10 ps. Therefore, it is difficult to treat tattoos of all sizes with a 1064 nm Q-switched laser or currently released subnanosecond laser with a 450–750 ps pulse duration.

For reference, the size of the smallest tattoo particles is known to be less than 10 nm. These small tattoo particles are not yet treatable by laser, but it is so small that it is not visible to our eyes by scattering, so there is no need to treat it [16].

Let's consider the therapeutic effect of subnanosecond laser in consideration of TRT and SRT of melanosomes, which is the goal of pigmentation treatment. The sizes of the melanin granules and melanosomes are 15 nm and 0.5 μm, respectively, and TRT is 400 ps and 0.5 μs, respectively [18]. The pulse duration of Q-switched Nd:YAG laser is 5–10 ns, which, in terms of thermal confinement, can treat melanosomes but cannot treat melanin granules. Because subnanosecond lasers have pulse durations of 450–750 ps, melanin granules can also be treated. However, since both lasers belong to the stress confinement zone, TRT cannot be applied. On the other hand, the SRT of melanin granules and melanosomes are 10 and 300 ps, respectively [18], and in terms of stress confinement, both lasers cannot treat melanin granules or melanosomes. In summary, both the Q-switched Nd:YAG laser and the subnanosecond laser are lasers in the stress confinement zone, but the pulse duration is longer than that of the SRT of some of the melanin granules and the melanosome so that the perfect stress confinement is not achieved. Then what is the difference between these two lasers?

The difference between the two lasers can be explained by peak tensile stress. Peak tensile stress is expressed by the following formula [17]:

$$\sigma = -3\gamma\mu F\left(\frac{\tau_a}{\tau}\right)^2$$

σ: the peak tensile stress, obtained at the center of the tattoo target.
F: the laser irradiance (fluence).
τ_a and τ: the acoustic transit time and laser pulse duration, respectively.
μ: the absorption coefficient of the target material at the laser wavelength.
γ: a constant that depends only on the properties of the target.

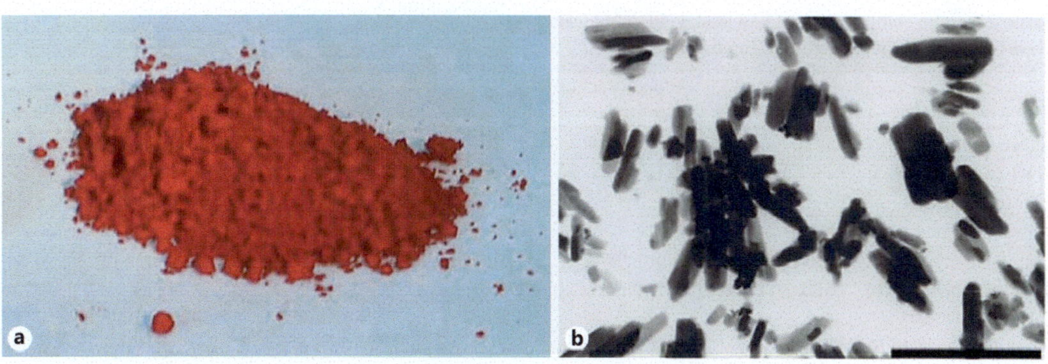

Fig. 2.11 (**a**) Azo pigment PR.22 powder. (**b**) Electron microscopy image of the disazo-diarylide pigment PY.82 powder (Scale bar, 1 μm). (Reproduced from [17])

The peak tensile stress formula shows that the absorption coefficient and fluence are also important, but the pulse duration has a very significant effect. For example, in a subnanosecond laser with 600 ps pulse duration, the pulse duration is ten times than that of a Q-switched laser having 6 ns pulse duration and the tensile stress is 100 times than that of a Q-switched laser. In other words, the subnanosecond laser breaks 100 times better than the Q-Switched laser. However, since the pulse duration is longer than SRT, there are side effects. But due to the low fluence, the range of side effects is less than that of the Q-switched lasers.

For example, when treating melasma with Q-switched Nd:YAG lasers, in terms of thermal confinement, the pulse duration should be shorter than the melanosome's TRT so that the melanosomes coagulate and have no side effects. However, because Q-switched Nd:YAG lasers are in the stress confinement zone, the coagulation effect is not large and the main effect is destroying the melanosome with a shock wave. Since the pulse duration of the Q-switched Nd:YAG laser is longer than the SRT, the possibility of side effects is high while the effect of destroying melanosomes is low. Subnanosecond lasers also belong to the stress confinement zone, so when treating melasma, melanosomes are broken by shock wave like the Q-switched laser. Since the pulse duration of the subnanosecond laser is longer than the SRT, there are side effects, but the pulse duration is shorter than that of the Q-switched Nd YAG laser, so side effects are less likely to occur and the melanosomes are broken well (Table 2.4).

Table 2.4 The comparison of Q-switched Nd: YAG laser versus subnanosecond laser targeting melanosome

	Q-switched Nd:YAG laser	Subnanosecond laser
Pulse duration	5–10 ns	450–750 ps
TRT of melanosome (500 ns)	TRT > PD	TRT ≫ PD
Tissue reaction	Stress confinement	Stress confinement
SRT of melanosome (300 ps)	SRT ≪ PD	SRT ≤ PD
Peak tensile stress	Lesser	Greater
Spatial extent of the shock wacve	Large	Small

2.7 Photothermal Effect

Let's review the photothermal effect. Photothermal effect has a pulse duration of 1 ms to 100 s and a power density of 1–10^6 W/cm^2. When a molecule absorbs a photon, the temperature is raised as light energy is converted into kinetic energy. The phenomena of photothermal effects vary with temperature and time by Arrhenius equation (see "Chap. 3"). Four typical phenomena are coagulation, vaporization, carbonization, and melting. In a situation where phase does not change, these phenomena appear sequentially as the temperature changes (linear change) [4]. Therefore, temperature plays the most important role in photothermal effect (Table 2.5).

When temperature exceeds 60 °C, protein and collagen are denaturized, resulting in coagulation and necrosis. Collagen melting is the desired reaction in skin rejuvenation. This is because collagen fiber shrinks, making a noticeable skin tightening, and new collagen is regenerated (collagen remodeling). However, when the temperature exceeds 80 °C, membrane permeability is impaired and the chemical equilibrium of the cell is destroyed [3]. This phenomenon is likely to be a phenomenon we do not want. Thus, the temperature we want is between 60 and 80 °C. This will be explained later in "Chap. 9."

Photothermal effect is mainly used in dermatology. Among the photothermal effects, mainly coagulation and vaporization are used since

Table 2.5 Response of skin tissue to temperature [8]

Temperature (°C)	Thermal reactions
42–45	Beginning of hyperthermia, conformational changes, and shrinkage of collagen
50	Reduction of enzymatic activity
60	Denaturation of proteins, coagulation of the collagens, membrane permeabilization
100	Tissue drying and formation of vacuoles
>100	Beginning of vaporization and tissue carbonization
300–1000	Thermoablation of tissue, photoablation, and disruption

carbonization and melting may cause serious side effects. These include argon lasers, pulsed dye lasers (PDLs), CO_2 lasers, Nd:YAG lasers, Er:YAG lasers, ruby lasers, and diode lasers. Treatment targets include laser hair removal, vascular therapy, pigmentation treatments, and skin rejuvenation [4].

Next, let's take a closer look at the four phenomena of the photothermal reaction.

First, coagulation is the ideal phenomenon described in the selective photothermolysis theory (Fig. 2.12). Applying the concept of TRT and having a pulse duration equal to or less than TRT (TRT $\geq$ PD) can cause damage target without affecting surrounding tissues. However, I think that the disadvantage of coagulation is that the therapeutic window is very narrow. In Fig. 2.12, the treatment range is from 75 to 100 °C [19], but other texts view the range of treatment from 60 to 80 °C when the above-mentioned coagulation begins [3].

Second, vaporization is used for ablative rejuvenation to ablate tissue using CO_2 laser or Er:YAG laser. The mechanism of ablative rejuvenation is thought to vaporize skin tissue, but it is not. When energy is accumulated in the skin in a very short time, the temperature of the water in the skin becomes high, so that the volume of the water is increased by vaporization and the pressure is increased. At 300 °C, the water rises to 1000 atm. As the water pressure increases in the tissue, the water in the tissue explodes due to the pressure difference with the atmosphere, and the skin tissue is removed together (explosive removal). Therefore, the mechanism of skin rejuvenation is not to vaporize all skin tissues, but to forcibly eject the skin from the surface using water [6]. Therefore, it would be correct to describe ablative skin rejuvenation as "cutting" or "digging" rather than "burning."

Ablation due to vaporization is an explosive removal reaction that damages the surrounding tissue and causes side effects (Fig. 2.13). Therefore, CO_2 laser and Er:YAG laser are in non-confinement zones, not thermal confinement and stress confinement zones (Fig. 2.10). In the treatment of epidermal pigmentations, CO_2 lasers are known to have the highest side effects than long-pulsed lasers and Q-switched lasers [20]. Since vaporization is caused by pressure, it is similar to the photomechanical effect, so the term thermomechanical effect is used [3].

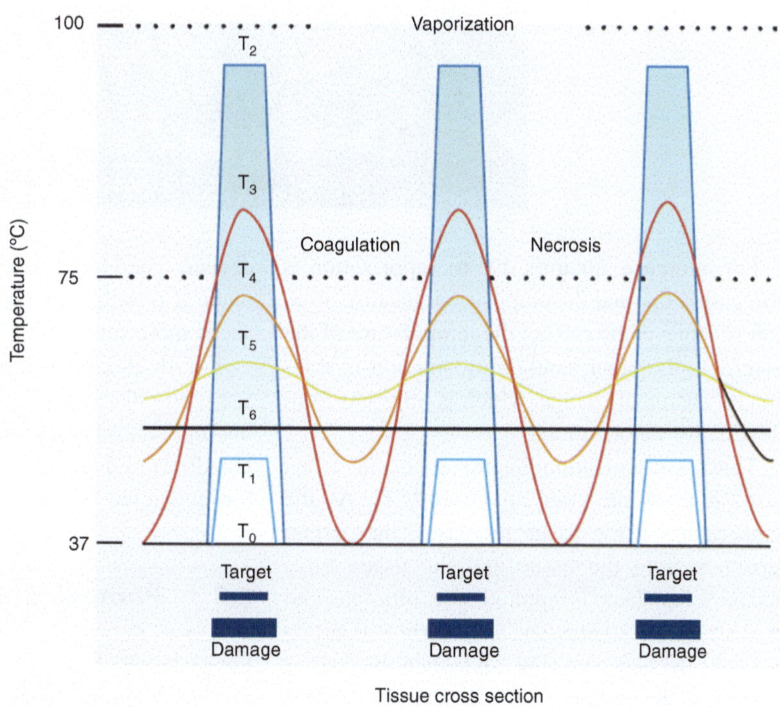

Fig. 2.12 Schematic temperature profiles during selective photothermolysis: T_0, before laser exposure (uniform body temperature); T_1, during laser exposure (selective rapid target heating); T_2, at the end of laser exposure (targets irreversibly damaged); T_3, one thermal relaxation time after laser pulse (targets cooling, surrounding tissue warming); T_4, two thermal relaxation times after laser pulse; T_5, five thermal target relaxation times after laser pulse; and T_6, tissue slowly returning to ambient thermal equilibrium. (Modified from [19])

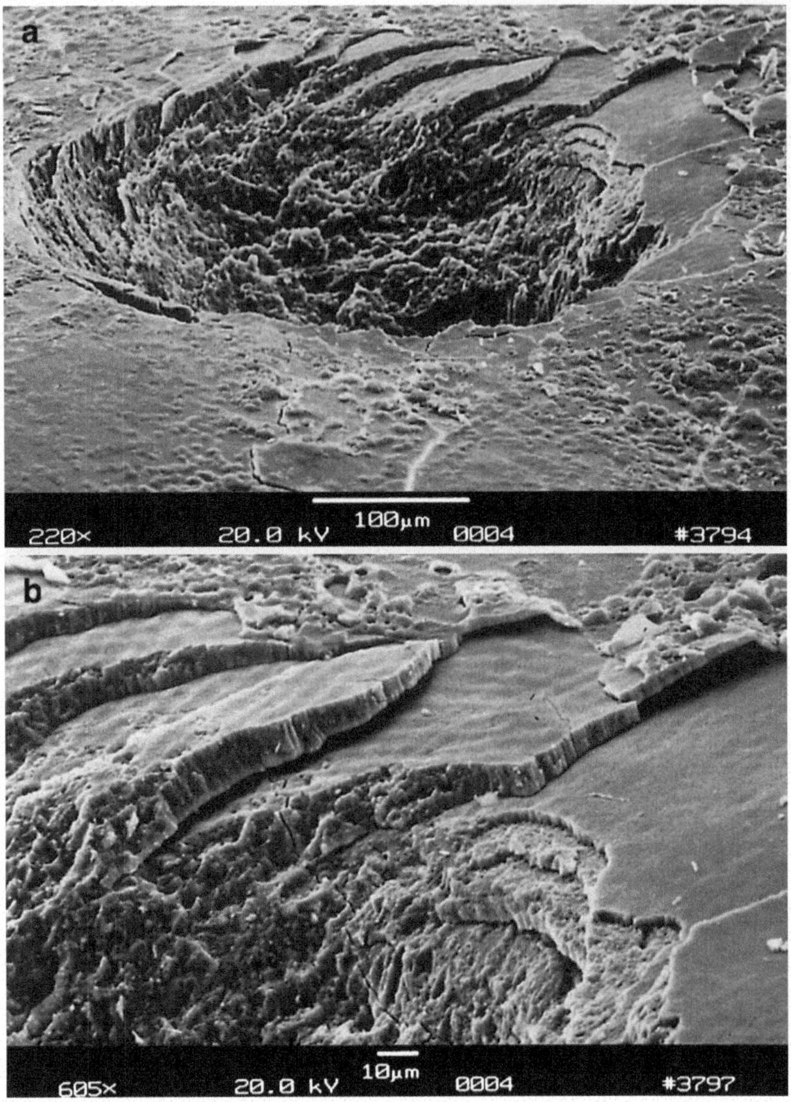

Fig. 2.13 (**a**) Human tooth vaporized by 20 pulses from an Er:YAG laser (pulse duration: 90 μs. Pulse energy: 100 mJ, repetition rate: 1 Hz). (**b**) Enlargement showing the edge of ablation. (Reproduced from [9])

For reference, ablation due to vaporization is also called thermal decomposition because ablation is achieved by raising the temperature of the water. On the other hand, photoablation is ablation by chemical change, which is different from ablation by vaporization.

Third, carbonization begins to occur when tissue temperature rises above 100 °C. As the temperature of the tissue increases, the carbon separates from the tissue and the tissue turns black. When heat is applied, the ultimate end product of all living tissue is carbon. Carbon becomes the new heat sink, and when the laser is irradiated, the temperature rises sharply to 300–600 °C and the residual thermal damage becomes deeper. Therefore, carbonization should not be made if possible, as damage to surrounding tissue is more severe [6].

Fourth, melting is a phenomenon in which tissue melts like lava. Gas bubbles form and melting and solidification of the tissue are observed. Hundreds of degrees of temperature are required for human teeth to melt.

2.8 Photoablation

Let's take a look at photoablation. Only the 308 nm excimer laser corresponds to photoablation in the dermatology field, so I'll go over it briefly.

Photoablation produces a chemical effect that breaks bonds between molecules, creating an ablative effect. In terms of laser parameters, the pulse duration is in nanoseconds and the power density corresponds to 10^7–10^8 W/cm^2. A laser with a pulse duration of 10 ns is the 308-nm excimer laser [4]. Because of the chemical changes, photoablation is sometimes included in the photochemical effect, but I believe that photoablation should be separated into independent reactions because it exhibits a completely different reaction from the photochemical effect such as photodynamic therapy (PDT).

The energy required to break the chemical bonds of molecules in the tissue is shown in Table 2.6. At least 3.0 eV of energy is required. However, in Table 2.7, the wavelength showing photon energy of more than 3.0 eV is less than 355 nm. A typical laser in this area is the 308-nm excimer laser. CO_2 lasers have pulse durations of 10 ns and can also produce pulse durations of nanoseconds, but they can't break molecular bonds with a photon energy of 0.1 eV [3].

Due to photoablation, tissue evaporates and liquefies as the molecular bonds break. The irradiated energy is used to vaporize and liquefy tissues and some energy is converted into kinetic energy and used to discharge the liquefied materials. The tissue response by photoablation appears very quickly and there is little time left for heat damage because there is little leftover energy [4]. Laser used for photoablation is also known as "cold lasers" because it ablates without heat damage. Ultraviolet wavelength also plays a role in not having deep penetration depth. In one laser text, the tissue response of photoablation was described as "very clean exact process with excellent predictability and little thermal damage" [4]. A similar expression was used in plasma-induced ablation. In other words, photoablation is very safe without side effects. Unfortunately, there is no laser available in esthetic dermatology.

Examples of the laser include ArF (193 nm), KrF (249 nm), XeCl (308 nm), XeF (351 nm), etc. In dermatology, 308-nm excimer laser is used for psoriasis, vitiligo, white stretch marks, etc. In ophthalmology, it is used to correct hyperopia, myopia, and astigmatism. In dentistry, 2780 nm ErCr:YSGG laser or Er:YAG laser is used.

Table 2.6 Dissociation energy of selected molecular bonds

Molecular bond	Dissociation energy (eV)	Molecular bond	Dissociation energy (eV)
C=O	7.5	C–O	3.6
C=C	6.4	C–C	3.6
O–H	4.8	S–H	3.5
C–H	4.3	C–N	3.0
N–H	4.1		

Reproduced from [11]

Table 2.7 Wavelength and photon energy of selected UV laser systems

Laser type	Wavelength (nm)	Photon energy (eV)
ArF excimer	193	6.4
Nd:YAG (5υ)	213	5.8
KrF excimer	248	5.0
Nd:YAG (4υ)	266	4.6
XeCl excimer	308	4.0
N_2	337	3.7
Nd:YAG (3υ)	355	3.5

Reproduced from [11]

2.9 Photochemical Effect

Photochemical effects and biostimulation have been studied extensively, but because there are many controversies and have no definite effect, I will review these briefly.

Photochemical effect refers to a reaction that causes chemical change without changing tissue with very low energy for a very long time. A typical example is photodynamic therapy (PDT). This corresponds to laser parameters with a long pulse duration of 10–1000 s and a very low-power density of 10^{-3} ~ 1 W/cm^2 [4]. It shows a low-temperature change below 45 °C so that hyperthermia does not occur. Theoretically, ultraviolet or violet wavelengths should be used, but the wavelength of visible light is used because of the effect or depth of penetration. For example, in PDT, when photosensitizer is applied to the skin and irradiated with a laser, cytotoxic reactants such as single oxygen are generated which have an effect on the skin. The lifetime of singlet oxygen is very short, 10–40 ns, and diffuses about 10–20 nm. PDT is also known to synthesize heat shock protein (HSP).

PDT uses blue LED (405–420 nm), red LED (635 nm), PDL (585 nm), IPL (500–1200 nm), argon-pumped dye lasers (630 nm), and diode (633 nm). The US FDA approved PDT for the treatment of nonhyperkeratotic actinic keratosis (AK) in the face and scalp. Clinically, it is used for photorejuvenation such as capillary vasodilatation, dyschromia, and skin texture. The most common indication is acne.

2.9.1 Biostimulation

There are still many controversies regarding biostimulation. It is sometimes considered as a reaction belonging to the photochemical effect or as an independent reaction [4]. Biostimulation uses a very low energy of 1–5 mW, 1–10 J/cm^2. There is no change in temperature. Some define biostimulation as a reaction with no thermal mechanism. It is known to have wound healing and anti-inflammatory effects. Red and infrared wavelength lasers are used such as 633-nm helium neon (HeNe) laser and 850 nm GaAs laser. Promoting cell proliferation is thought to be the mechanism of biostimulation. Biostimulation is discussed in detail in Sect. 9.8 in "Chap. 9."

2.10 Conclusion

So far, we have examined various physical phenomena and tissue responses by lasers (Fig. 2.1). Let's review our purpose once again. First, our purpose is to give energy to the target tissue. Second, there should be no damage to the surrounding tissue. In particular, when it comes to safety, more emphasis should be placed on the second purpose. What is the most appropriate reaction for this purpose?

First, plasma-induced ablation creates plasma and is considered as a safe reaction that is "very clean and well-defined without evidence of thermal or mechanical damage." On the other hand, photodisruption is unsafe because it causes adverse effects such as shock wave generation, cavitation, and jet formation in addition to plasma. Thus, when plasma-induced ablation is compared with photodisruption, plasma-induced ablation may be a reasonable response, but no corresponding laser has yet been released. Both picolaser (subnanosecond laser) and Q-switched lasers are included in the photoacoustic effect area. However, picolasers are safer than Q-switched lasers, but they are not without any side effects.

Second, both photoablation and vaporization of the photothermal effect cause ablation, but vaporization of the photothermal reaction has high side effects. Photoablation, on the other hand, is thought to be a reasonable response with "very clean exact process with excellent predictability and little thermal damage," but unfortunately there are no lasers available in the dermatology area.

Third, photothermal effect using coagulation is known to be a safe reaction by selective photothermolysis. It is also the only reaction that can be realistically selected from the five laser–tissue interactions. However, treatment is not easy because the therapeutic window is narrow. It is safe to repeat the treatment with a lower energy.

In conclusion, I believe that theoretically there are no lasers without any side effects, i.e., perfect lasers in dermatology.

References

1. Stratigos A, Dover JS (2000) Overview of lasers and their properties. Dermatol Ther 13(1):2–16
2. Jelínková H (2013) Lasers for medical applications: diagnostics, therapy and surgery. Elsevier
3. Niemz MH (2007) Laser-tissue interactions. Springer, New York
4. Allemann IB, Goldberg DJ (2011) Basics in dermatological laser applications. Karger Medical and Scientific Publishers
5. Berlien H-P (2003) Applied laser medicine. Springer Science & Business Media
6. Goldman MP (2006) Cutaneous and cosmetic laser surgery. Mosby Elsevier, Philadelphia, PA
7. Keyvan N (2012) Lasers in dermatology and medicine. [S.I.]. Springer

8. Raulin C, Karsai S (2011) Laser and IPL technology in dermatology and aesthetic medicine. Heidelberg, New York
9. Niemz MH (2019) Laser-tissue interactions. Springer
10. Tanghetti EA (2016) The histology of skin treated with a picosecond alexandrite laser and a fractional lens array. Lasers Surg Med 48(7): 646–652
11. Vogel A, Venugopalan V (2003) Mechanisms of pulsed laser ablation of biological tissues. Chem Rev 103(2):577–644
12. Ross E (2017) The picosecond revolution and laser tattoo treatments: are shorter pulses really better? Br J Dermatol 176(2):299–300
13. Karsai S, Bäumler W, Weiss C, Faulhaber J, Raulin C (2018) Laser tattoo removal: do we already have picosecond lasers? J Dtsch Dermatol Ges 16(4): 468–470
14. Kasai K (2017) Picosecond laser treatment for tattoos and benign cutaneous pigmented lesions (secondary publication). Laser Ther 26(4):274–281
15. Jacques SL (1992) Laser-tissue interactions. Photochemical, photothermal, and photomechanical. Surg Clin North Am 72(3):531–558
16. Ho DDM, London R, Zimmerman GB, Young DA (2002) Laser-tattoo removal—a study of the mechanism and the optimal treatment strategy via computer simulations. Lasers Surg Med 30(5):389–397
17. Serup J, Bäumler W (2017) Diagnosis and therapy of tattoo complications: with atlas of illustrative cases. Karger Medical and Scientific Publishers
18. Strauss M, Amendt PA, London RA, Maitland DJ, Glinsky ME, Lin CP, et al. (eds). Computational modeling of stress transient and bubble evolution in short-pulse laser-irradiated melanosome particles. Laser-Tissue Interaction VIII; 1997: International Society for Optics and Photonics
19. Anderson RR, Parrish JA (1983) Selective photothermolysis: precise microsurgery by selective absorption of pulsed radiation. Science 220(4596):524–527
20. Kauvar A, Hruza G (2005) Principles and practices in cutaneous laser surgery. CRC Press

3 Important Laser Principles

3.1 Advanced Theory of Selective Photothermolysis

In "Chap. 1," we reviewed that the most important theory regarding lasers is the theory of selective photothermolysis. In practice, however, there are cases in which the theory of selective photothermolysis does not apply and sometimes it even deviates from the theory of selective photothermolysis [1]. Next, we will review three advanced theories developed from the selective photothermolysis theory (Table 3.1).

3.1.1 Thermal Kinetic Selectivity

Thermal kinetic selectivity (TKS) is a theory applied to determine pulse duration when large and small target tissues coexist [2].

Since pulse duration is proportional to the square of the diameter, large tissues will have a longer TRT (T_2) and small tissues will have a shorter TRT (T_1) ($T_1 < T_2$). If the pulse duration (PD) is between TRTs of large and small tissues ($T_1 < PD < T_2$), large tissues will be damaged because large tissues ($PD < T_2$) are TRT > PD. The problem is with small tissues. In the case of small tissues ($T_1 < PD$), because TRT < PD, according to theory of selective photothermolysis, surrounding tissues should become damaged and have side effects. In practice, however, side effects do not occur; rather, small tissues are preserved without any effect (Fig. 3.1).

When TRT < PD, if the pulse duration is long enough, the temperature of small tissues does not rise further but cools down during irradiation. Why did the phenomenon deviate from the theory of selective photothermolysis? There are three ways to lose heat in tissues: heat conduction, heat convection caused by blood flow, and

Table 3.1 Advanced theory of selective photothermolysis

1.	Thermal kinetic selectivity
2.	Extended theory of selective photothermolysis
3.	Subcellular selective photothermolysis

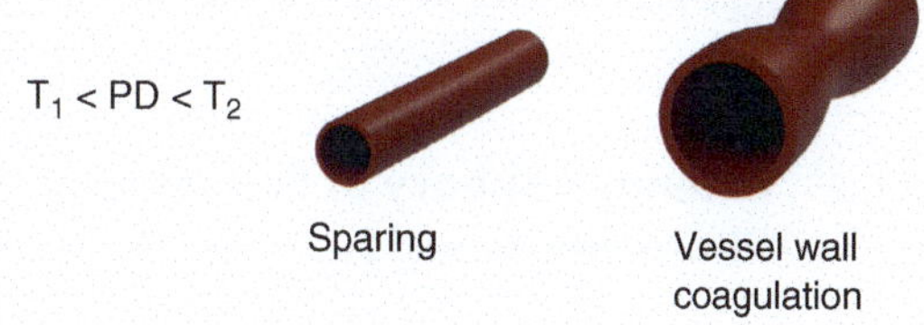
PD < T1 < T2
Vessel wall coagulation
Vessel wall rupture
T1 < PD < T2
Sparing
Vessel wall coagulation

Fig. 3.1 Two vessels in the skin (1 and 2), T_1 and T_2: thermal relaxation times (TRT) of 1 and 2, respectively. *PD* pulse duration

J. D. Lee et al., *Principles and Choice of Laser Treatment in Dermatology*,
https://doi.org/10.1007/978-981-15-6556-4_3

heat radiation [3]. Heat conduction, which transfers heat to the surroundings, is the main method of heat dissipation. However, if the pulse duration is long enough, small tissue cools down due to the latter two phenomena (heat convection and heat radiation). It is as if water is poured down slowly into a bucket with holes. For example, during the treatment of large tissues as in vascular therapy, small tissues such as melanosomes show no change. Also, during laser hair removal, even without epidermal cooling, pulse durations longer than the epidermal TRT (1–10 ms) such as 30 ms does not damage the epidermis. TKS is also applied to a variety of situations.

Then, at what pulse duration does TKS occur? I believe that TKS occurs at long pulse durations of milliseconds. In particular, I think it is a phenomenon that occurs in the photothermal effect below 100°C.

Let's think about pulse duration in large and small tissues again. In the situation where (T_1 < PD < T_2), large tissues are treated while small tissues are preserved. On the other hand, if the pulse duration (PD) is shorter than the TRTs of large and small tissues (PD < T_1 < T_2), both large and small tissues will be damaged because of TRT > PD. In this case, temperatures of large tissues can rise to temperatures that are too high, causing side effects [2]. Therefore, (T_1 < PD < T_2) is safer than (PD < T_1 < T_2). Then how do we treat small tissues? After removing large tissues first with PD < T_2, the pulse duration should be reduced, less than the TRT of the small tissue (PD < T_1), and the small tissues can be removed sequentially.

In conclusion, in long pulse durations of milliseconds, it is safe to remove large tissues and small tissues later.

3.1.2 Extended Theory of Selective Photothermolysis

Much of what is described in "Chap. 1" is based on the assumption that the target tissue and chromophore match. In practice, however, target tissue and chromophores do not match [1]. An example is the laser hair removal. The target tissues of laser hair removal are hair germ cells and follicular stem cells in the hair bulb and hair bulge, respectively, and the chromophores are the hair matrix and hair shaft, respectively. Hair germ cells and follicular stem cells do not have melanin.

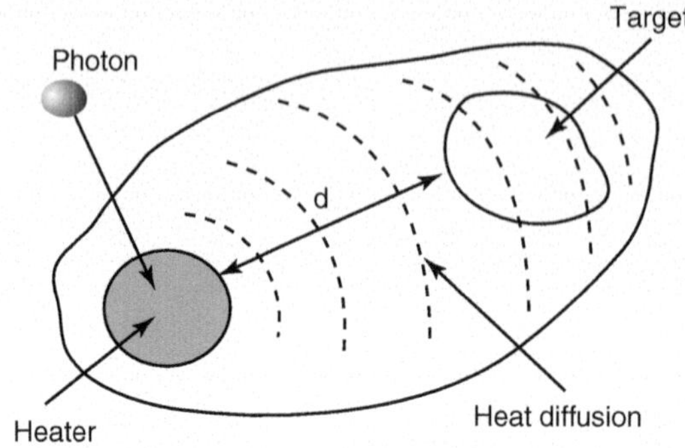

Fig. 3.2 General structure of biological target tissue with space separation between target and absorber (heater). (Reproduced from [4])

Extended theory of selective photothermolysis (extended theory) is a theory that damages target tissues when the chromophores and target tissues do not match. In the aforesaid example of laser hair removal, irradiation with the laser raises the temperature of the hair shaft, the chromophore, and the temperature is transferred to the follicular stem cells through heat diffusion and the cells are destroyed. The extended theory is a principle that indirectly damages the target tissue through heat diffusion in a heat generating chromophore (heater) (Fig. 3.2). Therefore, the thermal relaxation time (TRT) described in selective photothermolysis does not apply to the extended theory, but instead the thermal damage time (TDT) is applied. TDT is defined as the time it takes from the heat-generating chromophore (heater) to the temperature at which the outermost layer of the target tissue is damaged through thermal diffusion. By definition, TDT is longer than TRT (TDT > TRT) and pulse duration must be between TDT and TRT (TDT ≥ PD > TRT).

What are the conditions for the extended theory to be applied? One laser text describes that the extended theory applies to "non-uniformly

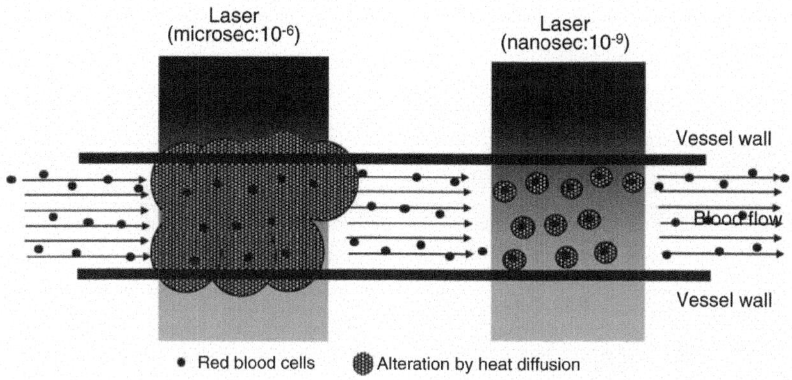

Fig. 3.3 A schema showing the difference in the treatment of vascular lesions between long (microsecond) and short (nanosecond) pulsed lasers. Nanosecond pulsed lasers can injure red blood cells, but not vessel walls, resulting in no effect on vascular lesions. However, microsecond pulsed lasers can injure not only red blood cells but also vessels walls. (Reproduced from [5])

absorbing target structure" [3]. The three major chromophores of the skin are melanin, hemoglobin, and water. Since water is uniform to the skin, the extended theory does not apply, but melanin and hemoglobin may not be uniform.

For example, RBC in blood vessels is uniform, but the blood vessel is composed of blood and vascular endothelial cells, so the entire blood vessel is not uniform. Irradiating a 532-nm Q-switched laser with a 10 ns pulse duration targeting an RBC with a TRT of 2–5 μs could damage the RBC but will not result in the treatment of blood vessels (Fig. 3.3). Therefore, vascular therapy is possible only by irradiating PDL with pulse duration corresponding to TDT (or TRT of the entire blood vessel) in which heat is transferred to the vessel wall, not with pulse duration corresponding to chromophores (hemoglobin and RBC). In the case of vessels with a TRT of 1.2–4.8 ms, a 450 μs 585 nm PDL corresponding to microseconds rather than nanosecond units should be used to achieve the desired effect. The same applies to melanin. Melanin in the melanosomes may be uniform, but melanocytes or keratinocytes with melanosomes, or the basal layer in which the keratinocytes are situated is not uniform.

Therefore, the extended theory is applied to laser hair removal, vascular treatment, and pigment treatment using long-pulsed laser.

3.1.3 Subcellular Selective Photothermolysis

Subcellular selective photothermolysis is a theory that became known by studying a method called "laser toning," a method used in private practice. In the past, lasers were contraindicated for melasma treatment since they aggravated melasma [6]. But, after the use of "laser toning" for melasma in private practice in East Asia, there were active researches on "laser toning."

To investigate the principle of laser toning, Kim et al. irradiated 1064-nm Q-switched Nd:YAG lasers on zebrafish and observed the change through microscope and biopsy [7]. They observed changes in melanosomes by irradiating fluence from 0.3 to 0.9 J/cm^2 with 7 mm spot size and pulse duration 5–7 ns. Melanosomes are broken even at 0.3 J/cm^2, but fluences of at least 0.4 J/cm^2 are required to clearly observe breaking of melanosomes (Fig. 3.4).

Figure 3.5 shows staining results; blue means normal nuclei and red means apoptotic cells, i.e., the cells that will soon die. Below 0.4 J/cm^2, the nucleus and the cells are both normal, but above 0.5 J/cm^2, apoptotic cells are observed despite normal nucleus.

Taken together, these results show that at 0.4 J/cm^2, only the melanosomes are broken and the cells are not damaged. In other words, there is

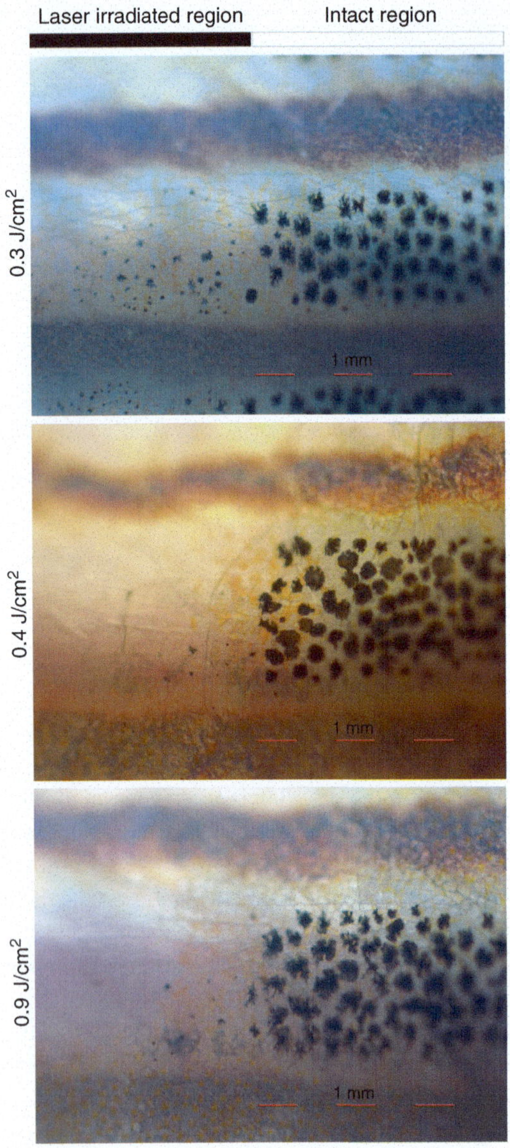

Fig. 3.4 Changes in melanosomes in the melanophores in the black stripes of zebrafish 5 days after Q-switched neodymium:yttrium–aluminum–garnet laser irradiation. At 0.4 and 0.9 J/cm^2 laser irradiation energy, most melanosomes in the beam path were absent by day 5 and the ablated region was pigment-free. In contrast, a number of pigmented spots remained at 0.3 J/cm^2 fluence. Bar = 1 mm. (Reproduced from [7])

an "energy level that can break only the melanosomes without damaging the cells." For example, laser toning in melasma does not affect melanocytes or keratinocytes and does not cause side effects and it is effective in treating melasma by eliminating only the melanosomes contained in melanocytes and keratinocytes.

After 2 months, the melanosomes all regenerated regardless of fluence.

The theory of subcellular selective photothermolysis originally corresponds to the theory of selective photothermolysis because the TRT of melanosomes is 250–1000 ns, and the pulse duration of Q-switched Nd:YAG laser is <10 ns, which is the same nanosecond unit. However, in the past, using the photomechanical effect of Q-switched lasers, the treatment of breaking cells (melanocyte TRT is 1–30 μs) was defined as the theory of selective photothermolysis. Thus the "theory of breaking only the melanosomes without damaging the cells" is just defined as "the theory of subcellular selective photothermolysis."

Let's think about the method of irradiating multiple passes, one of the parameters of laser toning. "Laser toning" which is frequently performed in private practice irradiates more than 1000 shots to the face at 10 Hz. Why irradiate so much at 10 Hz? Although not shown in this paper, Professor Ilhwan Kim's poster at the 60th Korean dermatological association fall conference in 2008 suggests that one shot (one pulse) was irradiated [8]. Also, if there is an "energy level that can break only the melanosomes without damaging the cells," isn't one shot enough? So, I perform the so-called one shot toning where melasma are shot one by one.

What is the essence of the theory of subcellular selective photothermolysis? There is an "energy level that can break only the melanosomes without damaging the cells." In other words, there is a concept of a therapeutic window. The concept is that it is ineffective at low energy and has side effects at high energy and that there is an adequate energy that is effective without side effects.

If we go one step further down from this concept, wouldn't there be an "energy level that only damages cells without affecting the surrounding cells?" Thus, for treatments of lentigines or PIHs without inflammation, I use higher energy for one shot toning. There will also be an "energy level that break down not only the cells but also

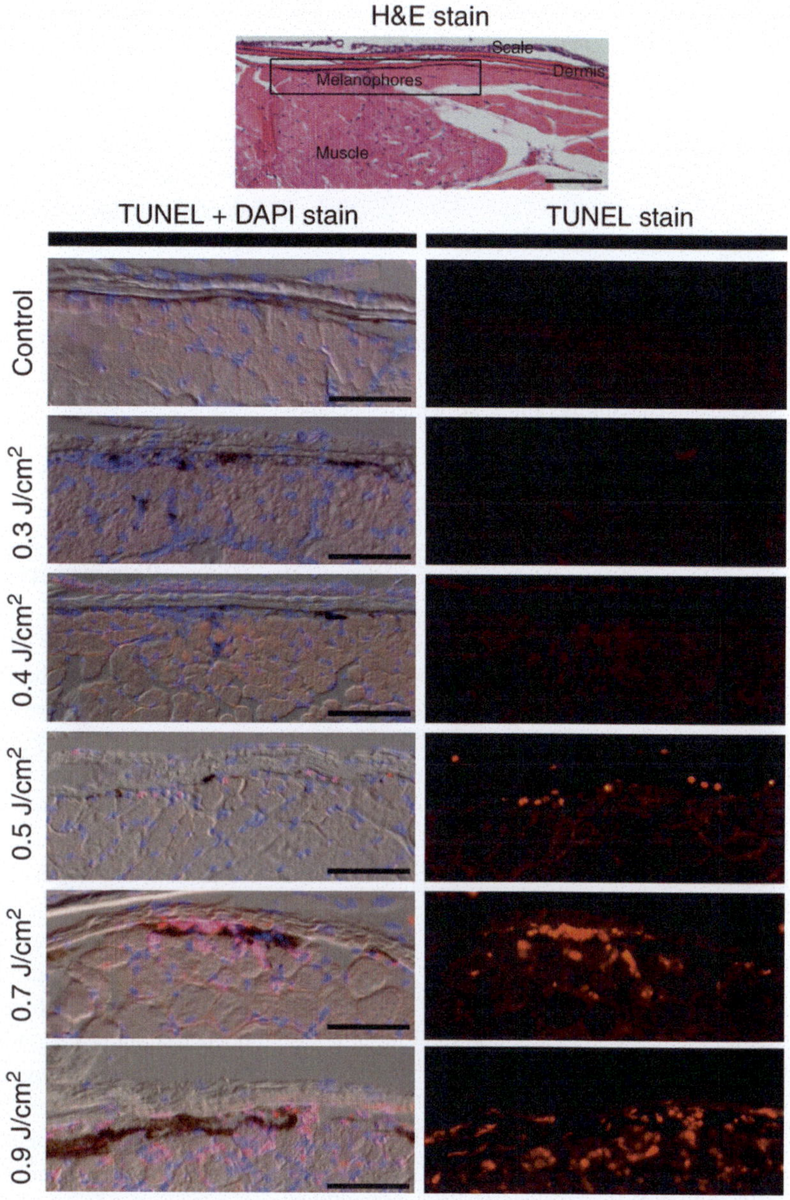

Fig. 3.5 TUNEL and 4′,6-diamidino-2-phenylindole staining of zebrafish skin 1 day after 1064-nm Q-switched neodymium:yttrium–aluminum–garnet laser irradiation. 4′,6-Diamidino-2-phenylindole staining (blue) shows that there were no differences in the distribution and number of normal nuclei in samples subjected to the different laser irradiation energies. In contrast, TUNEL staining (red) shows that apoptosis occurred after laser irradiation and with a clear laser irradiation energy dependency. At 0.5 J/cm^2 fluence, apoptotic cells are confined to the uppermost part of the hypodermis. At 0.7 and 0.9 J/cm^{-2} fluence, apoptosis is widespread in the entire hypodermis and muscle layer. Bar = 100 mm. (Reproduced from [7])

the surrounding blood vessels." That is why petechia occurs during the treatment of tattoo and ABNOM.

Then, what is the standard energy for "energy level that can break only the melanosomes without damaging the cells," "energy level that only damages cells without affecting the surrounding cells," and "energy level that break down not only the cells but also the surrounding blood vessels." After reviewing fluences for pigmented lesions in various papers, I concluded that:

In 1064-nm Q-switched Nd:YAG laser, a fluence of 4 J/cm^2 and 6 J/cm^2 with a 4 mm spot size should be the standard energy for one shot toning.

Thus, I recommend that with one shot toning, laser must be used below 4 J/cm^2 for melasma, which is an "energy level that can break only the melanosomes without damaging the cells." And for treatments of lentigines or PIHs without inflammation, energy level between 4 and 6 J/cm^2 should be used, which is an "energy level that only damages cells without affecting the surrounding cells." And for treatments of tattoos or melanocytic nevi, energy levels should be above 6 J/cm², which is an "energy level that break down not only the cells but also the surrounding blood vessels."

3.1.4 Fluence Calculation for Melanosomes

Let's calculate the actual "energy level that can break only the melanosomes without damaging the cells." The temperature at which melanosomes break up and photoacoustic effect appears is unknown, but the temperature at which the melanosomes coagulate is known. Because 1064-nm Q-switched Nd:YAG laser exists not in a thermal confinement zone but in a stress confinement zone, I believe that melanosome will break even at the temperature at which the melanosome is coagulated (see Sect. 2.6.1 in "Chap. 2").

Let's calculate the fluence required for coagulation of melanosomes based on papers by Anderson et al. [9]. Although the coagulation temperature varies among laser texts, the papers by Anderson et al. considered 75°C as the temperature at which melanosomes are coagulated with the skin temperature of 35°C.

$$D_0 \cong \frac{\rho S \Delta T}{f\alpha}, \alpha d < 1$$

D_0—laser exposure dose (J/cm²), ρ—density (≒1.1 g/cm³), *S*—specific heat (≒4.2 J/g°C), ΔT—temperature change, *f*—decreasing factor, α—absorption coefficient, *d*—average target size.

In the case of wavelength 1064 nm, optical penetration depth is longer than the size of melanosome, which corresponds to $\alpha d < 1$.

$$\mu_a = 1.70 \times 10^{12}\,\text{nm}^{-3.48}\left[\text{cm}^{-1}\right] \text{for skin.}$$

Absorption coefficients also vary among laser texts, but if we substitute 1064 nm in the formula of absorption coefficients in one paper, the absorption coefficient is 49.7 cm⁻¹ [10]. Finally, there are no texts or papers showing decreasing factor values, but let's substitute 0.9 since the decreasing factor is 0.5 at 351 nm and 0.8 at 700 nm.

The results show 4.1 J/cm² in 1064 nm. In other words, melanosomes coagulate with fluence of 4.1 J/cm² in a 1064-nm laser. This is similar to the "energy level that can break only the melanosomes without damaging the cells," which is energy level below 4 J/cm², as mentioned earlier (quoted with the permission of director Sunwoong Hwang. Published with kind permission of © Sunwoong Hwang 2019. All rights reserved).

For reference, when the decreasing factor is 0.65 at 532 nm, the fluence required to coagulate melanosomes is 0.51 J/cm².

3.2 Selection of Parameters

3.2.1 Difficulty in Determining Parameters

At least three parameters must be selected respectively to complete the theory of selective photothermolysis [11]. These three parameters are often known as the "three parameters" of selective photothermolysis theory: wavelength, pulse duration, and fluence. First, wavelength that absorbs more chromophores than the surrounding tissue should be chosen. The depth of chromophore should also be taken into account when selecting the wavelength. Second, pulse duration should be less than or equal to the TRT of the target tissue in order to limit heat damage to surrounding tissues. Third, fluence should cause sufficient thermal damage to the target tissue and destroy it.

Since each of these three parameters must be selected, there are many number of cases. For example, if there are three options for wavelength, pulse duration, and fluence, respectively, there are 27 number of cases (3 × 3 × 3 = 27). Since the wavelength is determined when purchasing the laser, there are actually nine number of cases (1 × 3 × 3 = 9). Nine cases, though less than 27, are not easy choices. For example, suppose that there are a number of cases 1–9, in which 1–4 are ineffective, 5 is effective, and side effects occur in 6–9. The probability of effectiveness without side effects is about 10%. Therefore, determining the parameters of the laser is not easy.

3.2.2 Effect Versus Safety?

The laser physician must determine three or six parameters. The final decision, however, is choosing effect or safety (fluence). Choosing effect increases the likelihood of side effects and choosing safety increases the likelihood of no effect. Which shall we choose? Effect versus safety?

Some like to compare private practice to martial arts, and like novices and masters of martial arts, they say there are novices and masters in laser physicians. What is the difference between novices and masters in laser physicians? I think if the lasers are the same, there is no difference in effects between novices and masters. Because if the laser is irradiated with high power, it will be effective for both novices and masters. However, there is a difference in the probability of side effects occurring for novices and masters. I think a "master laser physician" is someone who creates similar effects with minimal side effects.

Thus, I believe that in order to become a "master," safety must be chosen over effect. Of course, safety without effectiveness is also undesirable. Through education and experience, safe and effective parameters must be found.

Readers will be able to reach the heart of laser surgery if they place more emphasis on safety than effectiveness while reading this book.

3.3 Wavelength

3.3.1 Absorption Coefficient

The method of measuring the absorption coefficient is as follows. Light of a monochromatic wavelength, such as a laser, is irradiated and passed through a cloudy cuvette containing chromophores. The remaining light is measured with a detector. The ratio of the light intensity (I_0) before the irradiation to the target cuvette and the remaining light intensity past the target (I) is the absorption rate (Fig. 3.6) [13].

This absorption rate decreases by the function of the natural index (see Sect. 1.3.2 in "Chap. 1"). Absorption rate is expressed by the following equation:

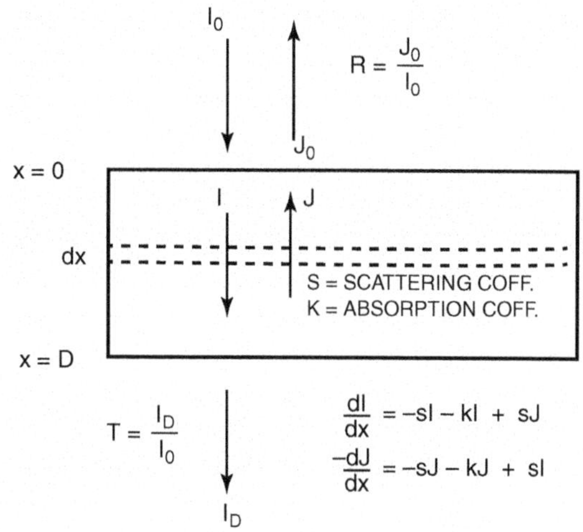

Fig. 3.6 The Kubelka–Munk model for radiation transfer in a turbid, absorbing medium. (Reproduced from [12])

$$\frac{I}{I_0} = e^{-\mu_a L}$$

$$\log \frac{I}{I_0} = -\mu_a L$$

Absorption rate is composed of target depth (length L) and the elements other than the target depth. The elements other than the target depth can be defined as the absorption coefficient (μ_a). Based on the light intensity where $\mu_a L$ is 1, the equation is summarized as follows:

$$\mu_a = \frac{1}{L}$$

Absorption coefficient is (1/length) and unit is cm^{-1}. Therefore, the definition of the absorption coefficient can be defined as the possibility or the probability of photons of a specific wavelength being absorbed per unit length [1].

If the absorption coefficient = 1/length is interpreted differently, it can be interpreted that "photons penetrate shallowly with the laser with the high absorption coefficient and photons penetrate deeply with the laser with the low absorption coefficient." Examples include CO_2 lasers having a high absorption coefficient for water and Nd:YAG lasers having a low absorption coefficient for water. CO_2 lasers with high absorption coefficients penetrate shallowly and evaporate the epidermal layer to ablate the skin, but

Nd:YAG lasers with low absorption coefficients transfer heat to the depth of the dermis, which can cause deep burns at high energy.

Absorption coefficient is known to be changed by two variables [14]. First, absorption coefficient changes depending on chromophore. Second, absorption coefficient varies depending on wavelength. Thus, an absorption curve is created (Fig. 3.7). For example, 694-nm ruby laser has been found to have high absorption in melanin and low absorption in hemoglobin and the 1064-nm Nd:YAG laser has been found to have low absorption in melanin, hemoglobin, and water. In conclusion, absorption coefficient depends on two variables, wavelength and chromophore.

However, absorption coefficient is not constant for each chromophore. Even with the same chromophore, absorption coefficient depends on the concentration of the chromophore [2]. For example, assuming that the blood in the dermal layer is uniformly distributed, the absorption coefficient of the dermal layer should be calculated as follows [14]:

$$\mu_a \cdot \text{derm} = (\text{f} \cdot \text{blood})(\mu_a \cdot \text{blood}) + (1 - \text{f} \cdot \text{blood})(\mu_a \cdot \text{skinbaseline})$$

μ_a·derm: absorption coefficient of dermis layer, f·blood: blood ratio of the dermis layer, μ_a·blood: absorption coefficient of blood, μ_a·skinbaseline: absorption coefficient of dermis layer except blood.

Therefore, even if the chromophores have the same absorption coefficient, the absorption coefficient varies depending on the concentration. The chromophores we assume as targets are single targets but the actual chromophores are target groups. For example, when treating pigmentations, the single target is the melanosome, but melanosome concentrations are different for each melanocyte containing melanosomes, and the concentration of melanocytes are also different in each of the lentigines in which the melanocytes are gathered. Therefore, even though the same melanosomes are targets, light lentigines have a low absorption coefficient, while the dark lentigines have a high absorption coefficient. That's why we know empirically that we should irradiate "dark lesions weak and light lesions strong."

From these, we can draw two conclusions:

1. Different lesions have different concentrations, so energy must be controlled differently. In other words, we should irradiate "dark lesions weak and light lesions strong."
2. There is no absolute parameter.

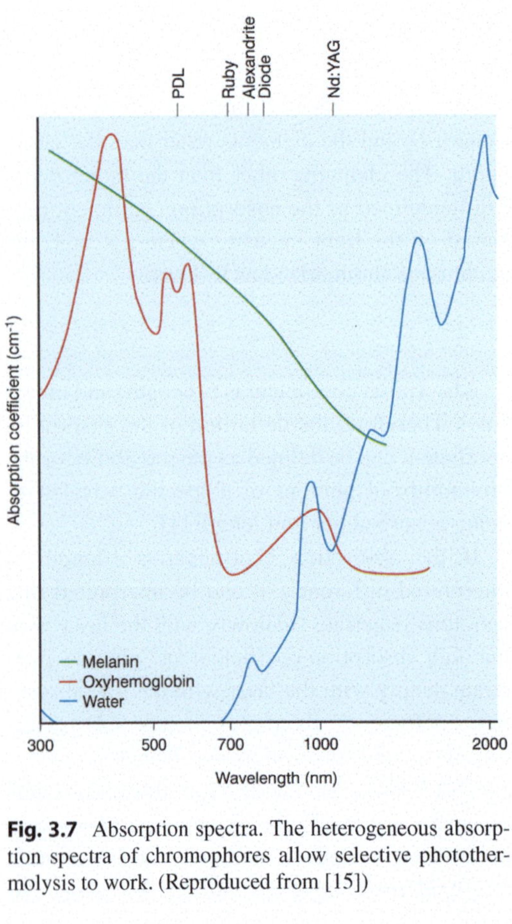

Fig. 3.7 Absorption spectra. The heterogeneous absorption spectra of chromophores allow selective photothermolysis to work. (Reproduced from [15])

3.3.2 Optical Penetration Depth

Skin can be thought of as a turbid medium made up of small substances such as blood, melanin, bilirubin, and collagen [1]. When photons encounter these materials scattering occurs due to the shape or size of the material, especially the difference in refractive index. However, at wavelengths above 2500 nm and below 250 nm, the absorption coefficients of water and melanin, respectively, are higher than that of scattering, resulting in no scattering [14]. Scattering only occurs between 250 and 2500 nm. (Of course, even at this wavelength, melanosomes and hemoglobin are absorbed.) Scattering occurs mainly in the dermis. Collagen is the main cause of scattering. As light enters the skin, scattering increases and the number of photons absorbed decreases. As the absorption coefficient increases, optical penetration depth decreases. Optical penetration depth also decreases by the scattering coefficient.

Thus, a more precise description of the formula (see "absorption coefficient") would be:

$$I_{(z)} = I_0 k e^{(-z/\delta)}$$

$$\delta = \frac{1}{\sqrt{3\mu_a\left(\mu_a + \mu_s(1-g)\right)}}$$

$I(z)$: the local surface fluence at some depth z.
k: constant that accounts for backscattered light.
δ: the wavelength-dependent optical penetration depth of light or the depth at which there is attenuation to 37% of the surface value (37% = $1/e$, where $e = 2.7$, the base of the natural logarithm).
g: anisotropy coefficient (a measure of the "mean" direction of the scattered photons). $g = 0.9$ for the skin.
μ_a: absorption coefficient.
μ_s: scattering coefficient.

The optical penetration depth decreases as the absorption coefficient and the scattering coefficient increase [14]. Scattering is easily observed in real life. When we cover the sun with our hand, "red" which has a long wavelength and is less scattered can be seen through the hand while "blue" cannot be seen. The same principle applies to the phenomenon of red sunset glow.

In particular, scattering coefficient has more influence on penetration depth than the absorption coefficient. In the visible region, 100 times of scattering occur before one photon is absorbed [1], and in the case of red light, the average travel length until absorption is 50 μm. The average travel length due to scattering is 5 mm, which is about 100 times [16].

3.3.3 Backscattering

Scattering can occur in all directions [17]. It is mistaken that there are more backscattering, but in the case of Mie scattering, forward scattering is known to be the main scattering [16]. When backscattering occurs, more photons accumulate on the surface of the skin and higher energy accumulates on the surface than intended. Therefore, shorter wavelengths with more accumulate more energy than longer wavelengths. Let's assume the following for the sake of understanding. Suppose that four photons out of ten photons are absorbed at 0.1 mm corresponding to the thickness of the epidermis and photons that are at a depth of 0.2 mm from the surface are backscattered resulting in one more photon absorption at 0.1 mm. In this case, at the depth of 0.1 mm, there are four photons resulting in a fluence of 4 J/cm^2, but due to backscattering there are a total of five photons resulting in an energy rise to 5 J/cm^2. As a result, lasers with shorter wavelengths accumulate more energy than actual energy on the skin surface. For example, even if both 532 and 755 nm lasers are irradiated with the same energy, 532-nm laser shows higher energy accumulation on the actual skin surface, resulting in an increased likelihood of side effects.

Also, due to backscattering, the "real" penetration depth is deeper than the optical penetration depth (OPD) [1]. Suppose four of ten photons penetrate at 2 mm depth and two penetrate at 2.5 mm, using a 1064-nm Nd:YAG laser. The depth of penetration is the depth at which photons are reduced to e^{-1}, i.e., the depth at which ten photons become four photons. The OPD by definition is 2 mm deep, but if the two remaining photons past the depth of 2.5 mm are backscattered back to the 2.5 mm point, there are four photons at 2.5 mm. Thus, "real" penetration depth is 2.5 mm. Real penetration depth is deeper than the OPD.

If no absorption occurs, the real penetration depth will be deeper. In case of pigmented tissue,

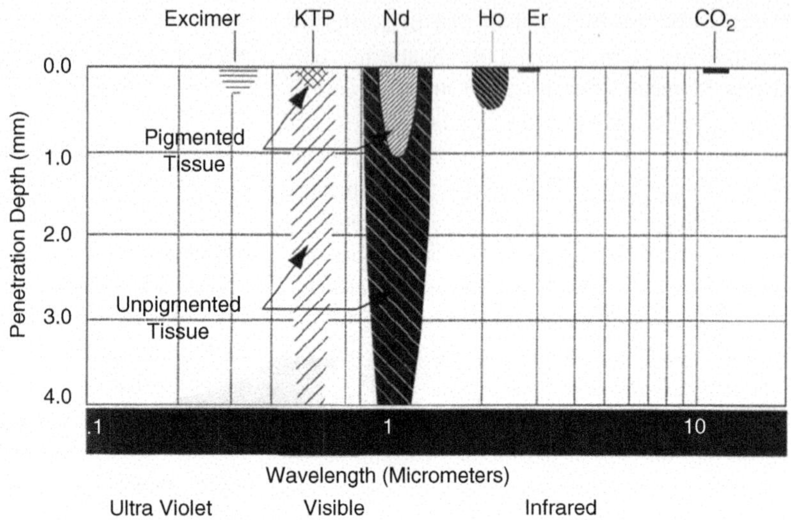

Fig. 3.8 Laser penetration depth with the presence of pigmented/unpigmented tissue. (Modified from [18])

532 nm absorbs all photons in the pigmented tissue, resulting in a shallow penetration depth (Fig. 3.8). However, in the absence of pigmented tissue, absorption does not occur and the real penetration depth becomes deeper.

In conclusion, OPD is a fixed value calculated mathematically or physically. In practice, however, OPD is deeper and may vary depending on the presence of an absorptive tissue and also on the amount of collagen.

Also, when treating the dermis (e.g., vascular therapy, hair removal, and tattoo removal), treating the pigment in the epidermis and then treating the dermis allows laser physicians to treat deeper portions of the skin (Fig. 3.8). Thus, a sequential procedure is useful when treating the dermis.

3.4 Pulse Duration

3.4.1 Thermal Relaxation Time

There are three ways to lose heat in tissues: heat conduction, heat convection caused by blood flow, and heat radiation [3]. The latter two phenomena are only meaningful in long pulse durations, and in short pulse duration, heat conduction, which transfers heat to the surroundings, is the main method of heat dissipation. The formula of thermal penetration depth due to heat conduction is as follows [19]:

$$z_{\text{therm}}(t) = \sqrt{4kt}.$$

$Z_{\text{therm}}(t)$—thermal penetration depth, k—heat conductivity, t—time.

The formula for thermal relaxation time is made by the formula for thermal penetration depth. The theory of selective photothermolysis states that “if a small amount of light energy is irradiated for a short time, the light energy received by the target tissue is used only to raise the temperature of the target tissue and does not transmit heat to surrounding tissues.”. Therefore, the thermal penetration depth should not be longer than the target diameter of the target tissue and should be the same or shorter (target diameter ≥ thermal penetration depth). Therefore, thermal relaxation time can be defined as the time of thermal penetration depth when the thermal penetration depth and the target tissue diameter are the same. Changing the thermal relaxation time using the formula for thermal penetration depth results in the thermal relaxation time (TRT) formula.

$$\tau = \delta^2 / g\kappa$$

δ—optical penetration depth for homogeneously absorbing layers.
κ—thermal diffusivity, a quantity based on the thermal conductivity and specific heat of the medium.
g—a constant based on the geometry of the target (slab, cylinder, or sphere).

Let's examine the definition of δ in this formula. In "Chap. 1," δ is the diameter of target tissue, but the original definition is optical penetration depth for homogeneously absorbing layers [14]. Why did this definition come about?

When laser is irradiated at the small target tissue (target diameter < OPD, $\alpha d < 1$) all the photons are able to pass through it [9]. But when target tissue is very large (target diameter > OPD, $\alpha d > 1$), the photons only irradiate part of the target tissue (Fig. 3.9). At this time, the length of part of the target tissue affected by the laser is OPD. In other words, when "target diameter < OPD," the thermal penetration depth is equal to the diameter of the target tissue. But when "target diameter > OPD," the thermal penetration depth is not equal to the diameter but is equal to the OPD (thermal penetration depth = optical penetration depth). In addition, in both situations, the heat conductivity (*k*) must be the same in order to apply the formula of the thermal penetration depth. In other words, the target tissue affected by laser should be a homogeneous tissue.

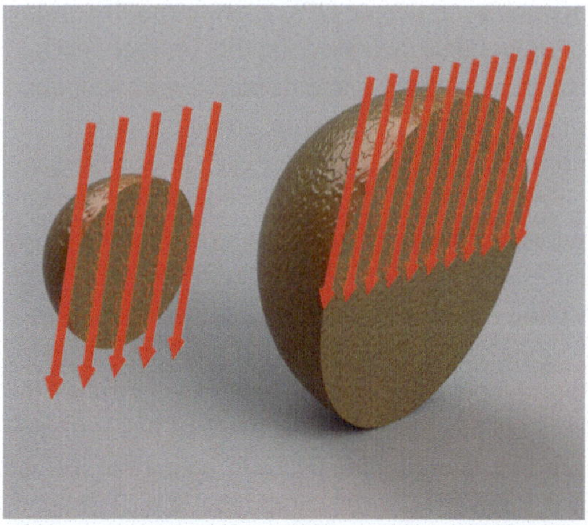

Fig. 3.9 Relationship between target tissues and OPD. Left (target diameter < OPD, $\alpha d < 1$), Right (target diameter > OPD, $\alpha d > 1$). (Published with kind permission of © Jin Kwon Cho 2019. All rights reserved)

To summarize the common parts in both situations, first, heat must be generated within the OPD. Second, the target tissues should be homogeneous. Therefore, δ is defined as follows: "optical penetration depth for homogeneously absorbing layers."

Because the definition of δ has two premises, there are two concepts of TRT [1]. First, since OPD is different depending on wavelength, TRT may vary depending on the wavelength. Second, skin has various components and chromophores, but in terms of thermal conductivity, skin is a homogeneous tissue with the same thermal diffusivity. In liquid water and most tissues, the thermal diffusivity is 1.4×10^{-7} m²/s [19] or 1.3×10^{-3} cm²/s depending on texts [1]. At this time, the factor that determines the thermal penetration depth is time, i.e., pulse duration. Therefore, TRT may vary depending on pulse duration.

Let's review this in detail.

3.4.2 TRT Determined by Wavelength

TRT can be varied depending on the wavelength. In the case of chromophores located everywhere in the skin, such as water, the OPD does not depend on the skin structure (epidermal layer, basal layer, melanosomes, etc.), but on wavelength [1]. For example, a laser of 1540 nm has a low absorption coefficient for water and penetrates deeply, with an OPD of several hundred micrometers. Thus, TRT is several hundred seconds. In contrast, CO_2 lasers with a high absorption coefficient for water have a shallow OPD with a TRT less than 1 ms. Er:YAG lasers even have a higher absorption coefficient of water compared to CO_2 lasers, with a TRT of 1 μs. Thus, the shallower the OPD, the shorter the TRT. In regards to water, TRT varies depending on the wavelength. Therefore, when describing the TRT of water, both wavelength and laser should be mentioned such as "<1 ms in CO_2 laser" or "1 μs in Er: YAG laser."

3.4.3 TRT Determined by Skin Structure

TRT may depend on skin structure. For example, melanosomes have a TRT of 347.2 ns with a size of 1 μm, and the basal layer of the epidermis where keratinocytes with melanosomes are has a TRT of 0.1 msec with a thickness of 10 μm, and the epidermal layer which is the sum of keratinocytes with melanosomes is has a TRT of 10 ms with a thickness of 100 μm.

Why do TRTs vary with skin structure? In the case of the Q-switched lasers, the heat is confined to only the melanosome, i.e., unevenly distributed. Thus, after the laser is irradiated, heat is transferred to the upper layer of the epidermis, while the melanosomes and the basal layer cool down. On the other hand, in the case of a long-pulsed lasers, for example, when irradiated with 10 ms, the heat of melanosomes is transmitted to the basal layer or the entire epidermal layer for a relatively longer pulse duration than the Q-switched laser, resulting in uniform heat distribution. Thus, although histologically not uniform, heat distribution is uniform. Therefore, even at the same wavelength, adjusting the pulse duration can change TRT and change the desired target. An example is a long-pulsed laser using millisecond units such as epidermal pigmentations, blood vessels, and hair removal.

This phenomenon can be explained by the aforementioned extended theory of selective photothermolysis. The situation in which the extended theory applies is when the tissue is not uniform, but when the heat distribution is uniform.

In Table 3.2 (mentioned in "Chap. 1"), we can see that TRT varies depending on the skin structure or the wavelength of laser. Also, one more thing to think about in this table is that there are no TRTs for melanin and hemoglobin, which are both components of three major chromophores. Why is this so? I think that is because first, melanin and hemoglobin have a TRT that is too short, so it is not yet possible to make a laser with a pulse duration suitable for this TRT. Second, the theory applied to actual laser treatment is not selective photothermolysis but the extended theory of selective photothermolysis.

Table 3.2 TRT to remember [1, 3, 13, 20, 21]

TRT to remember	
Melanosome	<1 μs (250–1000 ns)
Tattoo pigment	20 ns ~ 3 ms
Melanocyte	1–30 μs
Basal layer	0.4 ms
Epidermis	2ms (1–10ms)
Capillaries	4.5 ms (100 μm:100 μm corresponds to the size of the smallest visible blood vessel)
Hair follicle	40 ms (10–100 ms)
Water	<1 ms in CO_2 laser, 1 μs in Er:YAG

Table 3.2 shows that the TRTs for melanocytes are 1–30 μs, but likewise, the laser with this pulse duration does not exist yet. Therefore, at present, we cannot treat cells such as melanocytes in accordance with the TRT and can only treat cell layers such as the basal layer. However, it is possible to treat cells using a photomechanical effect without applying TRT.

3.5 Spot Size

3.5.1 Rule of Thumb in Spot Size

Let's review how to adjust the spot size when treating the dermal layer. For example, since the blood vessels are located at various depths of the dermal layer, deeper OPD is preferred. If so, spot size should be increased so OPD becomes deeper. But even with the same fluence, larger spot sizes require more photons to irradiate, so higher power is required. But since each laser has a limitation in power, it cannot maintain a certain fluence beyond a certain spot size. Therefore, it is necessary to find a suitable spot size. How large should the spot size be?

One laser text suggested that the "rule of thumb spot size" should be about ten times the target depth, "based on the depth of target tissue" [2]. For example, the depth of epidermal lesions is 0.1 mm so spot size should be 1 mm. The depth of port wine stain (PWS), tattoos, and hair is 1, 2, and 3 mm, respectively, so spot size should be 10, 20, and 30 mm, respectively. However, I think the spot size presented in this text is too large. I think that five times the target depth is the maximum spot size. For example, in case of laser hair removal, because 10 mm spot size is thought to be enough for hair removal, 15 mm, which is five times the depth of 3 mm, is probably the maximum size. Dr. Minho Lee suggested the "Half rule" because in a spot size of less than 10 mm, half of the spot size corresponds to the target depth (two times the target depth) and the target at this depth can be treated (Published with kind permission of © Minho Lee 2019. All rights reserved). On the other hand, Ross et al. stated that the spot size should be at least four times greater than the OPD [22].

3.5.2 Spot Size Effect

Let's take a closer look at the spot size effect described in "Chap. 1."

In "Chap. 1," we supposed that there is a large spot size of 1 cm^2 and a small spot size of 0.5 cm^2, 10 and 5 photons were shot respectively, and one photon is in the area outside the OPD. Eight photons will be absorbed by the large spot size and 3 by the small spot size (Fig. 3.10). Fluence is the number of photons per unit area, so the fluence of the laser is 10 J/cm^2 in both spot sizes, but inside the skin, the fluence is different (8 J/cm^2 and 6 J/m^2, respectively). In other words, the larger the spot size, the higher the actual energy in the skin. The reason for this is because photons that are deviated from the laser direction, and thus not absorbed is a "constant" and the fluence is an energy density, which is a "ratio."

In summary, the energy in the skin is relatively low at small spot sizes and relatively high at large spot sizes. So, what should we you do when converting the spot size in the same fluence? Reducing the spot size at the same fluence will result in lower energy absorbed resulting in no side effects, but less efficacy. If the spot size is increased, the actual energy becomes higher than the original energy, so there is a high possibility of side effects. Therefore, when increasing spot size, fluence should be reduced.

So, what should we do to get equal energy in the skin at different spot sizes? Figure 3.11 shows the number of photons converted to fluence from Fig. 3.10. Previously, at 10 J/cm^2 of the handpiece, the fluence in the skin was 8 J/cm^2 for the large spot size and 6 J/cm^2 for the small spot size. To create the equivalent energy in the skin with small spot sizes, the fluence of handpiece should be increased. To create the same energy at 8 J/cm^2 in the skin with a small spot size, the energy should be raised above the original handpiece's energy of 10 J/cm^2, for example, it should be raised to 12 J/cm^2. It is important to note that scattering occurs mainly in dermis. Scattering does not occur in epidermal layer. The energy of

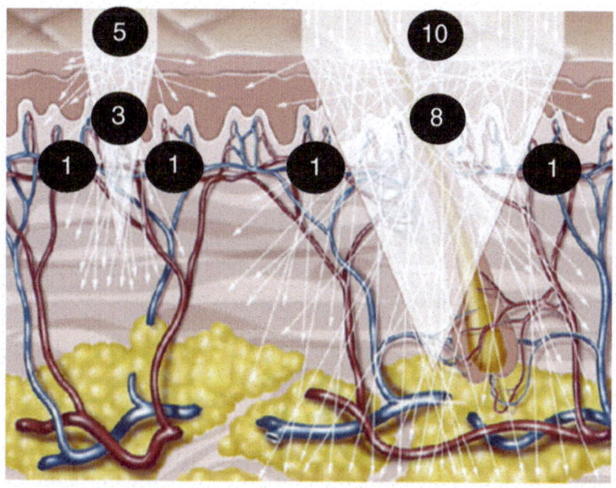

Fig. 3.10 Number of photons by spot size. When assuming that the spot size is 1 cm^2, 0.5 cm^2 and the fluence is the same at 10 J/cm^2, the number of photons is assumed to be 10 and 5, respectively (Modified from [23])

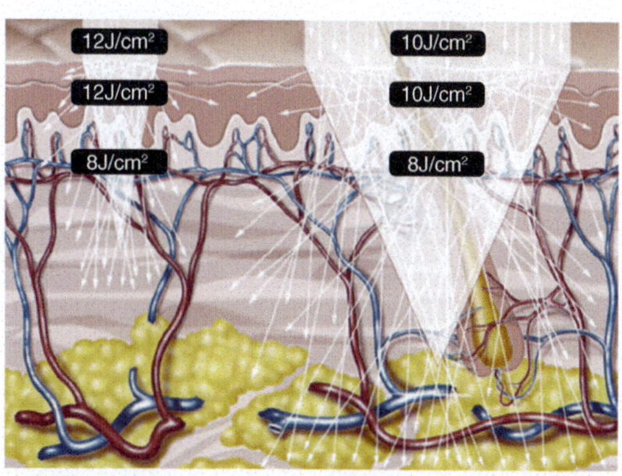

Fig. 3.11 The number of photons is converted to fluence from Fig. 3.10. The value of the "small spot size" is the assumed value of the fluence needed for the epidermis and the handpiece when adjusting the fluence of the dermis to 8 J/cm^2. (Modified from [23])

the large spot size in the epidermal layer is therefore 10 J/cm^2 but the energy of small spot size is 12 J/cm^2. In other words, small spot sizes have a relatively high epidermal energy compared to large spot sizes and are more likely to cause side effects on the epidermal layer. Therefore, in order to create the same effect in the dermal layer, increasing the spot size is a method to protect the epidermis.

The spot size effect can be summarized as follows.

1. The larger spot size, the deeper the penetration depth of laser.
2. When increasing spot size at the same fluence, the fluence should be reduced.
3. When treating the dermis, large spot sizes should be used to protect the epidermis.

Lee et al. used a long-pulsed Nd:YAG laser and a long-pulsed alexandrite laser and observed the temperature changes of epidermis and dermis when the spot size and fluence were 5, 8, 10 mm and 26, 30, 36 J/cm^2, respectively [24]. The results showed that the epidermal temperature difference was not large with changes in spot size, but epidermal temperature increased with increase in fluence. On the other hand, in the dermal layer, as in the epidermal layer, the higher the fluence, the higher the temperature of the dermis. But it was observed that the larger the spot size than the fluence, the higher the temperature. This is in line with the spot size effect described earlier.

Then, what kind of treatment can the spot size effect be used for? Spot size effect can be used for any treatment that targets the dermis. For example, large spot sizes are recommended for vascular therapy, hair removal, nonablative rejuvenation, dermal pigmented lesions, etc. Among these, we will examine how the spot size effect is applied when performing tattoo removal.

There are many challenges in laser tattoo removal but let's look at a few. First, laser should penetrate as deep as possible because tattoo pigments may be in a very deep layer of the dermis. Second, when the tattoo is applied twice or three times (retattooing), blisters or scars may occur even with mild fluence. Third, paradoxical darkening may occur. Paradoxical darkening refers to a phenomenon in which white, peach, pink, and red tattoo pigments turn black when they are treated with lasers, making it difficult to treat and increasing the number of treatments [3]. It is known to occur frequently in semipermanent tattoos, due to chemical changes from red-toned ferric oxide (Fe_2O_3) to black ferrous oxide (FeO). In addition, titanium dioxide, which is used for white or bright color tattoos, is also known as the cause. Beute et al. found the following phenomena during treatment of blue, green, and red tattoos with a 532-nm Q-switched laser [25]. Paradoxical darkening occurred in the center of the spot while tattoo was erased on the outside of the spot. The energy is weak in the outside of the spot due to scattering and Gaussian beam. Therefore, treatment with low energy can remove the tattoo with less paradoxical darkening.

Considering the three points mentioned above with the spot size effect, for laser tattoo removal, it is necessary to treat the skin with a large spot size to remove deep tattoo pigments and protect the epidermal layer. Low energy should be used first to keep the skin safe from overlaid tattoos or paradoxical darkening. And then, energy should be sequentially increased. In conclusion, a large spot size must first be used and energy must be sequentially increased from low energy [1].

Specifically, I treat tattoos as follows: Select clinical end point as "immediate whitening with marked petechia" and use a 1064-nm Q-switched Nd:YAG laser with parameters of 8-mm spot, 2.6 J/cm^2. The reason I use 2.6 J/cm^2 is because my Q-switched Nd:YAG laser has a maximum energy of 2.6 J/cm^2 at an 8-mm spot. Irradiate only one point and if clinical end point does not appear, reduce it to a 7 mm spot and raise the energy to the maximum which is 3.4 J/cm^2. Subsequently, the energy is increased by reducing the spot size: 6 mm spot size, 4.6 J/cm^2 → 5 mm spot size, 5.5 J/cm^2 → 5 mm spot size, 6.6 J/cm^2. When clinical end point is observed, the entire tattoo is treated with the corresponding energy. In the next treatment session, the same energy is tested again, and if the clinical end point cannot be observed, the spot size is reduced and the energy is increased. The reason for gradual reduction in spot size is because there is a limit to the energy that can be raised at a given spot size.

3.6 Fluence

The goal for laser treatment is to selectively raise the temperature of a specific chromophore and eventually induce a change in temperature of the target tissue. We will now look at temperature.

3.6.1 Relation Between Fluence and Pulse Duration

$$\Delta T = \frac{F_z \mu_a}{\rho c}\left(\frac{\tau_r}{\tau_r + \tau_p}\right)^{g/2}$$

ΔT: Temperature increase of a desired target
μ_a: absorption coefficient
Fz: local subsurface fluence
ρ: density
c: specific heat
g: geometric factor (one for planes, two for cylinders, and three for spheres)
τp: laser pulse duration
τ_r: thermal relaxation time of the target (TRT)

The equation above applies to temperature. From the equation above, we can see that the previously mentioned "irradiate dark lesions weak, light lesions strong" is correct. In other words, if absorption coefficient (μ_a) is high, a low fluence (F_z) must be irradiated to reach the temperature increase of a desired target. On the contrary, if absorption coefficient is low, high fluence must be irradiated to reach the temperature increase of a desired target.

What about pulse duration? What is the relationship between fluence and pulse duration? The equation above shows pulse duration (τ_p). However, since it is part of the denominator under the exponential function, it is difficult to know the correlation at first glance. But if you put numbers in the equation, you can see that pulse duration and temperature are inversely related. Conversely, fluence and pulse duration are proportional if the temperature is the same.

Trafeli et al. used a 755-nm long-pulse alexandrite laser to measure the fluence of similar clinical endpoints, i.e., the same temperature, depending on the pulse duration [26]. Based on the results and figures of this paper, two conclusions can be drawn. First, pulse duration and fluence are proportional. In other words, to see the same effect, fluence should be increased to increase pulse duration and fluence should be lowered to shorten pulse duration. Second, pulse duration and fluence are proportional, but there is no significant difference in fluence. Thus, if there is a clinical end point that is appropriate for a particular fluence at a given pulse duration, there is no need to adjust fluence whether the pulse duration is reduced or increased. Of course, in order to safely perform the procedure, it would be better to reduce the fluence when reducing pulse duration.

3.6.2 Epidermal Cooling in Epidermal Pigmentation

Another point to remember in this paper is that it is better not to cool the epidermis during epidermal treatment.

Table 3.3 is a table calculated by setting virtual values. Assuming that the normal skin temperature is 35°C, the temperature difference due to epidermal cooling is −10°C, and the target

Table 3.3 A hypothetical value assuming normal skin temperature is 35°C, the temperature difference due to epidermal cooling is −10°C, and the target temperature is 75°C, and the product of fluence and absorption coefficient is the temperature difference (ΔT)

Fluence	Target tissue ($\mu_a = 10$)	Normal tissue ($\mu_a = 1$)
5 J/cm² (with DCD)	(5 × 10) + 35 − 10 = 75°C	(5 × 1) + 35 − 10 = 30°C
4 J/cm² (without DCD)	(4 × 10) + 35 = 75°C	(4 × 1) + 35 = 39°C

(fluence × absorption coefficient) + normal temperature − cooling temperature = final temperature

temperature is 75°C, and the product of fluence and absorption coefficient is the temperature difference (ΔT), the final temperature is [(fluence × absorption coefficient) + normal temperature − cooling temperature = final temperature].

Cooling the epidermis will reduce the temperature by the same temperature difference (ΔT) for both epidermal pigment lesions and surrounding normal tissue. Normal tissues have a lower temperature than normal, so there is no possibility of side effects, but pigmented lesions will also have a low temperature and we cannot see the desired effect. In order to see the effect, the fluence needs to be increased (5 J/cm^2) while cooling the epidermis, so that the temperature of the epidermal pigmented lesion is higher (75°C), resulting in desired effect. The temperature of surrounding tissue is below normal temperature (30°C), resulting in safety. On the other hand, when epidermal cooling is not performed, the temperature of the epidermal pigmented lesion is the same as that of the epidermal cooling, but the temperature of the surrounding tissue is higher than that of the epidermal cooling (39° C).

Therefore, although the result is the same, because the temperature of the surrounding tissue decreases when epidermal cooling is performed, and the temperature of the surrounding tissue increases when epidermal cooling is not performed, epidermal cooling seems desirable. However, neither 30°C nor 39°C cause problems to the skin. Fluence is more a problem than temperature. In Table 3.3, the fluence difference seems to be minor, but if the laser is a low-power laser that cannot raise the fluence by more than 4 J/cm^2, the pulse duration must be increased to make 5 J/cm^2. And because the pulse duration cannot be reduced, small tissues are difficult to treat. Therefore, epidermal cooling is not meaningful in epidermal pigmented lesions because epidermal cooling has more disadvantages than advantages.

3.6.3 Arrhenius Equation

When the photon of the laser finally meets the chromophore, the temperature rises. As reviewed in "Chap. 2," as the temperature rises, phenomena such as plasma, shock wave, cavitation, and jet formation occur in the photomechanical effect. In the photothermal effect, coagulation, vaporization, carbonization, and melting occur. Among these phenomena, the Arrhenius equation is applied below 100°C where no vaporization occurs. Next, let's look at Arrhenius formula.

The Arrhenius formula is derived from the following formula:

$$2N_2O_5(g) \rightarrow 4NO_2(g) + O_2(g)$$

Reaction velocity = $k\,[N_2O_5]^n$.

k: rate constant.

When N_2O_2 is converted to NO_2 and O_2, the rate of change is proportional to the concentration of N_2O_2 and rate constant (k). In other words, the rate of change of a substance is primarily higher at higher concentrations of the substance. A variable other than the concentration of a substance is defined as a rate constant (k). This rate constant is independent of concentration and physicists have found that it varies with the temperature of material and the catalyst. Since we don't use a catalyst [27], let's focus on temperature. Physically calculating the rate constant, the equation is expressed as:

$$k = Ae^{-Ea/RT}$$

$$\log k = \log A - \frac{E_a}{R}\left(\frac{1}{T}\right)$$

k: rate constant of reaction
A: constant, depending on the reaction
E_a: activation energy
R: molar gas constant
T: temperature

Since the equation above is difficult to understand when drawn in a graph, it was expressed using the logarithmic function and equation like "$y = ax + b$." The original Arrhenius formula is a formula for determining the activation energy (E) corresponding to the slope (a) and the frequency factor (A) corresponding to the y-axis intercept (b) by measuring the rate constants according to two temperatures (Activation energy and fre-

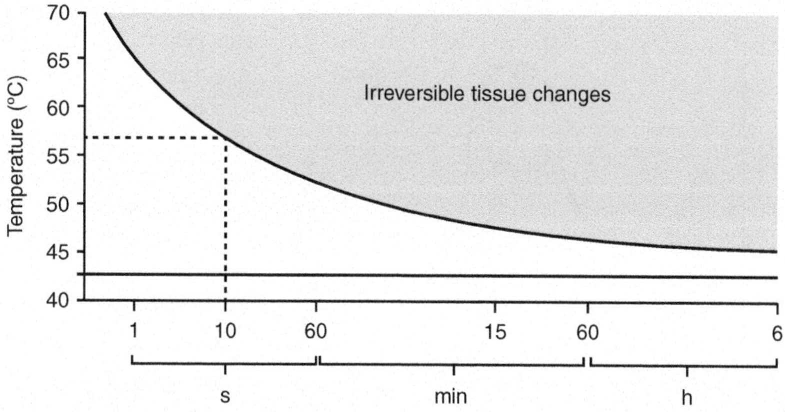

Fig. 3.12 Influence of temperature and exposure time on the irreversible destruction of tissues. (Reproduced from [28])

quency factors are called Arrhenius' constant [19]). However, since we only need to know the relationship between temperature and skin tissue, we can summarize the meaning of Arrhenius formula as follows:

First, the higher the temperature, the faster the reaction rate. In other words, materials change fast at higher temperatures. Conversely, materials change slowly in lower temperatures. Second, there is what is called activation energy. In other words, if there is a threshold and this threshold is not exceeded, tissue degeneration does not occur. Let's take a closer look at these two conclusions.

First, let's find out about temperature and time. Figure 3.12 plots the Arrhenius formula as a function of temperature over time, not rate. For tissue denaturation, not only temperature but also time is important. For example, tissue degeneration occurs at more than 10 s at 57°C, but does not occur at 5 s at 57°C. Also, tissue degeneration occurs at 1 s at 65°C but does not occur at 0.5 s. There is no absolute temperature for tissue degeneration or coagulation. Time as well as temperature must be considered. It is known that when the temperature decreases by 5°C, ten times the time is required [1].

Because temperature varies over time, the temperature at which tissue degeneration occurs is 50–70°C in some texts and 57–65°C or 60°C in others [16, 29]. To prevent this confusion, Pearce and Thomsen defined the critical temperature (T_{crit}) as the temperature at which 100% damage occurs in 1 s [1]. The critical temperature of human tissue is known to be between 60 and 85°C depending on tissues.

Table 3.4 Two methods of nonablative rejuvenation

Method	Time and temperature	Therapeutic window	Drawback
A	Short time and high temperature	Narrow	Pain, side effect
B	Long time and low temperature	Wide	Long procedure time

According to the Arrhenius formula, there are two methods to cause the coagulation phenomenon (Table 3.4). First method is using high temperature in a short time (A), and the second is using low temperature in a long time (*B*). Which is better? This will be explained in detail in "Chap. 9."

$$HI + HI \rightarrow H_2 + I_2$$

Second, what is activation energy? For HI and HI to react and change to H_2 and I_2, certain energy is required (Fig. 3.13). Change does not take place unless this energy is exceeded. In other words, activation energy is required to change reactants to products. Conversely, if activation energy is not exceeded, reactants are not able to create products. In other words, there is a threshold. For example, tissue degeneration occurs at 57°C at more than 10 s (Fig. 3.12). Looking at 45 and 55°C at 10 s, 55°C is higher than 45°C, but it has not exceeded the threshold of 57°C, so there is no change in both 45 and 55°C. It can be seen as an all-or-none phenomenon, but this phenomenon occurs because tissue degeneration progresses rapidly when the threshold is exceeded due to its exponential nature [1].

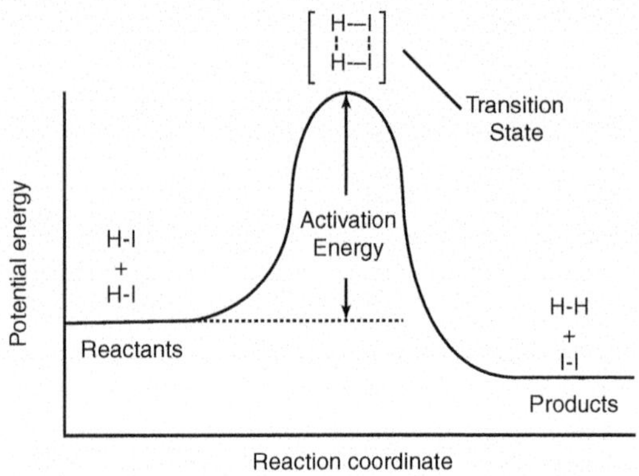

Fig. 3.13 Potential energy diagram for the decomposition of HI. (Reproduced from [30])

A specific example would be, in nonablative rejuvenation, 100 shots weekly using the genesis technique would not be effective because the procedure time is too short and it does not exceed the threshold. Rather, 10,000 shots at a single treatment session would be effective because it exceeds the threshold.

3.7 Frequency

3.7.1 Optical Thermal Model

Optical thermal models have been developed to determine appropriate laser parameters [31]. The optical thermal model is divided into three stages in order of laser-induced tissue reactions. First is the optical phase, where photons are absorbed by the target tissue. In order for the laser to be selectively absorbed by the target tissue, it is necessary to select a wavelength having a higher absorption coefficient in the target tissue than the surrounding tissue. Thus, the optical phase is the phase of selecting the wavelength. In addition, since the OPD is determined according to the wavelength, the depth of the target tissue should also be considered at this stage.

Second is the thermal phase where photons turn into heat. In order to minimize damage to the surrounding tissue, the thermal stage should be determined in accordance with the theory of selective photothermolysis so that the target tissue does not transfer heat to the surrounding tissue. Thus, the thermal phase is the phase of selecting the pulse duration.

Third is tissue denaturation process. When heat is applied to target tissue, the optical properties of the tissue change. For example, after irradiating IPL in lentigines, darkening is examined to determine whether the fluence is appropriate (clinical endpoint). This stage corresponds to the tissue denaturation process. Therefore, the order of selecting laser parameters is as follows. First, select the wavelength. Next, determine the pulse duration. Finally, tissue response should be observed to control fluence.

Wavelength → pulse duration → spot size → fluence.

I think that spot size should be added to these orders of selecting three laser parameters. Spot size should be added before fluence. When performing laser treatment, spot size determination is essential, especially when treating the dermis, because fluence varies with spot size (spot size effect). Therefore, laser parameters should be determined in order of wavelength, pulse duration, spot size, and fluence.

3.7.2 Tissue Degeneration Process

Let's take a closer look at the tissue degeneration process. The tissue degeneration process occurs after several tens to hundreds of milliseconds after laser irradiation. In the tissue denaturation process, the absorption coefficient of most tissues is increased by three to four times. For example, after irradiating IPL on lentigo, the lentigo turns to black, which has a higher absorption coefficient than the original brown lentigo. In addition, vascular treatment with long-pulsed Nd:YAG laser results in clot formation in red blood. This also looks darker and the absorption coefficient is increased.

After tissue degeneration process, the absorption coefficient of the target tissue is increased, and the ratio of absorption coefficient of the target tissue to the surrounding tissue is increased. Therefore, target tissue can be treated more selectively. For example, a multiplex laser (Cynergy™, Cynosure, Chelmsford, Massachusetts, USA), which irradiates 595-nm PDL first, followed by 1064-nm Nd:YAG laser, uses the principle of tissue degeneration process [16]. In addition, the laser can be repeatedly irradiated immediately after the initial laser irradiation (stacking, repeat pulse method).

3.7.3 Pulse Sequence

Repeat pulse method can be divided into two: uniform pulse sequence and nonuniform pulse sequence [31]. Uniform pulse sequence is a method of irradiating the pulse with the same pulse duration and the same fluence at the same time interval. With this method, the temperature rises gradually with repeated pulse irradiation (Fig. 3.14). In nonuniform pulse sequence, the first pulse is strong and the next pulse is weak to maintain a constant temperature for the total pulse duration (Fig. 3.15). Nonuniform pulse sequences are ideal, but they require accurate calculations so that laser machine must be preset, not adjusted by the operator. We will focus on the uniform pulse sequence that the operator can control.

Jia et al. applied uniform pulse sequence and repeated irradiation of 1064-nm Q-switched Nd:YAG laser on capillary glass tube with internal diameter of 1 mm and thickness of 0.1 mm to measure temperature change [32]. The parameters

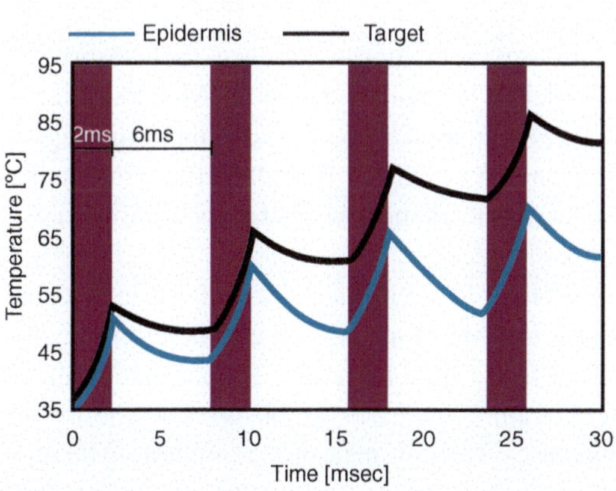

Fig. 3.14 Temperature change of target tissue and epidermis in uniform pulse sequence. (Modified from [31])

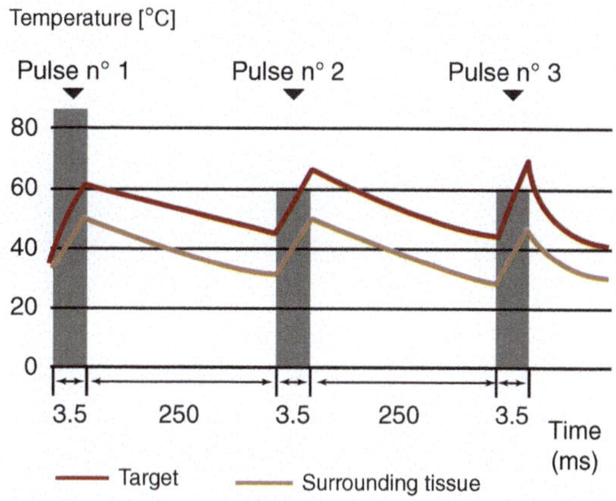

Fig. 3.15 Temperature changes in target and surrounding tissues in nonuniform pulse sequence. (Modified from [31])

were 2-mm spot size and 0.3-ms pulse duration (genesis mode). The result is as follows. When blood coagulation temperature is about 73°C, the skin temperature exceeded the blood coagulation temperature when irradiated four times at 30 J/cm^2, 4 Hz, and the skin temperature exceeded the blood coagulation temperature when irradiated twice at 40 J/cm^2, 2 Hz (Fig. 3.16).

From the results of this paper, it can be seen that when repeatedly irradiated with a uniform pulse sequence, the temperature rise varies depending on the three parameters: fluence, frequency, and pulse count.

Then how can we actually adjust these three parameters? Next, let's take a look at how to use the tissue degeneration process in vascular therapy and how to adjust three parameters.

3.7.4 Tissue Degeneration Process in Vascular Therapy

Can tissue degeneration process be used in vascular therapy? First, let's look at the phenomena in blood vessels during tissue degeneration process. Laser irradiation of blood produces MetHb and clot during tissue degeneration process. In particular, absorption curve of the clot rises above the original blood absorption curve. Irradiating multiple passes on the clot is possible because the absorption curve does not shift to the right like

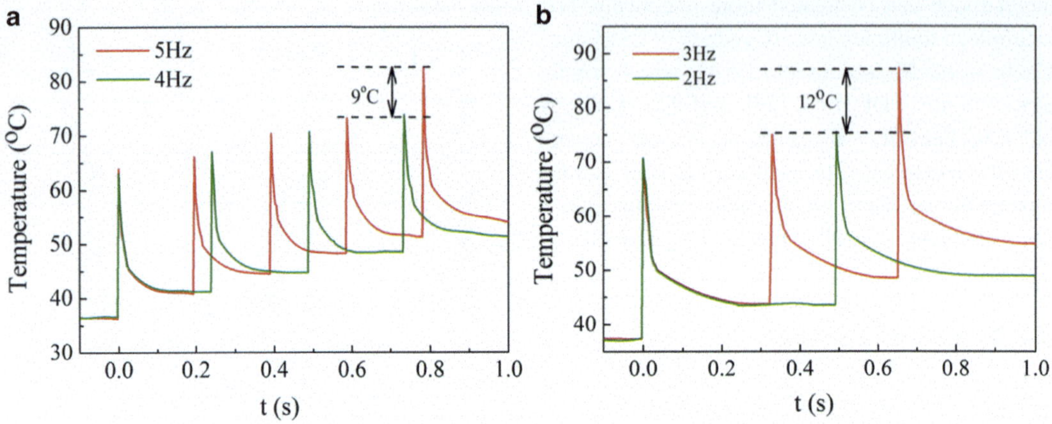

Fig. 3.16 Thermal response of blood samples in 1 s at (**a**) 30 and (**b**) 40 J/cm². (Reproduced from [32])

metHb (bathochromic shift or red shift [14], see Sect. 6.1.2 in "Chap. 6.") but rather rises upward. Typical methods are the stacking method that repeatedly irradiates 585-nm PDL at the same spot and the multipulse method of IPL. However, the 1064 long-pulsed Nd:YAG laser should be used with caution because the use of the stacking method can cause burns due to a rapid increase in absorption coefficient due to the occurrence of metHb.

Myhill et al. repeatedly irradiated IPL on live pig skin and observed changes in skin temperature [33]. One group was repeatedly irradiated with 16 J/cm² with 8 s intervals and the other group at 18 J/cm² with 9 s intervals. The reason for this interval of 8 and 9 s is to completely cool the skin after IPL and to exclude the heat accumulation effect due to repeated irradiation. The temperature measurement results show that even after repeated irradiation, the temperature immediately before the laser irradiation is returned to the original temperature relatively consistently, but the maximum temperature gradually increases with repeated irradiation. The reason why the temperature gradually increases even when IPL is repeatedly irradiated at intervals of 8–9 s, which is a relatively long time, suggests that other factors exist in addition to MetHb and clot. Myhill et al. estimated that absorption coefficients increase as blood vessels expand, blood flow increase, and hemoglobin concentration increases due to sub-coagulative vascular damage at low temperatures in which coagulation cannot occur.

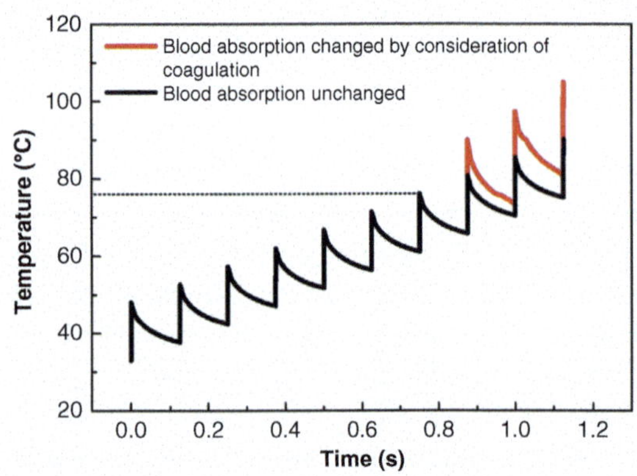

Fig. 3.17 Average temperature change of the target vessel with energy density of 53 J/cm² and pulse frequency of 8 Hz. (Reproduced from [34])

In summary, it can be seen that absorption coefficient is changed due to (1) MetHb, (2) clot, and (3) increased blood flow during tissue degeneration process. Then how does the temperature of the tissue change when the absorption coefficient changes?

MetHb and clot are formed during repeat pulse method or absorption coefficient increases when blood flow increases. In the same fluence, temperature increases as absorption coefficient increases. Li et al. measured temperature change by repeatedly irradiating a 1064-nm Q-switched Nd:YAG laser with pulse duration of 0.3 ms on a capillary tube containing blood (Fig. 3.17) [34]. The results show that during repeated irradiation, the temperature increases constantly but the temperature rises more rapidly from tissue degeneration process after clot formation.

Repeated irradiation of blood vessels initially results in constant temperature elevation but after tissue degeneration process, the temperature rises rapidly. Particularly, since MetHb increases its absorption coefficient by three times, a near-infrared laser such as the 1064-nm Q-switched Nd:YAG laser undergoes a rapid temperature change in the tissue degeneration process than vascular lasers of 500–600 nm wavelength. This phenomenon can be used for repeat pulse method, but care must be taken because abrupt temperature changes can cause side effects if the temperature passes damage threshold and rises beyond survival threshold (see Sect. 9.2.4 in "Chap. 9").

3.7.5 Repeat Pulse Method

Next, we will look specifically at repeat pulse method using clot and blood flow increase.

According to the papers of Jia et al. and Li et al., by using a 1064-nm wavelength, and repeatedly irradiating with a pulse duration of 0.3 ms, the blood temperature can be gradually increased. My own 1064-nm Q-switched Nd:YAG laser cannot raise energy above 100 J/cm^2 with 0.3 ms pulse duration, 2 mm spot size. I believe that fluence of at least 150 J/cm^2 is required, so I tried the repeat pulse method using a long-pulsed Nd:YAG laser rather than a Q-switched Nd:YAG laser. Currently, the parameters I use are 2 mm spot size, 0.3 ms, 150 J/cm^2, 3 Hz, and 3–4 shots. This method can be used to treat small vessels that are less than 5 ms TRT, which are ineffective by conventional long-pulsed Nd:YAG lasers. Since blood vessels with a TRT of 5 ms or more can already be treated with long-pulsed Nd:YAG lasers, these are not included in the treatment group.

I named the method of gradually raising the temperature by repeatedly irradiating with uniform pulse sequence as "repeat pulse method" to make it easier to understand. Although I do not yet have a sufficient command of this technique, I was able to treat not only blood vessels corresponding to TRT of 5 ms or more but also some blood vessels of TRT of 5 ms or less using the repeat pulse method with the long-pulsed Nd:YAG laser. Another advantage is that the purpura occurring in 585-nm PDL does not occur in the repeat pulse method by long-pulsed Nd:YAG laser.

The disadvantages of the repeat pulse method using long-pulsed Nd:YAG laser are as follows. First, the patient is uncomfortable due to pain, and second, the clinical end point is hard to see due to small blood vessel size. Third, even if the pulse count is four or five times, just one more shot may result in burns. Fourth, the procedure time is long because blood vessels need to be irradiated one by one. Fifth, although I have not tried it, flushing due to small blood veins not easily seen with a magnifying glass, is likely to be ineffective or is likely to cause side effects.

Then does the repeat pulse method apply only to vascular therapy? Can't the repeat pulse method be applied to pigmentation treatment? This will be explained in detail in "Chap. 7."

3.8 Strategy

There are three strategies for selectively raising the temperature in only one area spatially (Table 3.5) [14]. First, selective photothermolysis, second, epidermal cooling, and third, fractional photothermolysis. Let's review these three strategies one by one.

The first method is the theory of selective photothermolysis. The difference in absorption coefficients is used to increase the temperature of the target tissue while protect the surrounding tissue.

Table 3.5 Strategy of laser therapy

Spatially selective temperature elevation
1. Selective phototothermolysis A. Absorption coefficient (wavelengths), concentration of chromophore B. Pulse duration (thermal kinetic selectivity)
2. Epidermal cooling
3. Fractional photothermolysis

$$\Delta T = \frac{F_z \mu_a}{\rho c} \left(\frac{\tau_r}{\tau_r + \tau_p} \right)^{g/2}$$

ΔT: temperature increase of a desired target
μ_a: absorption coefficient
Fz: local subsurface fluence
ρ: density
c: specific heat
g: geometric factor (one for planes, two for cylinders, and three for spheres)
τ_p: laser pulse duration
τ_r: thermal relaxation time of the target (TRT)

Variables in this formula include fluence, absorption coefficient, TRT, pulse duration, shape parameter, density, and specific heat. At first glance, you might think that treatment can be done by adjusting fluence or pulse duration, but it is not. For example, suppose there are a 5-mm lentigo and a normal tissue surrounding the lentigo. If the laser is irradiated with a 10-mm spot size, in that spot there will be a temperature change of the lentigo (ΔT in lentigo) and a temperature change of the normal tissue (ΔT in normal tissue). There is no difference between fluence and pulse duration within the same spot. What is the difference between the two tissues? The first is absorption coefficient and the second is TRT. In other words, only the lentigo can be treated selectively by using the melanin absorption coefficient difference between lentigo and normal tissue or the concentration difference between lentigo and the normal tissue. In addition, thermal kinetic selectivity can be used to selectively treat one by one while sequentially decreasing from a long pulse duration to a short pulse duration.

The second method is epidermal cooling. For example, in laser hair removal, both the temperature of epidermal melanin and dermal hair is increased. When epidermal cooling forcibly reduces epidermal temperature, the temperature of dermal hair is selectively increased.

The third method is fractional photothermolysis. This method is a method of selectively treating only a partial portion spatially from the first irradiation. Lasers that use fractional photothermolysis are fractional lasers using Er:glass or CO_2 lasers. But is fractional photothermolysis only possible with fractional lasers? Fractional photothermolysis is effective not only with expensive fractional lasers but also with the pinhole method, where only one shot is shot with a regular CO_2 laser.

What kind of strategy should be applied in each situation? First, the theory of selective photothermolysis mainly applies to horizontal situations. This method is applied when target tissue and competition tissue are located horizontally. For example, this method is used to treat epidermal pigments such as lentigo. Second, epidermal cooling is applied in vertical situations. For example, it is applied when treating dermal lesions such as vascular therapy, hair removal, and nonablative rejuvenation. The third method is applicable to all situations.

Conversely, what is the situation in which these methods cause problems? First, in the theory of selective photothermolysis, problems arise when absorption coefficients are similar or the pulse duration is similar. For example, treatment is difficult when the original skin is dark so that the difference in absorption coefficient of the original skin and the lentigo is not large. On the contrary, treatment is difficult when the lentigo is bright and the original skin is light so that the difference in absorption coefficient of the original skin and the lentigo is not large. Second, in epidermal cooling, problems can arise if epidermal cooling is poor. The laser physician should always check the cooling machine. Third, in fractional photothermolysis, problems arise when fractional laser is too dense. In this case, regeneration from the normal tissue to the fractional irradiated tissue is not easy and may cause side effects.

References

1. Goldman MP (2006) Cutaneous and cosmetic laser surgery. Mosby Elsevier, Philadelphia, PA
2. Goldman MP (2013) Lasers and energy devices for the skin. Taylor & Francis. [S.I]
3. Allemann IB, Goldberg DJ (2011) Basics in dermatological laser applications. Karger Medical and Scientific Publishers

4. Altshuler GB, Anderson RR, Manstein D, Zenzie HH, Smirnov MZ (2001) Extended theory of selective photothermolysis. Lasers Surg Med 29(5):416–432
5. Watanabe S (2008) Basics of laser application to dermatology. Arch Dermatol Res 300(Suppl 1):S21–S30
6. Se YJ, Sung EC, Bak H, Choi JH, Kim I-H (2008) New melasma treatment by collimated low fluence Q-switched Nd: YAG laser. Korean J Dermatol 46(9):1163–1170
7. Kim JH, Kim H, Park HC, Kim IH (2010) Subcellular selective photothermolysis of melanosomes in adult zebrafish skin following 1064-nm Q-switched Nd:YAG laser irradiation. J Invest Dermatol 130(9):2333–2335
8. Kim JH, Jeong SY, Shin JB, Park H, Kim IH (2008) Subcellular selective photothermolysis in zebrafish: an electron microscopic evidence after Q-switched Nd:YAG laser ablation. Korean J Dermatol 46(20):187
9. Anderson RR, Parrish JA (1983) Selective photothermolysis: precise microsurgery by selective absorption of pulsed radiation. Science 220(4596):524–527
10. Jacques SL (1998) Melanosome absorption coefficient. Oregon Medical Laser Center; 7
11. Stratigos A, Dover JS (2000) Overview of lasers and their properties. Dermatol Ther 13(1):2–16
12. Anderson RR, Parrish JA (1981) The optics of human skin. J Investig Dermatol 77(1):13–19
13. Lee W (2008) Principles of IPL and its uses (Korean). Seoul, MDworld
14. Keyvan N (2012) Lasers in dermatology and medicine. Springer-Verlag, London
15. James WD, Elston D, Berger T (2011) Andrew's diseases of the skin E-book: clinical dermatology. Elsevier Health Sciences
16. Raulin C, Karsai S (2011) Laser and IPL technology in dermatology and aesthetic medicine. Heidelberg, New York
17. Niemz M (2019) Laser-tissue interactions. Springer International Publishing
18. (2000) Appendix. Laryngoscope 110(S95):31–37
19. Niemz MH (2007) Laser-tissue interactions. Springer, New York
20. Kauvar A, Hruza G (2005) Principles and practices in cutaneous laser surgery. CRC Press
21. Kang WH (2013) Treatment stratеties for pigmentation disorders in skin (Korean). Hansol Medical, Seoul
22. Ross EV, Ladin Z, Kreindel M, Dierickx C (1999) Theoretical considerations in laser hair removal. Dermatol Clin 17(2):333–355. viii
23. Gold MH (2007) Lasers and light sources for the removal of unwanted hair. Clin Dermatol 25(5):443–453
24. Lee JH, Park SR, Jo JH, Park SY, Seo YK, Kim SM (2014) Comparison of epidermal/dermal damage between the long-pulsed 1064 nm Nd:YAG and 755 nm alexandrite lasers under relatively high fluence conditions: quantitative and histological assessments. Photomed Laser Surg 32(7):386–393
25. Lee C, Bae E, Park J, Lim S (2009) Permanent makeup removal using Q-switched Nd: YAG laser. Clin Exp Dermatol 34(8):e594–e5e6
26. Trafeli JP, Kwan JM, Meehan KJ, Domankevitz Y, Gilbert S, Malomo K et al (2007) Use of a long-pulse alexandrite laser in the treatment of superficial pigmented lesions. Dermatol Surg 33(12):1477–1482
27. Lee JS (2011) Deep chemistry (Korean). Korea foundation for the advancement of science & creativity, Seoul
28. Berlien H-P (2003) Applied laser medicine. Springer Science & Business Media
29. Ortiz AE, Goldman MP, Fitzpatrick RE (2014) Ablative CO2 lasers for skin tightening: traditional versus fractional. Dermatol Surg 40(Suppl 12):S147–S151
30. Hoenig S (2001) Basic training in chemistry. Springer Science & Business Media
31. Mordon S, Brisot D, Fournier N (2003) Using a "non uniform pulse sequence" can improve selective coagulation with a Nd:YAG laser (1.06 microm) thanks to Met-hemoglobin absorption: a clinical study on blue leg veins. Lasers Surg Med 32(2):160–170
32. Jia H, Chen B, Li D (2017) Dynamic optical absorption characteristics of blood after slow and fast heating. Lasers Med Sci 32(3):513–525
33. Myhill J, Bäumler W, Hennings L, Bearden ED, Buckmiller LM, Shafirstein G (2008) The interaction of broadband intense pulsed light (IPL) and skin during a multi-pulse application. Med Laser Appl 23(2):71–78
34. Li D, Li R, Jia H, Chen B, Wu W, Ying Z (2017) Experimental and numerical investigation on the transient vascular thermal response to multi-pulse Nd:YAG laser. Lasers Surg Med 49(9):852–865

Part II

Lasers and PIH in Asian

4 Etiology and Treatment of Postinflammatory Hyperpigmentation

Although there are many side effects that can occur after laser treatment, the most common and problematic side effect in darker skin including Koreans is postinflammatory hyperpigmentation (PIH). Therefore, a full understanding and management of PIH are necessary. In this chapter, we go through PIH in detail.

4.1 Overview of PIH

The definition of PIH is "a common condition caused by numerous preceding cutaneous insults." The causes include drug reactions, phototoxicity reactions, inflammation, physical irritation or damage, allergic reactions, and inflammation diseases. The diagnosis of PIH is made when there is a hyperpigmented patch in the area of inflammation. PIH is prevalent and lasts longer in darker skin types (Fitzpatrick skin types III–VI). Wood's lamps can be used to distinguish epidermal and dermal PIH. Biopsy reveals "pigment incontinence" (epidermal pigment falling into the dermis, where they do not belong) and "melanophages" (dermal melanocytes or macrophages phagocytosing dermal pigments). Melanin is increased in both the epidermis and the dermis. The treatment of PIH is difficult. Spontaneous resolution is possible for epidermal PIH [1].

PIH is not frequently mentioned in dermatology texts and there are few papers about PIH. The lack of PIH content suggests that PIH is not a subject of interest in academics centered around the United States and Europe. On the other hand, in darker skin including Koreans, PIH occurs frequently and laser physicians should be familiar with PIH because it is the most problematic side effect during laser treatment. Fortunately, recent papers on PIH continue to be published. The following is a summary of the papers on PIH and my thoughts regarding them.

4.2 Epidemiology and Possible Etiology of PIH

PIH can occur at any age and in any skin type, and there is no difference in the incidence of men and women. However, it occurs more often in Fitzpatrick skin types IV, V, and VI. This may be due to hyperactive melanocytes, which are found in patients with darker skin types, which cause hypersensitivity to the same inflammation [2]. In summary, PIH occurs frequently in Koreans with Fitzpatrick skin types IV and V. Hyperactive melanocytes, which is also the cause of melasma, are considered to be a fundamental problem of PIH.

J. D. Lee et al., *Principles and Choice of Laser Treatment in Dermatology*,
https://doi.org/10.1007/978-981-15-6556-4_4

4.3 Risk Factor for PIH

PIH is caused by a number of underlying causes that can cause inflammation. Intrinsic causes include hereditary diseases that may cause “pigment incontinence,” skin diseases such as lichen planus, erythema dyschronicum persistans, and facial melanoses, and systemic diseases such as morphea, porphyria, and biliary cirrhosis. Extrinsic causes include physical damage (Fig. 4.1), sudden temperature changes, ionized and non-ionized radiation, phototoxicity reactions, laser resurfacing, and irritant contact dermatitis [3].

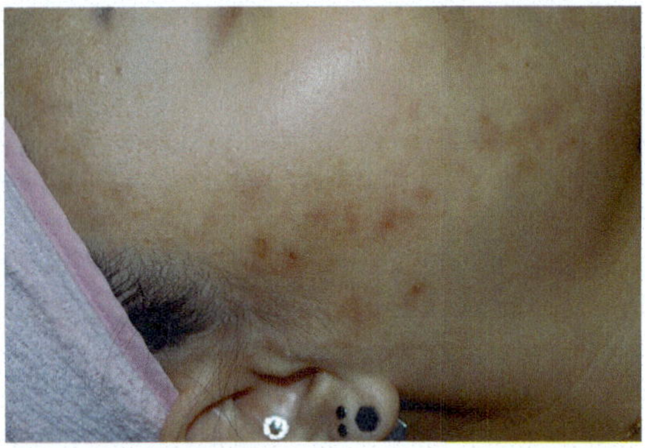

Fig. 4.1 PIH caused by excoriated acne

The important points here are: First, PIH may occur as a side effect after laser treatment (Fig. 4.2). Second, in addition to the causes described here, it is important to note that PIH can occur in “all situations that can cause inflammation” (Table 4.1).

4.3.1 Incidence of PIH Due to Cosmetic Procedures

Nonablative fractional lasers are known to be safe and effective in all skin types. However, darker skin types are known to have a high incidence of PIH when using nonablative fractional lasers. In a study of 18 patients with Fitzpatrick skin types IV and V, PIH was 43% when 1550-nm Er:glass laser was used with a lower-density parameter. However, when higher density parameters were used, PIH occurred in 71% despite hydroquinone

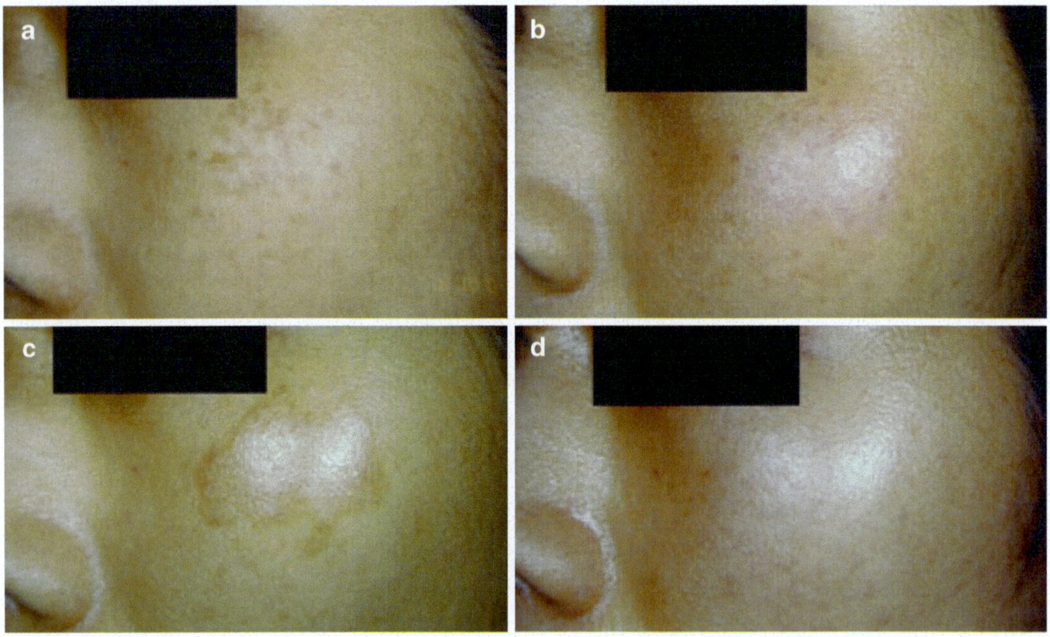

Fig. 4.2 A 24-year-old Thai–Chinese woman (skin phototype IV) with acquired bilateral nevus of Ota-like macules (Hori’s nevus). (**a**) Before treatment, (**b**) 1 week after treatment with a 1064-nm QS Nd:YAG laser, (**c**) postinflammatory hyperpigmentation developed at 2 weeks after laser treatment. The intensity of the pigmentation is usually darker than the color of the primary lesions, (**d**) 3 months after seven treatment sessions. (Reproduced from [4])

Table 4.1 Dermatologic conditions that can cause postinflammatory hyperpigmentation. (Reproduced from [5])

Inflammatory dermatoses	Acne/acneiform eruption
	Pseudofolliculitis barbae
	Eczema
	Atopic dermatitis
	Irritant contact dermatitis
	Allergic contact dermatitis
	Pigmented contact dermatitis
	Photoallergic contact dermatitis
	Lichen simplex chronicus
	Insect bites
	Papulosquamous disorders
	Psoriasis
	Pityriasis rosea
	Lichen planus/lichen planus pigmentosus
	Lichenoid dermatitis
	Erythema dyschromicum perstans
	Connective tissue disease
	Lupus erythematosus
	Vasculitis
	Morphea/scleroderma
	Atrophoderma of Pasini and Pierini
	Vesiculobullous disorders
	Pemphigus
	Bullous pemphigoid
	Dermatitis herpetiformis
Infections	Impetigo
	Viral exanthem
	Chickenpox
	Herpes zoster
	Dermatophytosis
	Syphilis
	Pinta
	Onchocerciasis
Drug reactions	Phototoxic dermatitis
	Morbilliform eruption
	Erythema multiforme
	Fixed drug eruption
	Stevens-Johnson syndrome/toxic epidermal necrolysis
	Lichenoid drug eruption
Dermatologic procedures	Chemical peel
	Dermabrasion
	Cryotherapy
	Laser treatment
	Intense pulsed light treatment
Miscellaneous	Mycosis fungoides
	Neurotic excoriation
	Sunburn
	Trauma
	Friction

pretreatment. A retrospective study using a 1540-nm fractional Er:glass laser in Asians showed 7.1% PIH in a low density/high energy parameter, but 12.4% in a high density/low energy parameter. Therefore, it is believed that the critical parameter for the generation of PIH in a fractional laser is treatment density. Another way to reduce PIH is to reduce the number of passes in one treatment, increase treatment intervals, and add cooling between passes [6].

Treatment of solar lentigines with a 532-nm Q-switched Nd:YAG laser showed that PIH occurred in 20.3% of patients with Fitzpatrick skin type III and IV [7]. In one paper, the treatment of solar lentigines in 193 patients with a 532-nm Q-switched Nd:YAG laser and 694-nm Q-switched ruby laser considered "obvious immediate whitening" as a clinical endpoint. In this case, the incidence of PIH was 23.18–33.33%. On the other hand, when "slight immediate whitening" was considered as the clinical endpoint, the incidence rate was 7.47–8.47% (Fig. 4.3). Therefore, using weak energy rather than strong energy can reduce the occurrence of PIH. But, solar lentigines did not disappear all at once when "slight immediate whitening" was a clinical endpoint [8].

It is known that the rate of PIH in an ablative laser is very high. In patients with Fitzpatrick skin type I-V, the use of dual-mode Er:YAG laser for moderate to severe acne scars showed 40% PIH. In a retrospective study of 500 patients (skin types I–IV) who underwent ablative skin rejuvenation with CO_2 laser, PIH developed in 37% of total patients. PIH developed in all (100%) patients with skin type IV and V [6].

The incidence of PIH for chemical peels increase as the depth of peels increases. Superficial chemical peels which are 20–30% salicylic acid (SA), 20–70% glycolic acid (GA), and 10–30% trichloroacetic acid (TCA) and Jessner's solution is known to have a very low incidence of PIH. In one study, Asians, Hispanics, and African-Americans with skin type III–V received 20–30% SA, and no PIH occurred. However, in a study of 35% SA in

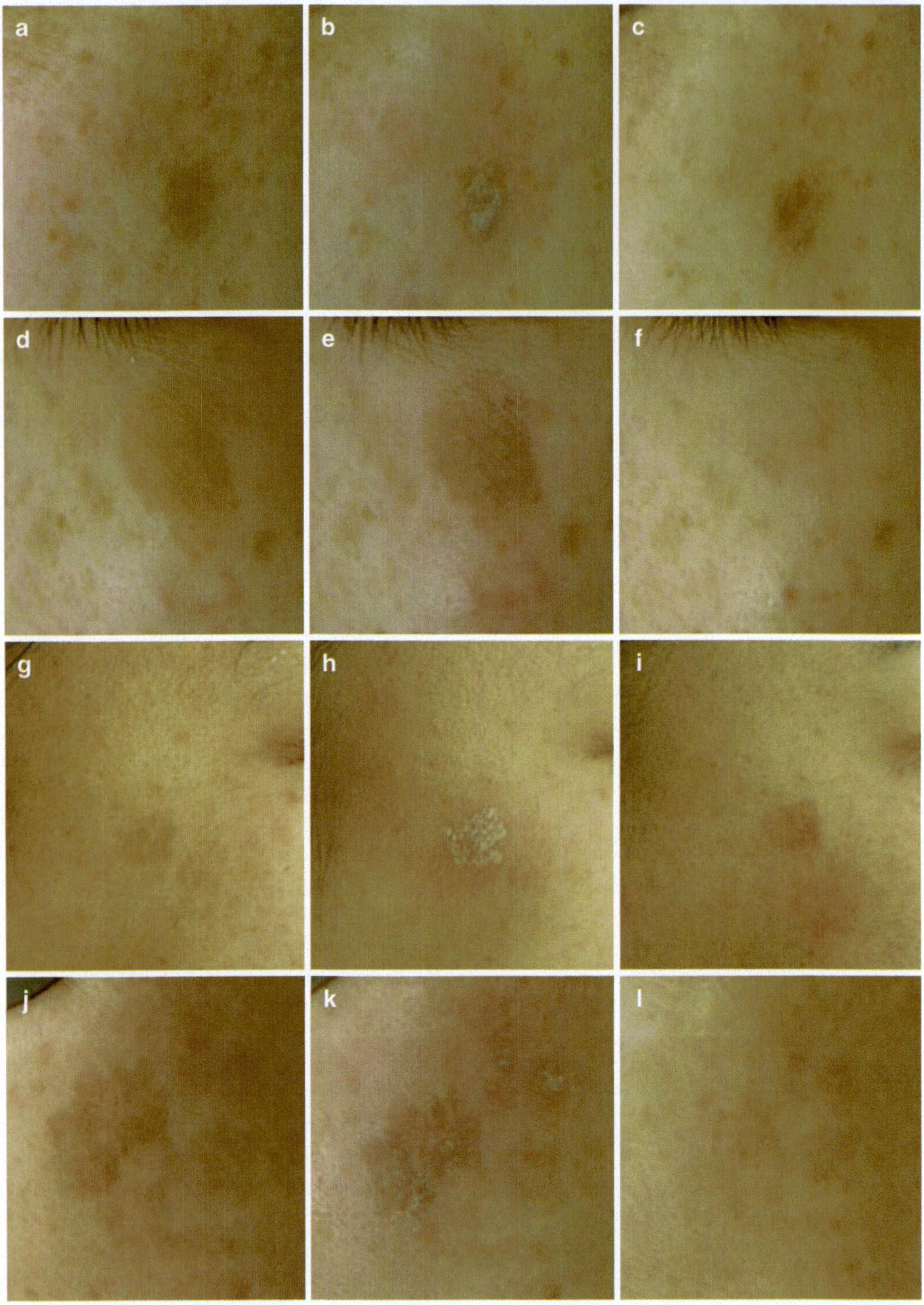

Fig. 4.3 Representative clinical cases from all four groups. A group 1 lesion aggressively irradiated with 6.0 J/cm^2 using the QS ruby laser. (**a**) before, (**b**) immediately after, and (**c**) 4 weeks after irradiation. PIH is evident. A group 2 lesion mildly irradiated with 4.0 J/cm^2 using the QS ruby laser. (**d**) before, (**e**) immediately after, and (**f**) 4 weeks after irradiation. Clearance is excellent. A group 3 lesion aggressively irradiated with 1.0 J/cm^2 using the QS frequency-doubled Nd:YAG laser. (**g**) before, (**h**) immediately after, and (**i**) 4 weeks after irradiation. PIH is evident. A group 4 lesion mildly irradiated with 0.8 J/cm^2 using the QS frequency-doubled Nd:YAG laser. (**j**) before, (**k**) immediately after, and (**l**) 4 weeks after irradiation. Clearance is excellent. (Reproduced from [8])

patients with skin type IV–VI, PIH occurred in 12%, although it disappeared after 7–10 days. 35-50% GA also showed a PIH incidence of 7.5–20% in darker skin types [6].

The incidence of PIH caused by microneedle therapy system (MTS, microneedling) has been controversial, and several studies have shown that PIH did not occur when MTS was used to treat acne scars. However, some studies have reported up to 14% of PIH [6].

4.4 Predicting PIH Occurrence

Since laser is also one of the underlying causes of PIH, people with a higher likelihood of PIH should be careful when using lasers. Is there a way to predict PIH occurrence in patients before laser treatment?

First, Fitzpatrick skin types IV and V can be distinguished through a questionnaire (This will be explained in detail in "Chap. 5"). Second, find out if any PIH has already occurred on the patient's skin. If the patient already has PIH, there is a higher likelihood of PIH after laser treatment. Third, if the skin tone of finger joints is darker than the surrounding skin, the probability of developing PIH is known to be high (Fig. 4.4) [9]. Fourth, if the patient's skin seems dark to the laser physician then PIH is more likely. More will be explained later in "Chap. 5". Care should be taken when performing laser procedures on these patients.

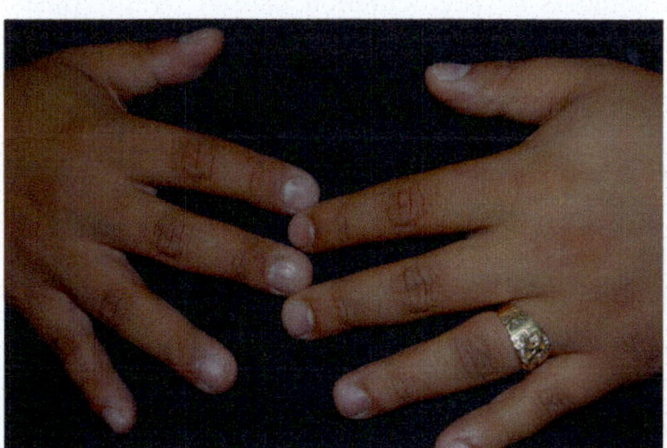

Fig. 4.4 Pigmentation observed in the finger joints of a 24-year-old male patient

4.5 Clinical Manifestations of PIH

PIH typically manifests as asymptomatic macules or patches in the same distribution as the initial inflammatory process. PIHs vary in size and shape, and they can vary in color from light brown to black. Epidermal PIH is pale brown with clear borders, and dermal PIH is darker gray with unclear boundaries [3]. However, the distinction between epidermal and dermal PIH is not easy.

Both PIH and melasma can be classified into epidermal, dermal, and mixed types. The treatment plan differs depending on whether the PIH is epidermal or dermal. How can we distinguish between epidermal and dermal pigments?

First, it can be distinguished by the color change caused by the Tyndall effect. Due to the Tyndall effect, the observer see the dermal pimgnets "blue" because the color blue has a short wavelength and is not absorbed in the dermis but is reflected by scattering and enters the observer's eye. Therefore, as pigments become deeper, it appears brown → gray → blue.

Second, Wood's lamp is used. Wood's lamp is a device that uses ultraviolet (UV) rays of 320 ~ 400 nm (360 nm). UV rays are highly absorbed by melanin and have a short wavelength, which makes them unable to penetrate the dermis. By Wood's lamp, the epidermal pigmentations appear darker than the original color (enhancement) because they absorb UV rays and do not reflect light. In contrast, there is no change in dermal pigmentations by Wood's lamp because UV rays are unable to reach the dermis. Thus, epidermal pigmentations appear darker and dermal pigmentations show no change by Wood's lamp. The disadvantage of Wood's lamp is that in the case of Fitzpatrick skin type VI, the color of the skin itself is dark, so the epidermal and dermal pigmentations cannot be distinguished by Wood's lamp. Fitzpatrick's skin type V is hard to diagnose by Wood's lamp. Mixed pigmentations with both epidermal and dermal pigmentations cannot be distinguished by Wood's lamp either [2].

Third, some authors suggest a skin stretch test, in which after the skin is stretched epidermal pigmentations become lighter and dermal pigmentations show no change [9].

Fourth, a biopsy can be performed. This is the most precise method. However, the biopsy is rarely used to distinguish between epidermal and dermal pigmentations. A biopsy is usually done to identify underlying causes [2].

There are various methods of distinguishing between epidermal and dermal pigmentations, but color changes due to the Tyndall effect is most commonly used. However, superficial dermal pigmentations such as ABNOM, melasma, and PIH are difficult to distinguish.

4.5.1 Diagnosis and Differential Diagnosis of PIH

PIH can be suspected and diagnosed by asking the patient if there has been a past inflammation at the location of hyperpigmentation. The diagnosis of PIH is made through a questionnaire. This also means that the diagnosis is difficult to make with the naked eye. Also, in many cases, the patients are unable to remember if they have had an inflammation before.

Is there a way to diagnose PIH with naked eyes? Although not written in texts or papers, I think this may be a diagnostic clue: Inflammation, the cause of PIH, will be more severe in the middle of the lesion and will become less severe as it goes to the periphery, resulting in darkest color in the center of the hyperpigmentation and lighter color with unclear boundaries on the periphery (Fig. 4.5). However, we must take notice that post-laser PIH often has a clear boundary.

There may be other causes of PIH in addition to inflammatory causes. Drugs are common non-inflammatory causes of PIH. Drugs that can cause hyperpigmentation include tetracycline, bleomycin, doxorubicin, 5-fluorouracil (5-FU), busulfan, arsenic, silver, gold, mercury, bismuth, lead, antimalarial drugs, hormones, clofazimine, and minocycline, etc. In particular, physicians should check whether acne medications such as tetracycline and minocycline are taken by dermatology patients and distinguish PIH by inflammatory causes (Fig. 4.6). In addition, the differential diagnosis of pigmentation caused by pityriasis versicolor is needed [3].

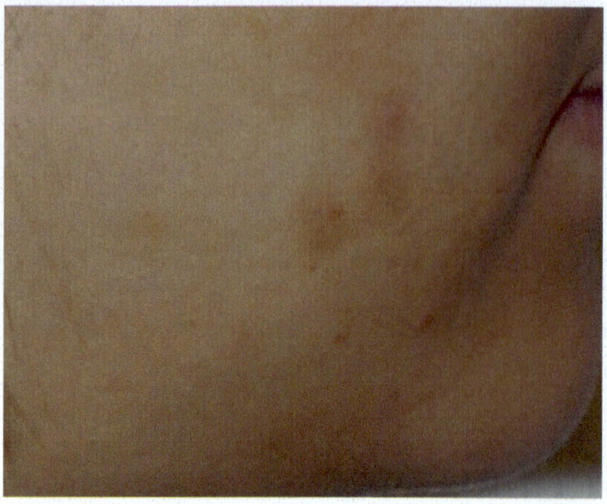

Fig. 4.5 Postinflammatory hyperpigmentation (PIH) with unclear boundaries

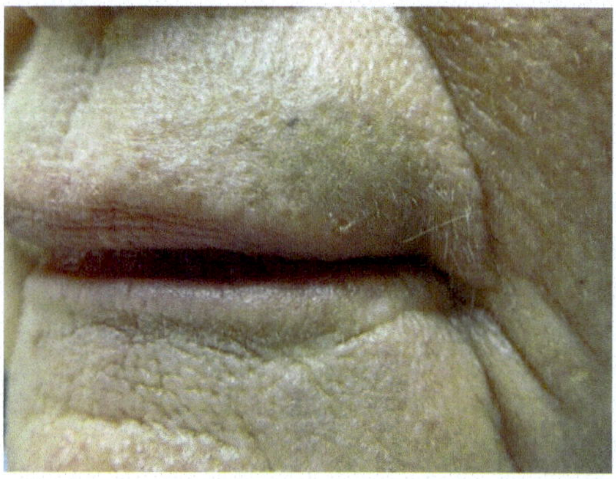

Fig. 4.6 Minocycline-induced hyperpigmentation. Note the violaceous discoloration on the lateral aspect of the upper lip. (Reproduced from [5])

4.6 Prognosis of PIH

Epidermal PIH disappears after 6–12 months, but it may take several years for dermal PIH resolution. PIH recovery time differs by site, in which the PIH of the face usually disappear after 6 months, while PIH of the body or upper limbs lasts 1–2 years, and the lower limb 3–4 years [9]. However, if the underlying cause is not resolved and inflammation persists, new PIH may occur even if the existing PIH disappears. This is why it is important to find and resolve the underlying cause of inflammation.

4.6.1 Prognostic Factors of PIH

The degree of PIH is known to vary depending on the color of the skin, degree and depth of inflammation, degree of damage to the dermo-epidermal junction, inflammatory state, and the stability of melanocytes. Takiwaki et al. reported that erythema and melanin index are directly proportional. That is, the more severe erythema, the darker the PIH [4].

Other prognostic factors of PIH are also being discussed. Kang et al. investigated PIH related factors in 516 Korean patients treated with 532-nm Q-switched Nd:YAG lasers [7]. The overall incidence of PIH was 20.3% (105/516 patients). Patients with erythematous lentigines presented with PIH more frequently compared with those without erythematous lentigines. And facial diffuse dyschromia, such as photoaging-associated mottled pigmentation (melasma, freckles, photoaging) was significantly associated with PIH. Furthermore, PIH occurred more frequently in patients with invisible pores and velvety skin. However, age, sex, Fitzpatrick skin type, and season of treatment showed little association with PIH.

Ruiz-Maldonado and Orozco-Covarrubias suggested the "individual chromatic tendency" hypothesis [5]. Individuals tend to have different pigmentation tendencies. Depending on the unique characteristics of the individual's melanocytes, after skin inflammation or injury, melanin production could be high, low, or normal. This is genetically determined and is not related to the patient's skin type.

Then how can we reduce PIH? First, inflammation should be prevented during the laser procedure, and procedures that do not damage the dermo-epidermal junction should be performed. And if inflammation develops, it should be quickly dealt with. In particular, severe erythema is a red flag of PIH. Therefore, if there is severe erythema after laser treatment, active actions should be taken. Despite these actions, PIH may occur because individuals tend to have different pigmentation development tendencies. Therefore, patients should be informed in advance of the possibility of developing PIH, and PIH should be treated safely for faster resolution.

4.7 Pathogenesis of PIH

PIH may be seen as the skin's "normal response" to inflammatory stimuli. In other words, it may be thought of as a normal process in which pigmentations are produced to protect the postinflammatory damaged skin from UV rays. What is the specific pathogenesis of PIH?

The following is the summary of the PIH pathogenesis in various papers, that I summarized. I would like to notify in advance that the mechanism for PIH has not yet been fully understood and there are many controversial issues.

First, due to the inflammatory response of the epidermal layer, arachidonic acid is secreted and oxidized to produce cytokines such as prostaglandin (PG) and leukotriene (LT). In vitro studies have shown that leukotriene C_4, leukotriene D_4, prostaglandin E_2, histamine, and thromboxane B_2 have properties that stimulate melanocytes. These cytokines increase the activity of melanocytes and immune cells, increasing melanin synthesis and increasing melanin delivery to surrounding keratinocytes. Arachidonic acid is present in the cell membrane (Fig. 4.7).

Second, the basal layer is destroyed due to inflammation. Melanocytes or keratinocytes with melanin in the basal layer drop to the upper dermis and is phagocytosed by macrophages. The phenomenon in which melanin, which should not be present in the dermis, is found in the dermis, is called "pigment incontinence" [3].

Third, keratinocytes, fibroblasts, endothelial cells, and inflammatory cells crosstalk with each other to regulate pigmentations. In other words, the epidermis and the dermis interact with each other to regulate pigmentations. For example,

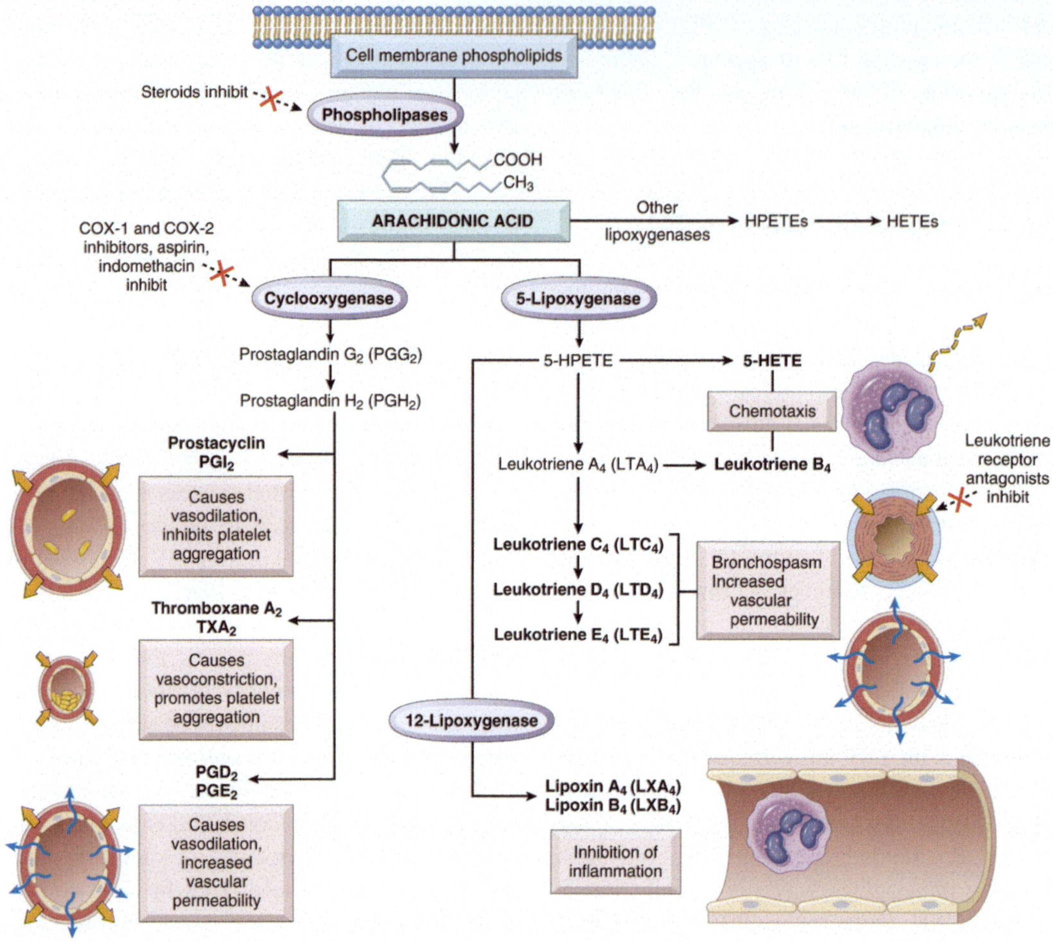

Fig. 4.7 Production of arachidonic acid metabolites and their roles in inflammation. (Modified from [10])

treatment with a very high-power Q-switched laser in nanoseconds results in photothermal and photomechanical effects on melanin. Undesired effects also take place: superficial vessels are damaged and inflammatory mediators from vascular endothelial cells and inflammatory cells crosstalk to activate melanocytes. An important inflammatory mediator from endothelial cells is nitric oxide (NO). NO is known to induce and enhance melanin formation after UV exposure. In addition, PIH after purpura by vascular lasers is known to be associated with hemosiderin infiltration [9].

The three pathophysiologies of PIH are summarized below, by location (Table 4.2).

Table 4.2 Pathophysiology of PIH by location

Pathophysiology of PIH	Location
1. Release and oxidation of arachidonic acid to PG and LT	Cell membrane
2. Pigment incontinence	Dermo-epidermal junction
3. NO from endothelial cells, hemosiderin	Vessels

Phenomena that take place while laser treatment occurs in the microscopic environment. Then how does PIH occur in this microscopic environment? For example, let's think about pigmentation treatment with a Q-switched laser. Melanosomes break and explode when the temperature of melanin rises sharply by the Q-switched laser. Due to the explosion, the melanosome fragments and shock wave break the nucleus and the cell membrane (first cause of PIH). If the explosive force is stronger, the dermo-epidermal junction below the basal layer is destroyed, resulting in keratinocytes with melanosomes or melanocytes dropping to the dermis (second cause of PIH). If the explosive force is much stronger, this will lead to the destruction of blood vessels in the upper dermis, leading to the release of NO and hemosiderin (third cause of PIH).

So how can we reduce PIH during laser treatment? First, less explosive force should be used to reduce surrounding damage. At first, low energy should be used, and if it isn't effective, it should be raised gradually. Second, long-pulsed lasers are safer than Q-switched lasers. I think if we coagulate the cells without breaking them, less arachidonic acid may be released. Third, the basal layer and the dermo-epidermal junction should be strengthened. I think the Genesis technique strengthens the basal layer and dermo-epidermal junction. The Genesis technique will be discussed in detail in "Chap 9." Fourth, purpura should be avoided during vascular treatment, and procedures that reduce flushing or telangiectasia should be added. Finally, procedures that may cause skin irritation should be avoided.

Out of these three, what is the most common pathogenesis for PIH? I think the first cause of PIH (breaking of cell membranes) is the most common mechanism because it occurs first. Therefore, avoiding high energy or procedures that may break cell membranes are the most important preventive measures in reducing PIH.

4.8 Treatment of Post-Laser PIH

PIH treatment can be divided into three phases by the treatment time. First, prevention. Second, treatment of the underlying inflammatory condition. Third, treatment of PIH itself (Table 4.3).

Table 4.3 Treatment of PIH by time

Treatment of PIH
1. Prevention
2. Treatment of the underlying inflammatory condition
3. Treatment of PIH itself

First, PIH prevention. We will not discuss details here because this has been described earlier, and throughout this book, I will be explaining which lasers and which parameters to choose.

Second, treatment of the underlying inflammatory condition is needed [11]. Because there are a number of underlying causes, appropriate treatment according to the underlying cause should be taken. For example, In the case of acne, the treatment of inflammation of acne should first proceed. In particular, the underlying cause of PIH we are interested in is PIH caused by side effects after the laser procedure. If PIH developed after the laser procedure, then the same laser procedure should not be repeated. If there is remnant inflammation or a possibility of developing PIH, the inflammation should be reduced as soon as possible.

The best medication for inflammation in the skin is steroids. Steroids are known to help restore and protect the epidermal barrier function by minimizing inflammation and protecting the skin in the inflammatory stage of the wound healing process. Also, steroids theoretically inhibit the release of prostaglandin (PG) and leukotriene (LT) derived from arachidonic acid. In other words, the steroid suppresses the first cause of PIH described earlier [9].

Cheyasak et al. treated 40 subjects with skin type IV and atrophic acne scars with an ablative fractional laser on both sides of the face [12]. Postoperatively, clobetasol propionate 0.05% ointment was applied to one randomly selected side of the face for the first 2 days, followed by an application of petrolatum jelly for the rest of the week. Petrolatum was applied to the other side for 7 days. The side of the face treated with petrolatum alone had a significantly higher incidence of PIH (75%) after laser irradiation than the side of the face treated with topical corticosteroids and petrolatum (40%). The PIH occurring on the petrolatum-treated sides had a significantly higher intensity and was spread over a significantly larger area, compared with the corticosteroid and petrolatum treated sides. In conclusion, a short-term application of topical corticosteroids postoperatively is associated with a decreased risk of PIH after the laser procedure.

But there are many concerns about the use of steroids. In Cheyasak et al. the authors address these concerns as follows. First, there is concern that the anti-proliferative effects of steroids may interfere with fibroblast activity and prevent new collagen formation, thus preventing scar improvement. But after 12 weeks, there was no difference in scar improvement between the two groups. Second, steroids may cause acneiform eruptions, but this is less likely because steroids were used short-term, for only 2 days. Third, postoperative infection occurred in two patients, but in these cases, the fractional coverage was increased by more than 80%. Higher coverage seems to be the cause rather than steroid use.

Based on this paper, I give a small amount of Group 1 steroids to patients with strong or long-lasting erythema after laser treatment and tell them to apply this generously three times a day for 2 days.

Third, the treatment of PIH itself. This can be divided into two phases, "inflammatory phase" and "non-inflammatory phase" depending on active inflammation. First, in the "inflammatory phase" there is active inflammation. For example, acne is still active and PIH is accompanied by inflammation. In this case, as in the second PIH treatment described above, acne treatment and inflammation treatment should be given priority. And since the primary cause of PIH is hyperactive melanocytes, I think that the rest of PIH treatment is the same as melasma treatment. For example, it is possible to apply the so-called laser toning to reduce the activity of melanocytes and eliminate melanosomes without side effects.

Cho et al. performed laser toning in three PIH patients after laser treatment (Q-switched ruby laser, IPL, and Q-switched Nd:YAG laser) [13]. Using a 1064-nm Q-switched Nd:YAG laser, three passes were performed at 1.9–2.6 J/cm^2 with a spot size of 6 mm, followed by three additional passes with the same fluence at the PIH site. After a total of five procedures at weekly intervals, all PIHs were improved. Kim et al. enrolled patients with acne and acne induced PIH [14]. Group A (20 patients) received laser toning, comedo removal, intralesional injection, and topical 4% benzoyl peroxide daily. Group B (20 patients) received only comedo removal, intralesional injection, and topical 4% benzoyl peroxide. Laser toning was applied with a Q-switched Nd:YAG laser with a spot size of 6 mm at 10 Hz. Fluence started at 3.3 J/cm^2 in the first session and was elevated 5.8 J/cm^2 in the last session. The clinical endpoint was whitening of downy hair and perilesional erythema. The procedure was performed five times weekly. The results showed that PIH was more improved in group A with laser toning, and also acne lesions were more reduced than group B. Laser toning will be discussed in detail in "Chap. 12".

In the "non-inflammatory phase" inflammation is completely reduced and there is no erythema. This is a very interesting period. PIH is caused by "temporarily" increased activity of melanocytes due to an underlying cause of inflammation. However, if there is no underlying cause of inflammation and if there is no active inflammation, then the melanocyte activity will be reduced, unlike melasma. I consider PIH in this phase as pigmentations, and pigmentation treatment is possible. Stronger laser toning, long-pulsed alexandrite laser, or even IPL may be used to treat this PIH. Various other whitening agents and chemical peels may be of help. Whitening agents and chemical peels are the same as in melasma treatment. This will be explained again in "Chap. 12".

For reference, Winhoven et al. reported a case in which a 23-year-old woman with acne and severe PIH took isotretinoin which resulted in a dramatic improvement of acne and PIH [15]. Although the paper aforementioned is just a case report, I too often observe significant improvement in PIH in acne patients taking isotretinoin at low-doses (10–20 mg/day).

4.9 Conclusion

PIH after laser treatment is troublesome and difficult for both patients and doctors. PIH prevention should first be taken into account. If post-laser PIH risk seems high, it is most important to get proper treatment as soon as possible. However, once PIH occurs, it does not disappear easily. I also went through many difficult situations due to PIH.

Finally, for physicians in trouble because of PIH, I would like to recommend "time," the most important method. Some say that dermal PIH may not go away, but most PIHs will go away because they are mostly epidermal. This is the biggest difference between melasma and PIH. In addition, in melasma, it is hard to know the exact cause, so there is no fundamental treatment. But PIH disappears when the temporary underlying cause (inflammation) disappears. The only question is when it will go away. Therefore, if you persuade your patient and take enough time to treat PIH, PIH will disappear.

Remember, "Time is on our side!"

References

1. Goldsmith LA, Katz SI, Gilchrest BA, Paller AS, Leffell DJ, Wolff K et al (2012) Fitzpatrick's dermatology in general medicine. McGraw-Hill Professional, New York
2. Callender VD, St Surin-Lord S, Davis EC, Maclin M (2011) Postinflammatory hyperpigmentation: etiologic and therapeutic considerations. Am J Clin Dermatol 12(2):87–99
3. Lacz NL, Vafaie J, Kihiczak NI, Schwartz RA (2004) Postinflammatory hyperpigmentation: a common but troubling condition. Int J Dermatol 43(5):362–365
4. Eimpunth S, Wanitphadeedecha R, Manuskiatti W (2013) A focused review on acne-induced and aesthetic procedure-related postinflammatory hyperpigmentation in Asians. J Eur Acad Dermatol Venereol 27(Suppl 1):7–18
5. Silpa-Archa N, Kohli I, Chaowattanapanit S, Lim HW, Hamzavi I (2017) Postinflammatory hyperpigmentation: a comprehensive overview: epidemiology, pathogenesis, clinical presentation, and noninvasive assessment technique. J Am Acad Dermatol 77(4):591–605
6. Kaufman BP, Aman T, Alexis AF (2018) Postinflammatory hyperpigmentation: epidemiology, clinical presentation, pathogenesis and treatment. Am J Clin Dermatol 19(4):489–503
7. Kang HJ, Na JI, Lee JH, Roh MR, Ko JY, Chang SE (2017) Postinflammatory hyperpigmentation associated with treatment of solar lentigines using a Q-switched 532-nm Nd:YAG laser: a multicenter survey. J Dermatolog Treat 28(5):447–451
8. Negishi K, Akita H, Tanaka S, Yokoyama Y, Wakamatsu S, Matsunaga K (2013) Comparative study of treatment efficacy and the incidence of post-inflammatory hyperpigmentation with different degrees of irradiation using two different quality-switched lasers for removing solar lentigines on Asian skin. J Eur Acad Dermatol Venereol 27(3):307–312
9. Committee C, SI C, Kim IH, Kang JS, Park SH, Chung KY et al (2016) Laser and light treatment in Asian skin. Koonja, Paju
10. Kumar V, Abbas AK, Aster JC, Robbins SL, Cotran RS (2014) Robbins and Cotran pathologic basis of disease. Elsevier, Philadelphia, PA
11. Davis EC, Callender VD (2010) Postinflammatory hyperpigmentation: a review of the epidemiology, clinical features, and treatment options in skin of color. J Clin Aesthet Dermatol 3(7):20–31
12. Cheyasak N, Manuskiatti W, Maneeprasopchoke P, Wanitphakdeedecha R (2015) Topical corticosteroids minimise the risk of postinflammatory hyper-pigmentation after ablative fractional CO2 laser resurfacing in Asians. Acta Derm Venereol 95(2):201–205
13. Cho SB, Park SJ, Kim JS, Kim MJ, Bu TS (2009) Treatment of post-inflammatory hyperpigmentation using 1064-nm Q-switched Nd:YAG laser with low fluence: report of three cases. J Eur Acad Dermatol Venereol 23(10):1206–1207
14. Kim S, Cho KH (2010) Treatment of facial postinflammatory hyperpigmentation with facial acne in Asian patients using a Q-switched neodymium-doped yttrium aluminum garnet laser. Dermatol Surg 36(9):1374–1380
15. Winhoven SM, Ahmed I, Owen CM, Lear JT (2005) Postinflammatory hyperpigmentation in an Asian patient: a dramatic response to oral isotretinoin (13-cis-retinoic acid). Br J Dermatol 152(2):368–369

5 Korean Skin and Types of Lasers

Many papers and dermatology laser texts usually describe lasers about white skin. In separate articles or chapters laser treatment of "darker skin" or ethnic, nonwhite, pigmented skin is described [1–4]. Here, the term "darker skin" refers to all races except Caucasians, including Chinese, Japanese, Indian, Pakistani, Hispanic, Latino, African, African-Caribbean, and African American. Fitzpatrick skin types are III, IV, V, and VI [5].

However, it should be noted that most of the patients I treat in private clinics are Koreans. Koreans are not white, but they do not have very dark skin like African blacks. Koreans belong to the yellow race, which is ethnically lighter in skin tone than Africans and Indians. In addition, Koreans do not have Fitzpatrick skin type IV and have only V or less [6]. This should be kept in mind while reviewing papers and texts. This should also be considered in the selection and treatment of lasers.

5.1 Characteristics of Darker Skin

5.1.1 Difference Between Caucasian Skin and Darker Skin

Darker skin is different from Caucasian skin (Table 5.1).

Table 5.1 Skin features of darker skin

1. High epidermal melanin content
2. Active melanocytes
3. Thicker dermis (increased mesenchymal reactivity)
4. Many pigmented disorders

First, the melanin content of the epidermal layer is higher than that of Caucasians. The reason of high melanin content compared to Caucasians is to protect the skin from strong ultraviolet rays. However, this high epidermal melanin content makes it difficult to treat dermal lesions with lasers [3]. For example, vascular therapy may be ineffective or less effective than Caucasians and even have side effects.

Second, melanocytes are activated. Melanocytes are activated so that melanin production is active even with a small stimulus or UV. Therefore, PIH, one of the side effects of laser, is a problem in darker skin [3]. On the other hand, if the laser is irradiated with a high energy intensity, which decreases the activity of melanocytes, melanin cannot be produced at all, causing hypopigmentation, and it becomes whiter than the surroundings and more noticeable. Also, there is more melasma in darker skin, suggesting higher melanocyte activation than Caucasians.

Third, darker skin has a thick dermal layer and high activity of mesenchymal tissue. Darker skin contains more melanin than Caucasian skin, resulting in thicker dermal layers and fewer facial

J. D. Lee et al., *Principles and Choice of Laser Treatment in Dermatology*,
https://doi.org/10.1007/978-981-15-6556-4_5

wrinkles. Wrinkles are the main symptom of photoaging in Caucasian skin, but pigmentation such as lentigo and liver spots are the main symptoms of photoaging in darker skin. In addition, darker skin has a higher activity of mesenchymal tissue, resulting in a higher incidence of hypertrophic scar or keloid than Caucasian skin, and erythema persists during wound regeneration [3]. However, Koreans do not develop as many hypertrophic scars or keloids as blacks.

Fourth, darker skin has many pigmented lesions. In particular, there are many nevus of Ota, ABNOM (Hori's macules), and melasma (Fig. 5.1) [5]. Caucasians receive skin lasers primarily because of vascular lesions and wrinkles, but patients with darker skin receive laser treatment mainly because of pigmented lesions. On the other hand, the incidence of melanoma, which is a type of skin cancer, is lower in darker skin compared to Caucasians [3]. So, there is less to worry while removing melanocytic nevi.

5.1.2 Absorption Curve of Melanin

Melanin absorption curve has a wide distribution from 200 to 1200 nm (Fig. 5.2). In the ultraviolet and visible region of the absorption curve, the absorption curve is high and is constantly decreased as the wavelength becomes longer. Thus, shorter wavelengths have higher absorption coefficients for melanin and longer wavelengths have lower absorption coefficients [3].

The broad distribution of melanin absorption curves in laser treatment is problematic for darker skin [5]. Since melanin has an absorption curve in a wide area, side effects may occur in most laser treatments. In particular, there are many side effects during vascular therapy using short wavelengths of 500 nm, and care should be taken during hair removal and pigmentation treatments.

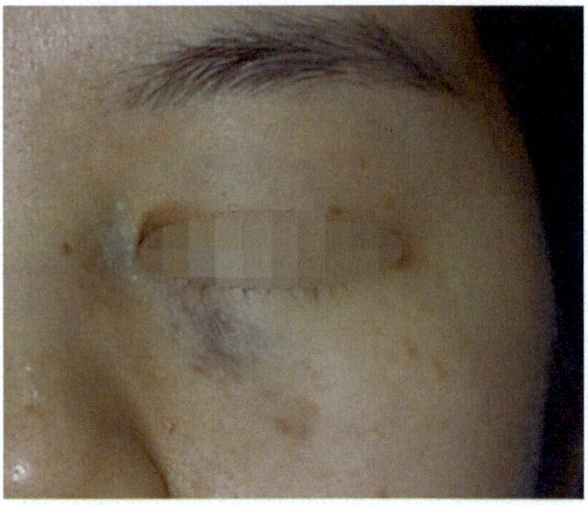

Fig. 5.1 Nevus of Ota, located near the medial and inferior orbital rim

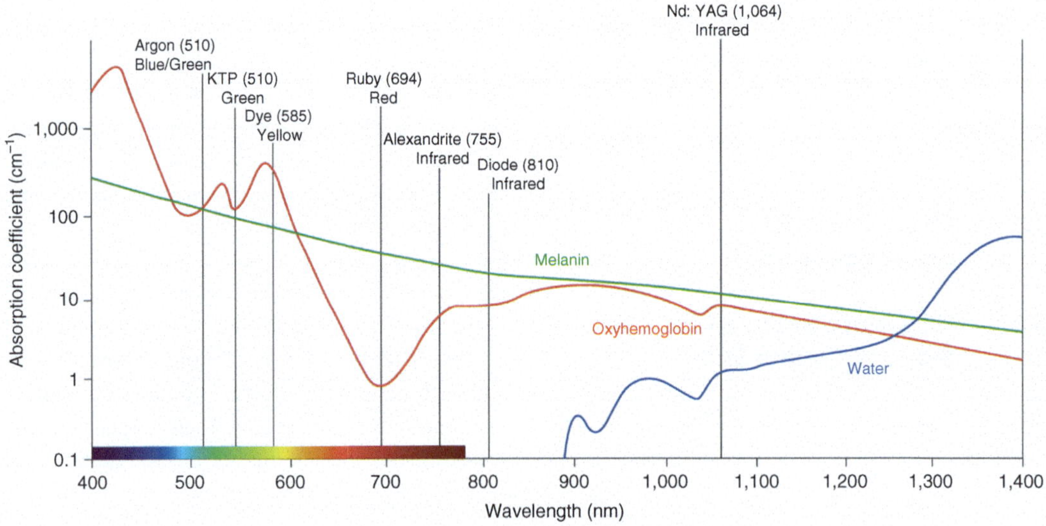

Fig. 5.2 Absorption curves for various wavelengths and chromophores. (Modified from [4])

5.1.3 Increased Epidermal Melanin Content

The reason why darker skin is particularly problematic in laser treatment compared to Caucasians is due to the high melanin content of the epidermal layer, as mentioned earlier. The specific problems are as follows.

First, for people with a very dark skin color Fitzpatrick skin type VI, it is known that the same fluence results in more than 40% higher energy than brighter skin types of Fitzpatrick skin types I and II [7]. There is also a high risk of side effects such as blistering, hyperpigmentation, and hypopigmentation. For reference, based on the fact that Fitzpatrick skin type VI results in 40% more energy than Fitzpatrick skin types I and II, I lower the fluence about 20% for patients with Fitzpatrick IV and V, compared to the usual fluence (usually used by Fitzpatrick III).

Second, epidermal melanin acts as a competing chromophore in laser treatment. For example, in vascular laser or laser hair removal, photons pass through the epidermis and into the dermis. Due to high epidermal melanin content, most of the photons are absorbed by melanin and the photons that reach the blood vessels or hair bulbs are reduced resulting in decreased therapeutic effect [4]. On the other hand, increasing fluence to make up for the lack of effect can result in too much energy in the epidermis, i.e., side effects.

Third, when treating epidermal pigment, due to a small difference in melanin between pigmented lesions and normal skin, low fluence is not effective. But if the fluence is increased, melanin in normal skin may react and hypopigmentation may occur. An example is the tiger print (footprint) caused by IPL (Fig. 5.3) [8].

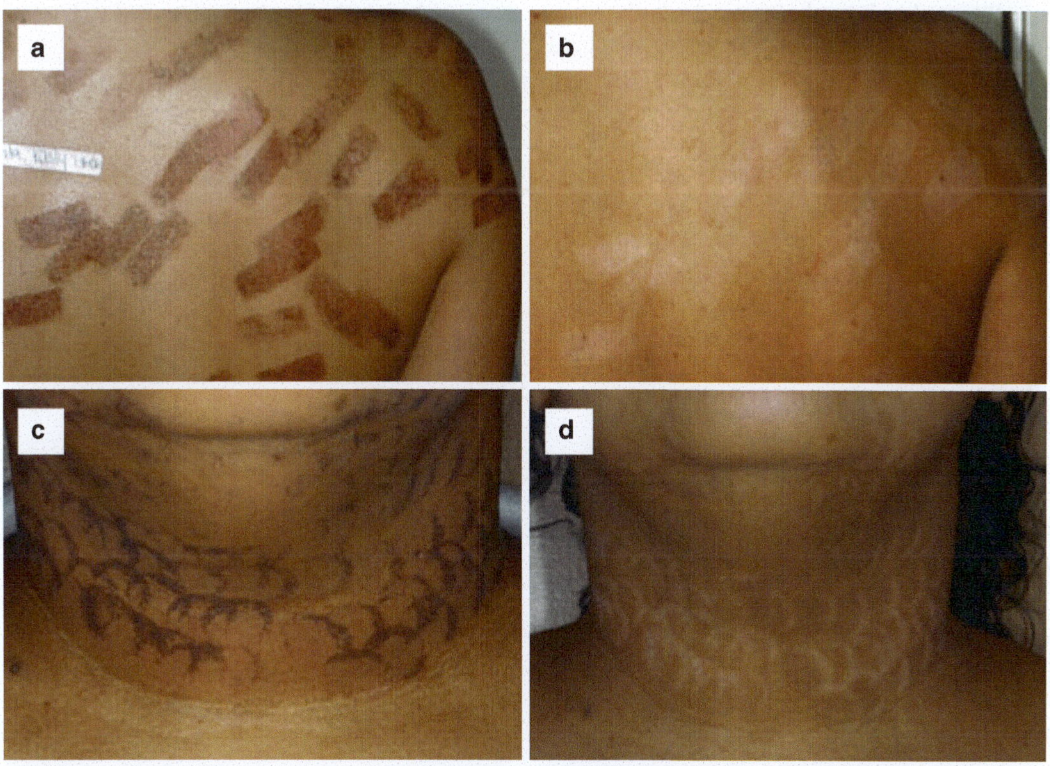

Fig. 5.3 Permanent hypopigmentation resulting from laser hair removal. (**a**) Temporary hyperpigmentation in a Fitzpatrick skin phototype IV treated with an intense pulsed light device for hair removal. (**b**) One month later, the hyperpigmented patches were replaced with persisting hypopigmented patches. (**c**) Temporary hyperpigmentation in a Fitzpatrick skin phototype VI patient treated with an Nd:Yag device. (**d**) Two weeks later, the annular hyperpigmented patches were replaced with persisting hypopigmented patches. (Reproduced from [9])

5.2 Safer Laser Treatment of Darker Skin

Several laser texts offer several methods in reducing side effects when treating darker skin (Table 5.2). Let's take a look at each of the methods to see if they are appropriate for Koreans.

5.2.1 Fitzpatrick Skin Typing System

There are several ways to distinguish the skin type of patients. The most used method is the Fitzpatrick skin typing system. Fitzpatrick skin type was first used after UVA treatment with Psoralen (PUVA) in patients with psoriasis, suggesting that some patients might develop pigmentation easily, while some patient's skins were vulnerable to burns.

In Fitzpatrick skin type, the skin type is classified into six types by surveying whether the skin is well tanned or burned (Table 5.3). In the treatment of psoriasis, Fitzpatrick skin type was used to investigate minimal erythema dose (MED) for each skin type and to determine an appropriate irradiation amount of PUVA for each skin type [10].

Table 5.2 Methods to reduce side effects in darker skin [2, 4]

To prevent adverse events when treating skin of color
1. Patient selection
2. Longer wavelength
3. Longer pulse duarion
4. Skin cooling
5. Test spot, preoperative procedure
6. Homecare. Strict sun avoidance, sun protection, and topical bleaching agents

Table 5.3 Classification of Fitzpatrick skin types by questionnaire. (Modified from [11])

Type	Sunburn	Tan
I	Burns easily	Never tans
II	Burns easily	Tans minimally with difficulty
III	Burns moderately	Tans moderately and uniformly
IV	Burns minimally	Tans moderately and easily
V	Rarely burns	Tans profusely
VI	Never burns	Tans profusely

Table 5.4 Classification of Fitzpatrick skin type by simple observation. (Modified from [11])

Skin phototypes	Typical features
I	Pale white skin; blonde or red hair; blue eyes; freckles
II	White fair skin; blonde or red hair; blue, green hazel eyes
III	Cream white skin; any hair or eye color
IV	Moderate brown skin, Mediterranean
V	Dark brown skin, Middle Eastern
VI	Deeply pigmented dark brown to black

Fitzpatrick's skin type was originally used for classification of Caucasian skin, and initially, there were only four types from I to IV. However, Fitzpatrick's skin type V and VI were later added, resulting in a total of six skin types [6].

Fitzpatrick skin type is also used simply as a way of describing the skin color of patients. In other words, this is also used to classify skin types just by observing the skin color, rather than asking whether the skin is well tanned or burned in the sun (Table 5.4, Fig. 5.4).

Fitzpatrick skin type can be divided into (1) Fitzpatrick skin type by questionnaire and (2) Fitzpatrick skin type by simple observation. In dermatology texts, Fitzpatrick skin types are often used to describe skin color, rather than describing the tendency for tan or burn. The reason why Fitzpatrick skin type is used as a method of expressing the skin color is probably that the skin color and the Fitzpatrick skin type matched to some extent because most of the early Fitzpatrick skin types were Caucasians. Another reason may be because most papers and dermatology texts that target Caucasians are mainstream in academia.

Fitzpatrick skin type has been applied in a wide range of areas including laser treatment as well as psoriasis treatment in the dermatology area, but two problems occurred in the process of applying Fitzpatrick skin types [10].

First, some authors challenged the prediction of MED by questionnaire. In one study, the Fitzpatrick skin type by questionnaire and MED did not correlate. Rather skin complexion such as the color of eyes and hair, the incidence of freckles, and the number of nevi and MED are correlated. Another study of Asian and Arabian

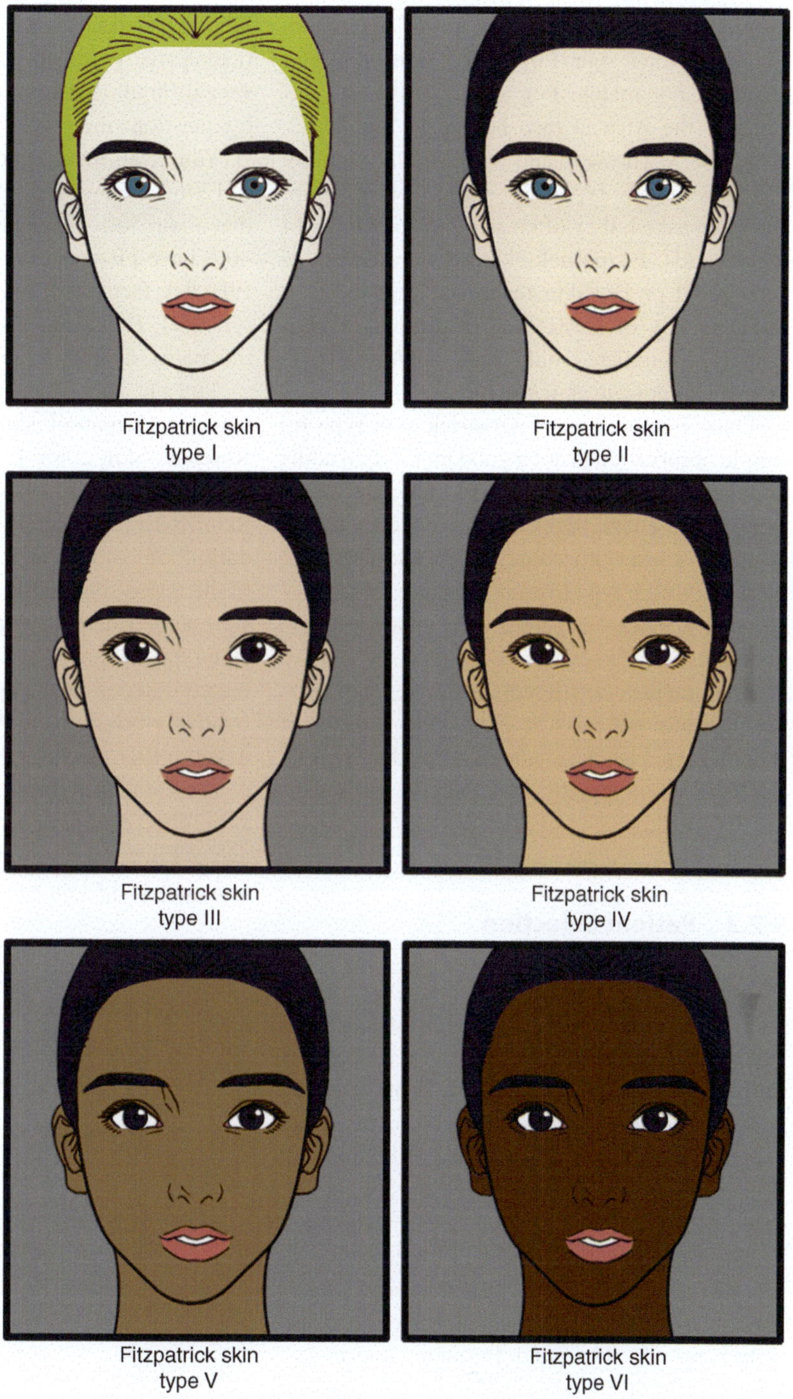

Fig. 5.4 Classification of Fitzpatrick skin type by simple observation. (Reproduced from [12])

patients found that Fitzpatrick skin type by questionnaire did not correlate with MED, suggesting that it is difficult to apply Fitzpatrick skin type in some ethnics. In other words, it means that Fitzpatrick's skin type by questionnaire cannot completely predict pigmentation and burn tendency. However, I believe that Fitzpatrick skin type by questionnaire is the most effective way to predict pigmentation and burn tendency than other skin classification methods.

Second, some authors have found that, especially in darker skin, Fitzpatrick skin type, and MED do not match. For example, the descendants of the African race belong to Fitzpatrick skin type V (brown) and VI (dark brown) by Fitzpatrick skin types by simple observation, but when asked, they often say they get burns. In other words, Fitzpatrick skin type by questionnaire is III or IV. Skin reactions (pigmentation and tendency of burns) due to ultraviolet light cannot be predicted only with epidermal pigments that indicate skin color.

Thus, I believe that Fitzpatrick skin type by simple observation is not a good method. In addition, since our main purpose is to use Fitzpatrick skin type to check pigmentation tendency of the skin after a laser procedure, we should prioritize Fitzpatrick skin type by questionnaire.

Finally, since Fitzpatrick skin type by questionnaire and Fitzpatrick skin type by simple observation have a different meaning, when writing dermatology texts or publishing a paper, it should be made clear whether the skin type is Fitzpatrick skin type by questionnaire or by simple observation.

5.2.2 Patient Selection

In one laser seminar, a physician once asked me, "how to screen patients with tendency for side effects, especially PIH, so that procedures in these patients can be avoided." This question raises two doubts. First, can we correctly select patients with the risk of developing PIH? Second, is it right to screen patients with the risk of developing PIH?

The problem is that dividing Fitzpatrick's skin types is not objective, i.e., cameras or machines are not used, but is rather subjective, because skin types are identified through "questions." For example, if you answer "No" to the question "Does your skin tan in summer?," your skin type is I, II, III. If you answer "Yes" to that question, the next question will be "Does it turn red and then black? (skin type IV), Or does it become black right away? (skin type V)." Fitzpatrick skin type is very inaccurate because it divides Fitzpatrick skin type by questionnaires. In particular, many use sunscreens these days, so it is very difficult to distinguish Fitzpatrick skin type by questionnaire.

Yun et al. investigated Fitzpatrick skin types in 1296 Koreans (Table 5.5) [6]. The results show that about 50% of Koreans have skin type III, and 40% have Fitzpatrick skin types IV and V (both PIH risk factors). There are no Fitzpatrick skin types VI. However, if you look more closely at this paper, another interpretation can be made.

Yun et al. investigated the relationship between Fitzpatrick skin types and skin color in Koreans. Skin color 1, 2, 3, and 4 are the skin color of the patient (Skin color 1: relatively light, Skin color 2: normal, Skin color 3: relatively dark, Skin color 4: very dark). Let's look at some of the interesting things about the results. First, in skin color 1 and 2, the percentage of Fitzpatrick skin types IV and V are 33.1%. In other words, it means that one-third of patients whose skin looks relatively bright when the doctor sees them may develop PIH. Second, the patients who visit and want treatment in laser clinics often have darker skin. Then excluding skin color 1, what percentage of Fitzpatrick skin types IV and V are in skin 2, 3, and 4? 49.1%, which is almost half. In other

Table 5.5 Korean Fitzpatrick skin type classification. Classification according to skin condition after sunbathing for 30–45 min without applying anything in spring-summer [13].

Fitzpatrick skin type classification	Percentage	Questionnaires
Skin type I	2.4	Not immediately reddened or darkened
Skin type II	8.8	Soon reddened and slightly darkened
Skin type III	48.8	Reddened and blacked
Skin type IV	22.2	Slight reddened or immediately darkened
Skin type V	17.8	Rarely reddened and necessarily darkened
Skin type VI	0	Never reddened and becomes very darkened

words, half of the patients who visit the clinic for laser treatment may have a risk of developing PIH. This means that it's a hit and miss. Third, although not statistically significant due to the small sample size (9 patients), all patients with very dark skin (skin color 4) correspond to Fitzpatrick skin types IV and V.

Let's go back to the second question. Is it right to screen patients with the risk of developing PIH? According to the survey above, at least 40–50% of the patients should not be treated. Is this possible in private practice? Then what should we do? I assume that "all patients can develop PIH." Therefore, first, a treatment method that produces less PIH should be chosen. Second, if PIH does occur, ways to get rid of it quickly should be found.

Table 5.6 Lancer ethnicity scale (LES)

Geography	Fitzpatrick skin type	LES skin type
African background		
Central East, West African	V	5
Eritrean and Ethiopian	V	5
North African, Middle East	V	5
Arabian background		
Sephardic Jewish	III	4
Asian background		
Chinese, Korean, Japanese, Thai, Vietnamese	IV	4
Filipino, Polynesian	IV	4
European background		
Ashkenazi Jewish	II	6
Celtic	I	1
Central Eastern European	III	2
Nordic	I-II	1
Northern European (general)	I	1–2
Southern European, Mediterranean	III	3–4
Latin/Central/South American background		
Central/South American Indian	IV	4
North American background		
Native American (including Inuit)	II	3

Risk factor: LES type 1 = very low risk, LES type 2 = low risk, LES type 3 = moderate risk, LES type 4 = significant risk, LES type 5 = considerable risk. Reproduced from [14]

5.2.3 Lancer Ethnicity Scale

Let's look at another skin type classification method.

Lancer Ethnicity Scale (LES) is a method of classifying skin types by ethnicity (Table 5.6). The numbers of skin types according to the ethnicities of paternal grandfather, paternal grandmother, maternal grandfather, and maternal grandmother are summed and then divided by 4, resulting in one's skin type [3].

The limitation of LES is that most Koreans are of one ethnic race. In recent years, multicultural families have increased, but most are of one ethnic race. Koreans have LES type 4. Paternal grandfather, paternal grandmother, maternal grandfather, and maternal grandmother all have LES type 4. As a result, I too have LES type 4. LES type 4 represents significant risks. In other words, Koreans all have "very dangerous" skin types for laser treatment.

5.2.4 Longer Wavelength (Epidermal Bypass Effect)

Figure 5.2 is the most common figure you see at a conference after you buy your first laser. This figure shows the absorption curves for the three chromophores. Physicians who have just started laser treatment often misunderstand this figure by thinking "the ruby laser is the best among Q-switched pigmentation lasers." Why the misunderstanding?

"The larger the difference in absorption coefficient between the two chromophores, the higher the temperature of the target tissue, so lowering the temperature of the surrounding tissue will be effective and will have fewer side effects." This is true. "Therefore, among Q-switched pigmentation lasers such as ruby lasers, alexandrite lasers, and Nd:YAG lasers, ruby lasers have a high absorption coefficient for melanin and low absorption coefficient for hemoglobin and may be considered as the best laser." Is this true?

Table 5.7 shows the absorption coefficients by wavelength [16]. Ruby laser (694 nm) is not

Table 5.7 Absorption coefficients for respective chromophores in interest. (Reproduced from [15])

	532 nm	595 nm	755 nm	800 nm	1064 nm
Hb	219 cm^{-1}	114 cm^{-1}	8.4 cm^{-1}	4.1 cm^{-1}	0.3 cm^{-1}
HbO_2	237 cm^{-1}	36 cm^{-1}	3 cm^{-1}	4.4 cm^{-1}	3 cm^{-1}
Blood (68% oxy, 32% deoxy)	231 cm^{-1}	61 cm^{-1}	4.7 cm^{-1}	4.3 cm^{-1}	2.1 cm^{-1}
Melanin (12% volume fraction)	67 cm^{-1}	46 cm^{-1}	21 cm^{-1}	17 cm^{-1}	7 cm^{-1}
Ratio (melanin/blood)	0.3	0.5	4.5	4	3.3

found in this table, so let's consider the 755 nm alexandrite laser with an absorption coefficient similar to a ruby laser. As mentioned earlier, the laser having the highest absorption coefficient ratio of melanin to blood is the alexandrite laser (4.5). So, shouldn't the best laser for blood vessels be a 532-nm laser with the lowest melanin absorption coefficient compared to blood (0.3)? In reality, however, 595-nm lasers are considered much safer than 532-nm lasers. Why is this so?

The most problematic side effect of laser procedure in darker skin is PIH. The problem is that we think the cause of this PIH is limited only to the cause of blood vessels. As explained in "Chap. 4," the breaking of cell membranes is a more common cause for PIH than the cause of blood vessels. This is because blood vessels can burst after the cell membrane is broken. Side effects can be reduced by weakening the explosive power.

Therefore, I think that the fact that the melanin absorption coefficient is exponential is more important than the absorption coefficient ratio. The y-axis units are increasing exponentially in units of 1, 10, 100, and 1000, rather than 1, 2, 3, and 4 (Fig. 5.2). In other words, we think that the ruby laser has a slightly higher melanin absorption coefficient than the alexandrite laser, but the absorption coefficient is twice as high. If the temperature is raised from 35 to 200 °C when treating lentigo with alexandrite laser, the temperature difference ΔT generated by the alexandrite laser is 165 °C. Ruby lasers have twice as much absorption coefficient as alexandrite lasers, so 330 °C, which is twice the temperature difference, is added to the original temperature of 35 °C, and the temperature is 365 °C. As the temperature rises sharply, the photomechanical effect becomes much larger. In other words, explosive power becomes larger. Therefore, lasers with lower absorption coefficients are safer. In Fig. 5.2, it becomes safer as you go to the right of the melanin curve. That's why longer wavelengths are considered safe in many laser texts [2, 4, 5].

However, in the equation below [17], even if the absorption coefficient is high, reducing fluence eventually results in the same temperature, so there is no difference in effects or side effects.

$$\Delta T = \frac{F_z \mu_a}{\rho c} \left(\frac{\tau_r}{\tau_r + \tau_p} \right)^{g/2}$$

ΔT: temperature increase of the desired target.
μ_a: absorption coefficient,
F_z: local subsurface fluence.
ρ: density,
c: specific heat,
g: geometric factor (1 for planes, 2 for cylinders, and 3 for spheres),
τ_p: laser pulse duration,
τ_r: thermal relaxation time of the target (TRT).

Table 5.8 shows simulated numbers I wrote for a better understanding. Assume that the temperature we want is 73 °C and the temperature at which PIH occurs is 75 °C. 532 and 1064 nm have a tenfold difference in the absorption coefficient. Therefore, the temperature of the target tissue is the same when 10 J/cm^2 is irradiated with a 1064 nm laser and 1 J/cm^2 is irradiated with a 532-nm laser. However, since 532 nm can raise energy at 0.1 J/cm^2 intervals, the temperature rises by 7 °C, 1 J/cm^2 is not effective, 1.1 J/cm^2 is effective but PIH occurs. On the other hand, 1064-nm laser can also raise energy at 0.1 J/cm^2 intervals, but the absorption coefficient is one-tenth, so the temperature increases

Table 5.8 Temperature change by fluence. The numbers are simulated

532 nm ($\mu_a = 70\ cm^{-1}$)		1064 nm ($\mu_a = 7\ cm^{-1}$)	
1.0 J/cm²	70.0 °C	10.0 J/cm²	70.0 °C
1.1 J/cm²	77.0 °C	10.1 J/cm²	70.7 °C
1.2 J/cm²	84.0 °C	10.2 J/cm²	71.4 °C
		10.3 J/cm²	72.1 °C
		10.4 J/cm²	72.8 °C
		10.5 J/cm²	73.5 °C
		10.6 J/cm²	74.2 °C
		10.7 J/cm²	74.9 °C
		10.8 J/cm²	75.6 °C

by 0.7 °C. Therefore, 1064-nm laser is effective at 10.5, 10.6, and 10.7 J/cm², and no PIH is generated.

Lasers with low absorption coefficients can raise temperatures little by little compared to lasers with high absorption coefficients, even if fluence intervals are the same. Shorter wavelengths may have little or no safe treatment range (therapeutic window) while the therapeutic window of longer wavelengths is wide.

There is one more thing to consider because Koreans have high levels of epidermal melanin. Depending on the wavelength, there is a wavelength that is better absorbed by epidermal pigmentations, and a wavelength that is better absorbed by the dermis. Wavelengths below 800 nm are better absorbed by epidermal pigmentations, and wavelengths above 800 nm are better absorbed by the dermis [3]. Why does this happen? Just like scattering occurring in the dermis, short-wavelengths often meets melanin and is absorbed well in the epidermis, resulting in relatively few photons entering the dermis. Longer wavelengths encounter less melanin in the epidermal layer (epidermal bypass) so that more photons enter the dermis. The boundary of these wavelengths is approximately 800 nm. So, we use 810-nm diode laser as for hair removal and 1064-nm laser to treat the dermal tattoo. 694-nm ruby laser or 755-nm alexandrite laser, even 532-nm lasers are used to treat epidermal pigmentations.

However, wavelengths above 800 nm are not entirely unabsorbed by the epidermis. Therefore, epidermal cooling is essential during laser hair removal with 810- and 1064-nm lasers. For the same reason, 1064-nm Q-switched Nd:YAG lasers are not entirely unabsorbed by the epidermis, but because the laser has low absorption, it is suitable for use in "laser toning."

In summary, the following conclusions are reached.

1. Lasers with lower absorption coefficients are safer. In the case of melanin, lasers with wavelengths to the right of the absorption curve are safer (longer wavelength).
2. Wavelengths of less than 800 nm are mainly used to treat epidermal pigmentations, while wavelengths of more than 800 nm are mainly used to treat dermal pigmentations (epidermal bypass).

From now on, I will define the two conclusions aforementioned as the "epidermal bypass effect" for the ease of explanation.

Where can the epidermal bypass effect be applied? This is highly applicable in the selection of pigment lasers. When selecting epidermal pigment lasers, a laser of 800 nm or less must be purchased, and the corresponding lasers are 532, 694, and 755 nm. The safest laser is 755-nm alexandrite laser, and the laser with the highest side-effect is the 532-nm laser. I, therefore, believe that alexandrite lasers should be chosen over ruby lasers for epidermal pigmentation treatments. The only dermal pigment laser is the 1064-nm Nd:YAG laser. Ruby lasers and alexandrite lasers are also able to treat dermal pigmentations and tattoos, but Nd:YAG laser is more effective because of the epidermal bypass effect.

So why did past papers and Kenichirou Kasai, author of the "Skin Spot Treatment Clinics" and "Q-switched ruby lasers," describe the ruby laser as the best laser for ABNOM treatment? [18] I think that in the past, the output of the laser was too low to increase fluence itself. Even if the absorption coefficient is low, high fluence can produce the same effect because it can be raised to the same temperature, but since the fluence itself cannot be increased, only a ruby laser with high absorption coefficient can achieve the effect by raising the temperature. This is why regardless of side effect, it was considered the best laser. However, because there are currently many lasers with high power outputs, it is right to choose a laser with fewer side effects if the effect is the same. Therefore, recent papers on dermal pigmentations such as ABNOM and Ota nevus has been treated with Q-switched Nd:YAG laser rather than ruby lasers [19–21].

5.2.5 Petechia Due to Q-Switched Lasers

Let's look back at the previously mentioned idea: "the ruby laser is the best among Q-switched pigmentation lasers." The concept is that Q-switched lasers, which have a high absorption coefficient for hemoglobin, are bad because they damage blood vessels, which increases the risk of PIH. A Q-switched laser is absorbed by hemoglobin, causing the RBC to explode, destroying the blood vessel wall. A typical laser is a 532-nm Q-switched laser with a high absorption coefficient for hemoglobin. I also believe that 532-nm Q-switched laser is a dangerous laser because of PIH due to vascular causes.

1064 nm wavelength is also irradiated with a Q-switch Nd:YAG laser, same as 532 nm. The absorption coefficient of melanin to blood is low, and petechia occurs frequently when treating ABNOM or tattoos so that 1064-nm wavelength can also be considered as a dangerous wavelength at which PIH is caused by vascular causes. However, I believe that the 1064-nm wavelength has a low risk of developing PIH due to vascular causes.

The reasons for this are as follows. First, as mentioned earlier, the ratio of the absorption coefficient of melanin to blood is as follows; 532 nm, 0.3; 595 nm, 0.5; 755 nm, 4.5; 800 nm, 4; 1064 nm, 3.3. 1064 nm wavelength has a relatively high ratio of melanin absorption to blood (3.3), although not as high as the alexandrite laser (4.5). Second, the treatment of ABNOM or tattoos with fluence 6 J/cm^2 using a 1064-nm Q-switched Nd:YAG laser can produce petechia. However, I observed that petechia hardly occurred when 6 J/cm^2 was irradiated to normal tissue without pigment in the dermal layer. I irradiated 1064-nm Q-switched Nd:YAG laser on the skin inside my left forearm with a 4 mm spot of up to 6, 7, 8 J/cm^2. Thirty minutes later, at 7 and 8 J/cm^2, mild petechia was observed (weaker than petechia after ABNOM or tattoo treatment), but at 6 J/cm^2, fine petechia was visible only with a magnifying glass (Fig. 5.5).

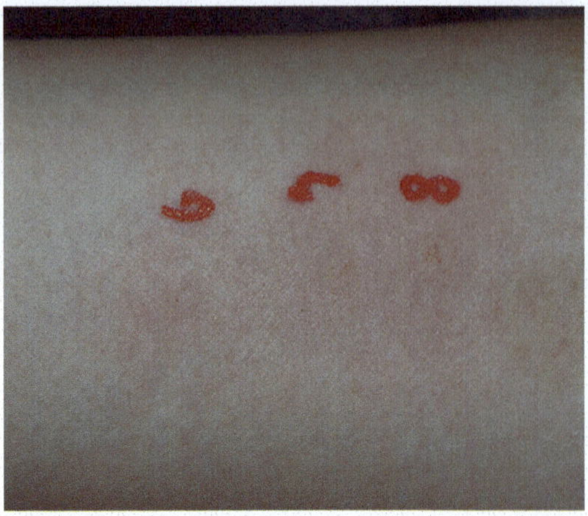

Fig. 5.5 Photograph 30 min after irradiating 6, 7, 8 J/cm^2 with 1064-nm Q-switched Nd:YAG laser on the inner skin of the left forearm. Mild petechia is visible at 7 and 8 J/cm^2, but petechia cannot be observed with 6 J/cm^2

Since the same energy was used when treating ABNOM or tattoos or irradiating normal tissue, the same pattern of petechia should occur if the 1064-nm Q-switched Nd:YAG laser was absorbed directly by the hemoglobin and damaged the vessel wall. But different results came out. Why is this so?

Thus, I believe that petechia, which occurs at 1064 nm when treating ABNOM or tattoos, is caused by the explosion of pigments and not by the explosion of RBCs, resulting in destruction of the blood vessel walls. In other words, I think that petechia occurs when melanocytes, melanin-containing phagocytes (melanophages), or dermal tattoo ink is exploded by Q-switched lasers and damages the blood vessels next to the dermis. On the other hand, in normal skin, petechia does not occur because there are few mediators such as melanocytes or melanophages. The reason for the petechia at 7, 8 J/cm^2 seems to be that the high energy level causes low dose melanosomes in the basal layer to explode, resulting in the destruction of blood vessels resulting in petechia.

So, to reduce PIH caused by vascular causes, I use the repeat pulse method to reduce fluence for 532 nm and use fluences between 4 and 6 J/cm^2 for 1064 nm when treating epidermal pigmentations with Q-switched Nd:YAG laser.

5.2.6 Longer Pulse Duration

In "Chap. 3," we reviewed thermal kinetic selectivity (TKS). In short, if there are two target tissues, the large target tissues should be treated first, and then the small target tissues should be treated next by reducing the pulse duration sequentially from long to short. This is TKS. Also, laser irradiation with a longer pulse duration than TRT of small target tissue does not cause side effects but rather cools quickly and spares the small target tissue. If you consider the meaning of TKS, there may be another meaning.

In one laser text, there were photographs of the skin after irradiating IPL at a pulse duration of 20 ms, 60 ms, and 100 ms with the same 20 J/cm^2 fluence [3]. The results show that the shorter the pulse duration, the more severe the side effects, and the longer the pulse duration the smaller the epidermal side effects. That is, the longer the pulse duration than TRT of the small target tissue (epidermal TRT = 10 ms), the "better" sparing of the small target tissue (epidermis).

For example, a hair removal laser called Super Long Pulse (Palomar, Burlington, Mass.) used this principle to increase the pulse duration from 200 to 400 ms [3]. However, this laser is currently not actively used. I suspect that the pain can be severe and there are technical problems with making a long pulse duration.

The use of longer pulse duration due to TKS is safer in darker skin with high pigmentation content in the epidermis. However, the principle of TKS states that lesions with TRT shorter than pulse duration are ineffective. Therefore, using only a long pulse duration for safety may result in ineffective treatment. Therefore, it is necessary to treat sequentially while reducing the pulse duration step by step from long to short.

5.2.7 Epidermal Cooling

Epidermal cooling is essential in "vertical situations," such as hair removal, vascular treatments, and nonablative rejuvenation. Darker skin in particular should have better cooling than Caucasians because of their high epidermal melanin content. This is because, if epidermal melanin content is high, the epidermal temperature caused by the laser may overwhelm the cooling temperature even after cooling, which may cause side effects. Then what cooling method is most effective?

There is an index called the cooling protection factor (CPF) that shows a cooling effect. CPF is an index proposed by RR Anderson using the concept of sun protection factor (SPF), sunscreen index [3].

$$\mathrm{CPF} = \frac{T_{\mathrm{c}} - T_{\mathrm{ic}}}{T_{\mathrm{c}} - T_{\mathrm{i}}}$$

T_{ic}: basal layer temperature before laser irradiation with cooling.

T_{i}: basal layer temperature without cooling.

T_{c}: critical temperature at which thermal injury occurs.

For example, assuming that normal skin temperature is 30 °C, skin temperature with contact cooling is 20 °C, and skin temperature with laser irradiation is 60 °C, the CPF value is (60–20)/(60–30) = 1.33. If cryogen spray cooling is used instead of contact cooling, the skin temperature is 0 °C. In this case, the CPF value is (60–0)/(60–30) = 2.0. That is, like the SPF index, the higher the CPF index, the better the cooling.

As described above, the CPF of contact cooling is 1.33, the CPF of cryogen spray cooling 2.0, and convective air cooling is known to have a CPF similar to contact cooling. Therefore, cryogen spray cooling is the most effective skin cooling. It is known that there are more side effects in contact cooling compared to cryogen spray cooling when treating port-wine stains of darker skin. Typical parameters for cryogen spray cooling in skin types III and IV are 40-ms spray time with 20-ms delay. To treat darker skin, the spray time can be increased to 50 ms [4].

But effective epidermal cooling is not always optimal. Each skin cooling method has advantages and disadvantages, so it is necessary to select an appropriate skin cooling method according to the situation. Nevertheless, it should be noted that for darker skins with high melanin content, cryogen spray cooling is the safest method of cooling. Therefore, if a laser is selected from the same type of laser, it is better to select a laser that is equipped with a cryogen spray cooling method.

5.2.8 Test Shot and Preoperative Procedure

Several papers and laser texts recommend that test shots to predict side effects in advance. However, the test results are not completely consistent with the final results, and even if there are no side effects during test shots, the risk of developing side effects cannot be completely excluded from the final results [4]. In addition, it is difficult to apply test shots in private practice. It is difficult to tell a patient to do a test shot today, and check the results at least 1 month later, and then perform the procedure. Therefore, in reality, there are not many cases of actually conducting test shots.

Other papers and books recommend preoperative procedures. The most common method of pretreatment is to treat epidermal pigmentations first by applying a whitening agent such as tretinoin or hydroquinone and perform the laser treatment later. I think the concept is theoretically correct. However, there is controversy over pretreatment procedures [2]. West and Alster et al. pretreated with tretinoin but this did not prevent PIH after laser treatment. They suggested that the reason for this is because while the superficial epidermis is suppressed with tretinoin, pigmentations remain in the deeper epidermis (basal layer, etc.). There is no evidence that the PIH is reduced by using tretinoin as a pretreatment procedure, especially in darker skin [22].

Hydroquinone can be used as a pretreatment. I do not recommend hydroquinone for pretreatment or posttreatment. Hydroquinone is the most powerful whitening agent against tyrosinase, which plays an important role in melanin synthesis. Foreign papers have cited hydroquinone as the primary treatment for melasma. However, hydroquinone may cause exogenous ochronosis, and animal studies with rodents suggest that hydroquinone may be a carcinogen. Therefore, in 2006, the US FDA excluded hydroquinone from over-the-counter (OTC) products [23]. I do not use it for the following reasons. Hydroquinone products have been reported to contain not only hydroquinone but also additives such as sodium metabisulfite, which can cause skin irritation and erythema, causing PIH [24]. I have also experienced PIH development and aggravation of melasma in patients using hydroquinone.

Is there a way to replace test shots and preoperative procedures? I recommend that laser procedure should be performed in multiple sessions rather than in a single procedure. You have to do what is called "ticketing." The advantage of "ticketing" is, first, a stepwise treatment is possible as pretreatment. For example, first, the epidermal pigmentations are treated, and later, the blood vessels in the dermis may be treated. Also, low fluences may be shot first and skin reactions are observed later to decide whether to raise or stop it. Second, posttreatment can be included in the course of treatment. If PIH occurs during the course of treatment, there is time to treat PIH itself.

5.2.9 Homecare

Patients visit the clinic at most once a week, and skincare is about 1–2 h. In addition, laser treatment takes only 10–20 min at most. The rest of the time is entirely dependent on the patient. In other words, no matter how good the laser treatment, the patient's exposure to sunshine for an hour can result in new pigmentation and aggravation of melasma.

I emphasize three things for homecare.

First, you must wear sunscreen. The most important thing in using sunscreen is the amount you apply. Because sunscreen is easily erased after friction, sweating, and especially swimming, the dermatology text, "Sixth Edition Text book of Dermatology (Korean)," recommends applying sunscreen every 2–3 h [25]. In reality, however, it is not easy to apply every 2–3 h, so I recommend applying it in the morning and applying it before going out, i.e., applying at least twice a day. I also recommend wearing a hat or a sunshade.

Second, moisturizers should be applied. The basic function of the skin is the "skin barrier" that protects the skin. In particular, it plays a role in confining moisture in our bodies. But due to aging, lipid contents drop resulting in a reduction of moisturizing power and ultimately breaking down the skin barrier. Therefore, intercellular lipids should be supplemented with the moisturizer.

Finally, the skin should not be irritated. Kenichirou Kasai, the author of the book, "Skin Spot Treatment Clinics," describes the causes of melasma as the breakdown of barriers caused by chronic hyper irritation [18]. Just irritating the skin can cause melasma and darken the skin. Therefore, when washing face, rubbing with a lot of friction should be avoided. A lot of soap bubbles should be made to gently "pump" them to the face so that the hands do not touch the face. Trying to remove all makeup should be discouraged and one should believe "It doesn't matter if there's makeup left." Cosmetics irritating the skin should be avoided and when applying makeup, irritation should be minimized by tapping on the skin rather than rubbing. Finally, skin irritation should be reduced by reducing the number and type of cosmetics applied to the face. Rather, it may be better not to put on makeup.

5.3 Conclusion

These are my recommendations for laser treatment for Koreans.

1. Assume that all patients can develop PIH, before initiating laser therapy.
2. Select the laser corresponding to the epidermal bypass effect (longer wavelength).
3. Start from longer pulse duration and low fluence.
4. Epidermal cooling is important for Koreans compared to Caucasians.
5. Ticketing is recommended (Stepwise treatment, postoperative procedure).
6. Homecare - sunscreen, moisturizers, and irritation avoidance.

Compared to Caucasians, Koreans can easily have side effects like PIH with laser treatment. Therefore, rather than selecting and treating patients, it is necessary to assume that PIH can occur in all patients. and to carefully select and perform laser treatment [26]. It is better to choose longer wavelengths in parameter selection and use a small spot size in darker skin because it may look cosmetically undesirable by hypopigmentation. The treatment plan should not be a one-time procedure but should be a package procedure for multiple treatments, followed by sequential and stepwise treatment. During stepwise treatment, the parameters should be controlled by observing the treatment response. Pulse duration should start from long to short and fluence should start from low to high.

In conclusion, laser treatment in Koreans should take a conservative approach [26].

5.4 Types of Lasers

Earlier, in "Chap. 1," we reviewed that there are wavelengths that absorb better depending on chromophore. Since the wavelength is determined when purchasing the laser, the type of laser is determined by the absorption curve of chromophore.

I think that there are five different types of lasers (Fig. 5.6). First, vascular laser with a high absorption coefficient of hemoglobin at 500–600 nm wavelength. Second, pigment laser with low hemoglobin absorption coefficient and high melanin absorption coefficient, third, hair removal laser that has a low hemoglobin absorption coefficient, a high melanin absorption coefficient, and long pulse duration, fourth, nonablative rejuvenation laser that penetrates deeply into the skin due to low absorption coefficient for water and generates heat, and fifth, ablative skin rejuvenation laser that ablates the surface of the skin due to a high absorption coefficient for water.

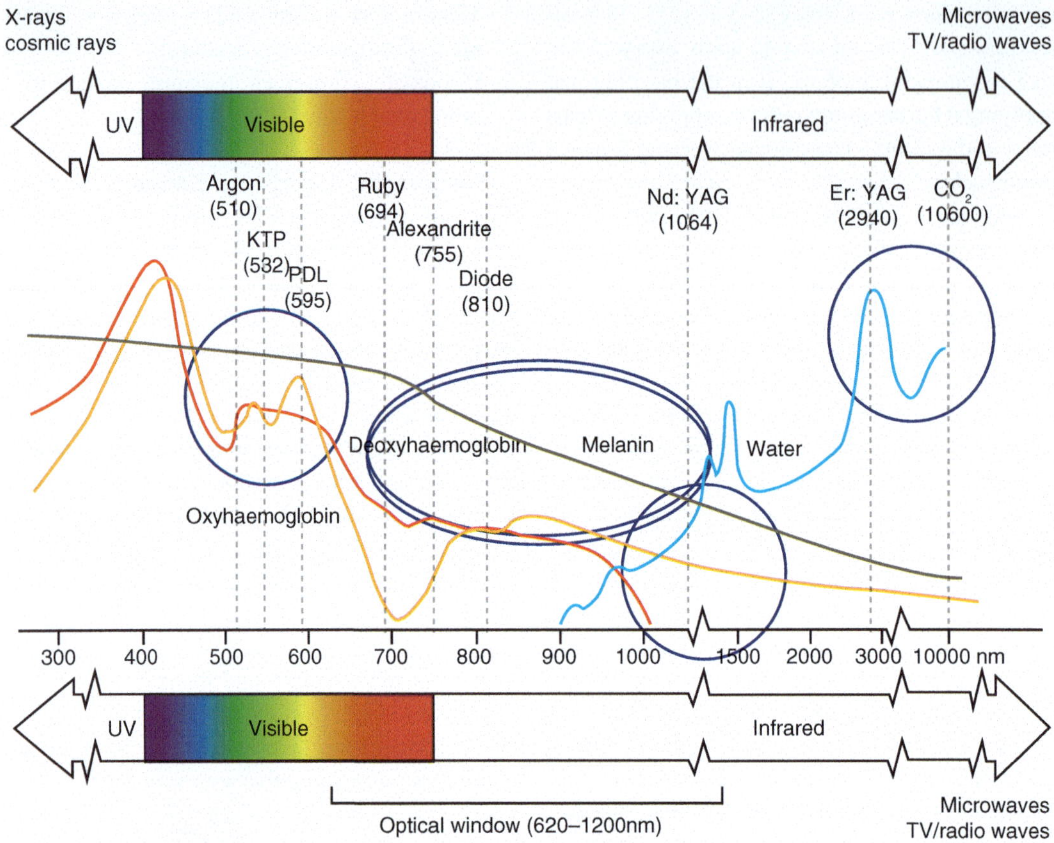

Fig. 5.6 absorption curve and type of laser. Vascular laser, pigment laser, hair removal laser, non-ablative laser, ablative laser in order from the left circle. Modified from [27]

Of course, there are vascular lasers with low hemoglobin absorption coefficients, such as the 1064-nm long-pulsed Nd:YAG laser, and 532-nm Nd:YAG lasers may be used for pigment treatment, and some lasers do not correspond to midinfrared (MIR) wavelengths, such as low-level light therapy (LLLT) in nonablative rejuvenation. Also, excimer laser used in vitiligo or acne laser using 400-nm wavelength corresponding to the Soret band is omitted. I simply divided into five lasers that are easy to explain.

In the following chapters, we will explain in detail the types of lasers that are applicable to each of these five lasers, and which lasers will be specifically selected for Koreans, how to set parameters, and which treatments are appropriate for each skin disease.

References

1. Tung R, Rubin MG (2010) Procedures in cosmetic dermatology series: chemical peels E-book. Elsevier Health Sciences
2. Kauvar A, Hruza G (2005) Principles and practices in cutaneous laser surgery. CRC Press
3. Goldman MP (2006) Cutaneous and cosmetic laser surgery. Mosby Elsevier, Philadelphia, PA
4. Allemann IB, Goldberg DJ (2011) Basics in dermatological laser applications. Karger Medical and Scientific Publishers
5. Hruza GJ, Tanzi EL (2018) Lasers and lights. Elsevier, Edinburgh
6. Youn JI, Choe YB, Park SB, Suh DH, Park YK, Ahn SK et al (2000) The Fitzpatrick skin type in Korean people. Korean J Dermatol 38(7):920
7. Shah S, Alster TS (2010) Laser treatment of dark skin: an updated review. Am J Clin Dermatol 11(6):389–397
8. Goldman MP, Weiss RA, Weiss MA (2005) Intense pulsed light as a nonablative approach to photoaging. Dermatol Surg 31:1179–1187

9. Ibrahimi OA, Avram MM, Hanke CW, Kilmer SL, Anderson RR (2011) Laser hair removal. Dermatol Ther 24(1):94–107
10. Baumann LS, Baumann L (2009) Cosmetic dermatology. McGraw-Hill Professional Publishing
11. Richter AL, Barrera J, Markus RF, Brissett A (2014) Laser skin treatment in non-Caucasian patients. Facial Plast Surg Clin North Am 22(3):439–446
12. Korean Aesthetic Surgery and Laser Society (2018) Introduction to laser (Korean). MDworld, Seoul
13. Korea Food & Drug Administration (2007) How do you use sunscreen cosmetics? (Korean). Korea Food & Drug Administration, Seoul
14. Shiffman MA, Mirrafati S, Lam SM, Cueteaux CG (2007) Simplified facial rejuvenation. Springer Science & Business Media
15. Ross E, Meehan K, Gilbert S, Domankevitz Y (2009) Optimal pulse durations for the treatment of leg telangiectasias with an Alexandrite laser. Lasers Surg Med 41(2):104–109
16. Grunewald S, Bodendorf MO, Paasch U (2011) Dermatologische Lasertherapie Band 2: Gefäßlaser: Indikationen-Einstellungen-Resultate: Kolster
17. Nouri K (2018) Lasers in dermatology and medicine: dermatologic applications. Springer International Publishing
18. Kasai K (2007) Skin spots treatment clinics (Korean edition). Shinheung Med Science, Seoul
19. Shah VV, Bray FN, Aldahan AS, Mlacker S, Nouri K (2016) Lasers and nevus of Ota: a comprehensive review. Lasers Med Sci 31(1):179–185
20. Cho SB, Park SJ, Kim MJ, Bu TS (2009) Treatment of acquired bilateral nevus of Ota-like macules (Hori's nevus) using 1064-nm Q-switched Nd:YAG laser with low fluence. Int J Dermatol 48(12):1308–1312
21. Committee C, Chun S, Kim IH, Kang JS, Park SH, Chung KY et al (2016) Laser and light treatment in Asian skin. Koonja, Paju
22. Wong JK (2011) Laser treatment of pigmented lesions for Asians. Facial Plast Surg Clin 19(2):417–422
23. Ball Arefiev KL, Hantash BM (2012) Advances in the treatment of melasma: a review of the recent literature. Dermatol Surg 38(7 Pt 1):971–984
24. Woolery-Lloyd H, Viera MH, Valins W (2011) Laser therapy in black skin. Facial Plast Surg Clin North Am 19(2):405
25. Textbook Compilation Committee in Korean Dermatological Association (2014) Text book of dermatology, 6th edn. (Korean). Daehanuihak, Seoul
26. Goldman MP (2013) Lasers and energy devices for the skin. [S.I.]. Taylor & Francis
27. Stewart N, Lim AC, Lowe PM, Goodman G (2013) Lasers and laser-like devices: part one. Australas J Dermatol 54(3):173–183

Part III

Lasers and Energy Devices in Cutaneous Disorders

6 Vascular Lasers and Treatment of Erythema

6.1 Choice of Wavelength

6.1.1 Absorption Curve of Hemoglobin

Hemoglobin (Hb) includes oxygen-bound oxyhemoglobin (HbO_2), oxygen-free deoxyhemoglobin (deoxyHb), and methemoglobin (metHb), which underwent protein denaturation by heat. The absorption curve of HbO_2 reaches a peak at 418 nm, reaches a small peak at 542 and 577 nm, then decreases, and finally forms a smaller peak at 940 nm. DeoxyHb reaches peaks at 430 and 555 nm and reaches a peak once again between 800 and 1200 nm (Fig. 6.1) [1, 2].

HbO_2 accounts for 99% of Hb in arterial blood and 60–70% in venous blood. DeoxyHb accounts for the rest of Hb. In other words, because deoxyHb does not occupy all of venous Hb, when actually using a vascular laser, the absorption coefficient of HbO_2 is mainly used in venous blood rather than the absorption coefficient of deoxyHb [4].

When choosing a wavelength (laser), the laser with highest absorption coefficient in the absorption curve of a particular chromophore may be mistaken as the best laser. However, considering the principles of laser, if there is only an absorption coefficient for a specific chromophore, even a laser having a low absorption coefficient can increase the temperature of the chromophore by significantly increasing the fluence. Therefore, any laser having an absorption coefficient for Hb can be used as a vascular laser.

Of course, selecting a laser having a wavelength higher in absorption coefficient of the target tissue than the surrounding tissue may selectively damage the target tissue. When interpreting the absorption curve of HbO_2, it can be misunderstood that only 500–600 nm wavelength (green–yellow light) lasers with higher absorption of Hb than melanin can be used as vascular lasers and near-infrared (NIR) lasers cannot be used as vascular lasers or have side effects.

In a selective photothermolysis paper, Richard R. Anderson stated that the absorption coefficients of the target and the surrounding tissues should be more than ten times different and at least two times different in order to be applied to the theory of selective photothermolysis [5].

Histologically, the surrounding tissue next to the blood vessels is not melanin but dermal layer without blood vessels. When the ratio of absorption coefficient between blood vessel and dermal layer is more than ten times or more than two times different, the 500–600 nm wavelength laser and NIR laser can both be used as vascular laser and even ruby laser with lowest absorption coefficient of Hb can theoretically treat blood vessels (Fig. 6.2). Of course, the photons of the laser move past the epidermis and into dermis, so the epidermal layer is also a competitive tissue. In

J. D. Lee et al., *Principles and Choice of Laser Treatment in Dermatology*, https://doi.org/10.1007/978-981-15-6556-4_6

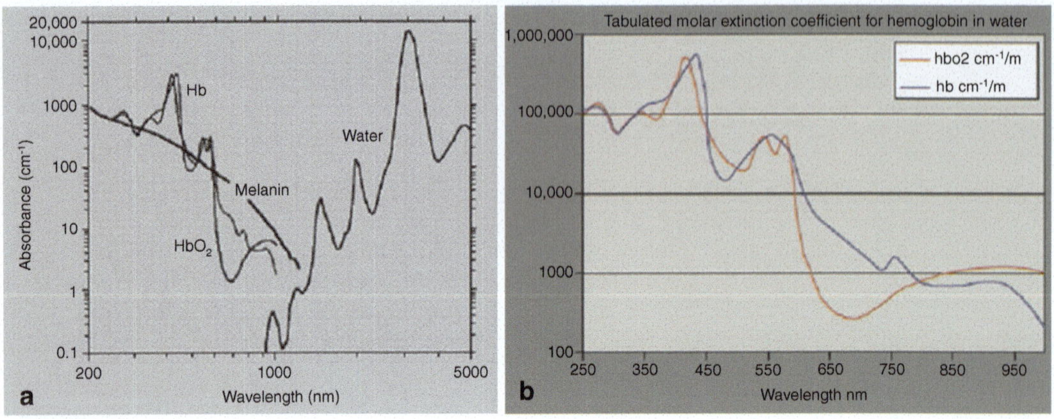

Fig. 6.1 Absorption curve for (**a**) hemoglobin, melanin, and water and (**b**) oxygenated (red) and deoxygenated (blue) hemoglobin. (Reproduced from [3])

Fig. 6.2 It shows the optical properties of blood, dermis, and light-skinned epidermis at 500–1100 nm. (Reproduced from [6])

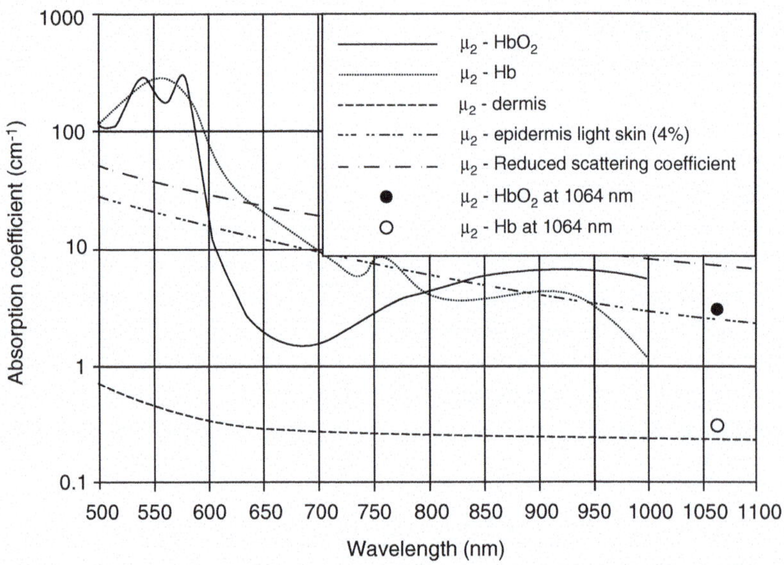

strict sense, however, the entire epidermal layer, including melanin, is competitive tissue. The absorption curve of the entire epidermal layer is represented by dotted line (- ·· - ·· -) in Fig. 6.2. Therefore, 500–600 nm wavelength lasers and lasers with a wavelength of 850 nm or more can be used for vascular treatment.

6.1.2 Absorption Curve of Methemoglobin

Laser irradiation of blood produces metHb [7]. The absorption curve of metHb is lower than HbO_2 and deoxyHb at 500–600 nm wavelengths and higher in near infrared (Fig. 6.3). This phenomenon of absorption curve shifting to the right is called bathochromic shift or red shift [8].

There are three methods of vascular therapy using the bathochromic shift. First, metHb is produced using a 595-nm laser and then 1064-nm laser in the near-infrared region with high absorption coefficient is irradiated. Lasers using this principle are multiplex lasers with wavelength of 595 and 1064 nm (Cynergy™, Cynosure, Chelmsford, MA, USA) [7]. Second, a recently released IPL uses metHb by reducing the spectral shift and creating two wavelength bands of 500–670 and 870–1200 nm (Icon™, Cynosure, Westford, MA). Third, 1064 nm long-pulsed Nd:YAG lasers treat blood vessels by using metHb rather than HbO_2. As long-pulsed Nd:YAG lasers are irradiated, metHb is produced and the absorption coefficient increases. Vascular treatment is possible with long-pulsed Nd:YAG lasers with low absorption coefficients for HbO_2 because of metHb. Originally, the absorption coefficient of HbO_2 is lower than that of melanin at 1064 nm, but when metHb is formed, the absorption coefficient is increased three times, resulting in higher absorption coefficient than melanin.

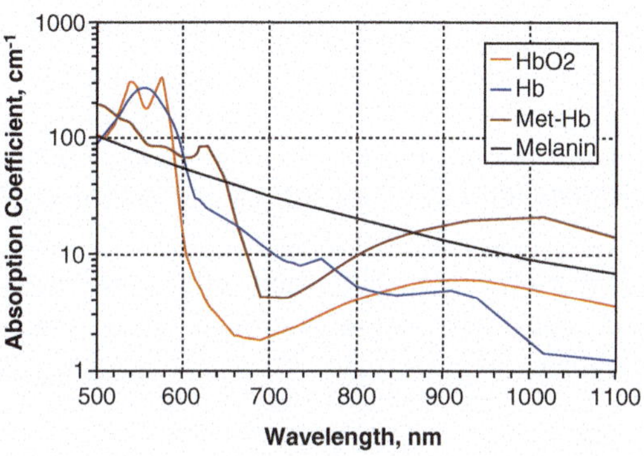

Fig. 6.3 Absorption coefficients for chromophores in the blood and epidermis. (Reproduced from [7])

An important point in the treatment with metHb is that the absorption coefficient by metHb is increased only when the pulse duration is at least 4 ms or longer (Fig. 6.4) [9].

In the case of multiplex lasers, metHb should be made by irradiation with 595 nm. If the pulse duration is less than 4 ms with 585 nm PDL, even if metHb is generated, the ratio does not increase enough to change the absorption coefficient, and the subsequent irradiation with 1064 nm, i.e., using a "multiplex laser" is pointless. Therefore, multiplex lasers have no great effect on erythema, corresponding to TRT 4 ms or less. In this case, only 0.45 ms of 585 nm PDL alone can be used as treatment methods.

6.1.3 Multiplex Lasers

For reference, let's look at multiplex lasers. The temperature of 0.5 ms PDL increases highest in 100 μm sized vessels corresponding to TRT

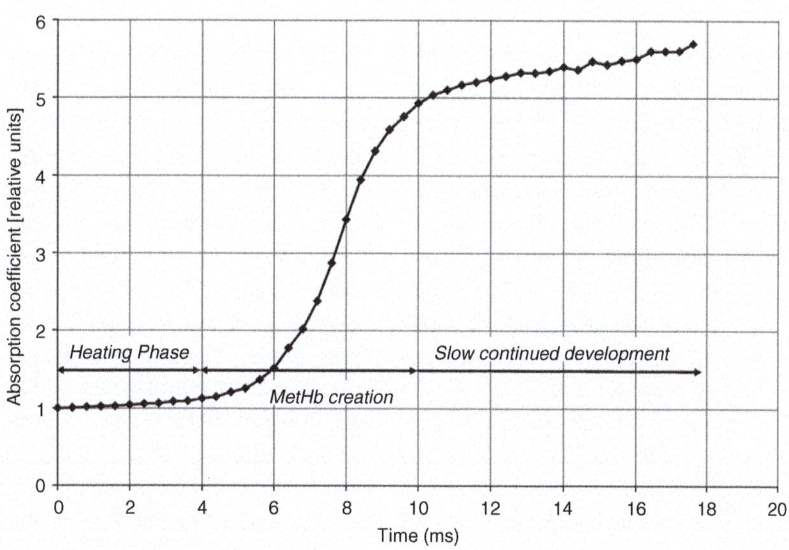

Fig. 6.4 Relative increase in the absorption coefficient of whole blood estimated from integrating sphere measurements at 633 nm, during and immediately after a 10 ms, 1064 nm, 100 J/cm^2 laser pulse. The slight increase during the first 4 ms can be attributed to the bathochromic shift of the absorption resonances of HbO_2. The more dramatic increase during the next 6 ms is due to the formation of metHb, which has an absorptivity about 30× greater than HbO_2. Some slow continued development of the absorption coefficient is seen as the blood cools post pulse. (Reproduced from [9])

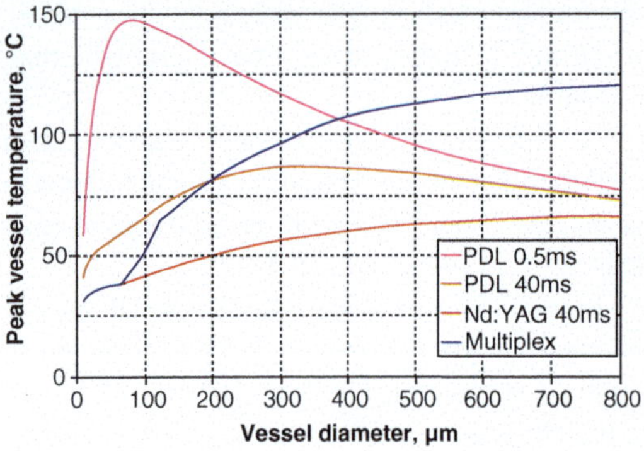

Fig. 6.5 Peak vessel temperature rise calculation based on analytical model published in Mirkov et al. [10]. Pulse dye laser (PDL) fluence is 12 J/cm^2 in 0.5 or 40 ms; neodymium:yttrium aluminum garnet (Nd:YAG) fluence is 50 J/cm^2 in 40 ms. In the multiplex PDL/Nd:YAG combination, the 40-ms PDL is delivered first. Reproduced from [7]

4.5 ms, and the multiplex temperature increases highest in vessels sized 300 μm or more corresponding to TRT 40 ms or more (Fig. 6.5). As mentioned earlier, the result is consistent with the fact that 595 nm PDL is effective for erythema and that "multiplex" laser is effective for visible blood vessels.

But is the laser with highest temperature elevation the best laser? Multiplex laser has the highest temperature rise and Nd:YAG laser has the lowest temperature rise in vessels over 300 μm with a TRT of 40 ms or more. Nd:YAG has the lowest rise in temperature, but it will have therapeutic effect if blood vessel is above coagulation temperature. Also, since blood vessels do not burst because the temperature is less than 100 °C, there will be less side effects. If the temperature does not reach coagulation temperature, then the power should be increased.

In the past, long-pulsed Nd:YAG lasers had insufficient power, so only the multiplex lasers using metHb were effective for vascular therapy. Now, however, the power of long-pulsed Nd:YAG laser is high, so long-pulsed Nd:YAG laser alone is sufficient for vascular therapy. Therefore, I think it is not necessary to buy expensive multiplex lasers. Also, since long-pulsed Nd:YAG lasers usually have pulse durations of 5 ms or more, inevitably, metHb is already produced.

6.1.4 Optical Penetration Depth by Wavelength

Blood vessels exist in a variety of locations, from very shallow vessels such as senile hemangioma to vessels located in deep dermal and subcutaneous fat layers and leg veins located several millimeters deep from the epidermal layer. To treat these various blood vessels, the laser must penetrate into various depths.

The optical penetration depth (OPD) of laser is the location where the fluence is reduced by 37%, which is 1/*e*. In dermal blood vessels located deeper than the OPD, the treatment efficiency is significantly decreased because the fluence reaches below 37%. Therefore, 532 nm and 595 nm lasers and IPL cannot treat dermal blood vessels located deeper than 1.2–2.0 mm. Conversely, 755, 800, and 1064 nm lasers can treat both shallow and deep blood vessels (Fig. 6.6) [7].

6.1.5 Thickness of Blood Vessels by Wavelength

Because deep blood vessels are thicker, blood vessels near the epidermal layer are thinner and longer wavelength has deeper OPD, 500–600-nm wavelength laser is used to treat thin blood vessels and the NIR laser is used to treat thick blood vessels. However, this is not the only reason that vascular therapy varies with wavelength.

The OPD of the laser is only a theoretical penetration depth. The actual penetration depth depends on the patient's skin condition (Fig. 6.7). For example, 532-nm laser is known to have OPD of about 1 mm. However, if a Caucasian is irradiated with 532 nm laser or if 532 nm laser is irradiated after removing epidermal pigmentations, the laser can penetrate up to 4 mm or more. Then can 532 nm treat thick veins? It is known that 532 nm long-pulsed lasers cannot cure thick veins. Why is this so?

Ross et al. measured the temperature of dermis using a mathematical model and a variety of lasers [13]. The best ideal vascular treatment is that the entire vessel wall coagulates and con-

Fig. 6.6 Depth of penetration of different lasers. (Reproduced from [11])

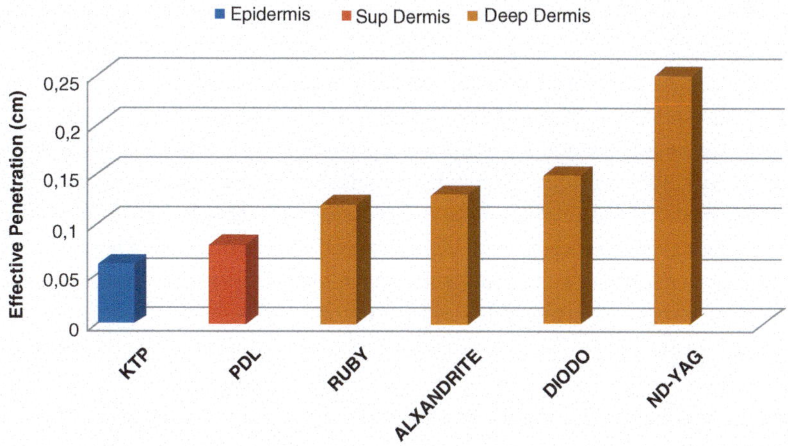

Fig. 6.7 Penetration depths by laser type. Penetration depth is different in the pigmented and nonpigmented tissues. (Modified from [12])

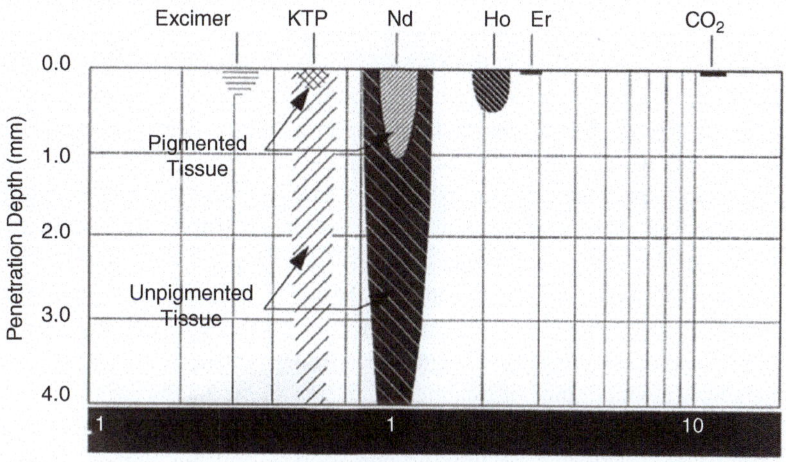

tracts, causing the vessels to disappear. If any part of the blood vessel does not coagulate, it will later recanalize and the blood vessel will not disappear. Therefore, the condition for contraction of blood vessels is first, since the number of photons decreases as the photon descends downward from the top of the skin, when viewed in cross section, the deepest wall of the blood vessel must be coagulated. Thus, our main concern is the deepest blood vessel wall. Second, since the blood vessels burst above 100 °C, the temperature of shallowest blood vessel wall close to epidermal layer should not exceed 100 °C.

Ross et al. measured the temperature change when irradiating a laser to a medium-sized vein of 500 μm thickness at a depth of 500 μm with various lasers and various pulse durations ((1) 532 nm, 20 ms, 10.5 J/cm^2, (2) 595 nm, 20 ms, 13.5 J/cm^2, (3) 595 nm, 0.45 ms, 8.9 J/cm^2, (4) 1064 nm, 20 ms, 89 J/cm^2). This paper considered that the coagulation temperature to be 70 °C. None of the lasers exceeded 100 °C, but only (4) Nd:YAG laser exceeded 70 °C, the temperature at which the deepest blood vessel wall coagulates. The other lasers cannot coagulate the blood vessel wall. In other words, the other lasers are ineffective in treating medium-sized vein. However, for blood vessels that are 120-μm thick, two lasers will be effective: (2) 595 nm with a pulse duration of 20 ms and (4) Nd:YAG laser. For blood vessels that are 60-μm thick, all four lasers will be effective.

Why does this phenomenon occur? The reason is the same as the reason why the CO_2 laser does not penetrate deep into the skin due to its high absorption coefficient for water. 500 to 600 nm wavelength lasers have high absorption for blood vessels and therefore cannot penetrate deeply into the vessels. When photons enter dermis, there are two factors that determine OPD: absorption coefficient and scattering coefficient. Of these, the scattering coefficient has an important effect on light penetration depth, but once the photon enters the blood vessel, the absorption coefficient has a more important effect than the scattering coefficient. (see Sect. 3.3.2 in "Chap. 3.).

In other words, when selecting the wavelength for vascular treatment, the thickness of blood vessels should be taken into account as well as the location of the blood vessels. In other words, 500–600-nm wavelength lasers cannot treat thick blood vessels because they not only have a shallow OPD, but also the absorption coefficient of Hb is high. However, NIR lasers can treat both thin and thick blood vessels because of the low absorption coefficient of Hb and the long OPD. Thus, considering wavelength alone, NIR lasers have a wider range of treatment than 500–600-nm wavelength lasers.

However, treatments of hypertrophic port-wine stains or large hemangioma are rarely performed in private practice. Usually thin blood vessels on the face are treated. Thus, 500–600 nm wavelength lasers can be used effectively.

6.2 Types of Vascular Lasers

6.2.1 500–600 nm Wavelength Vascular Laser (Green–Yellow Light and Laser) and Melanin

The types of vascular lasers can be broadly classified into 500–600-nm wavelength lasers and near-infrared (NIR) lasers. 500–600 nm wavelength lasers include 532-nm KTP, 585-nm PDL, 595-nm PDL, and NIR lasers include the 1064-nm long-pulsed Nd:YAG laser.

500–600 nm wavelength lasers have a high absorption coefficient for melanin, which is likely to cause side effects on epidermis. For example, the fluence required to treat 0.25 mm capillaries with a 532-nm KTP laser is 10 J/cm^2, but only 6–8 J/cm^2 fluence is required to treat lentigo with the same laser [13]. In other words, vascular therapy with KTP lasers can also cure lentigo, but it can cause side effects because the energy is too high for lentigo treatment. In addition, because many photons have already been absorbed by the lentigo, photons that reach the blood vessels are reduced and only low energy is absorbed resulting in ineffective treatment.

When treating dermal blood vessels in darker skin or recently sunburned skin, even if epidermal cooling is performed, heat generated from epidermis can overwhelm the cooling temperature, causing blisters or dermal burns. In the situation where the relationship between the target tissue and the competition tissue is vertical, the most appropriate method is epidermal cooling (see Sect. 3.8 in "Chap. 3"), but the following three methods may be attempted [7]. First, a test shot can be evaluated 24–48 h later to find an appropriate energy for treatment. Second, suntanned skin can be treated after waiting for 4 weeks for the melanin pigment to decrease. Third, an NIR laser with a low melanin absorption coefficient may be used. Of course, NIR lasers are not completely unabsorbed by melanin, so epidermal cooling must be sufficiently performed.

The first and second of the above three methods are not appropriate in private practice, as treatment must be delayed for 1–2 days or even a month. Therefore, for Koreans with a large amount of melanin in the epidermis (Fitzpatrick skin type ≥ IV), the third method, NIR laser, is the appropriate choice.

Also when treating with a NIR vascular laser, it would be better to apply the second method and treat with sequential procedure. In other words, epidermal pigmentations should be treated first and then dermal blood vessels should be treated [13]. Even in this case, it would be safer to use an NIR laser because epidermal pigmentation is higher than that of Caucasians.

6.2.2 Near-Infrared Vascular Laser

In addition to the long-pulsed Nd:YAG laser, near-infrared (NIR) lasers for vascular treatment include 755-nm long-pulsed alexandrite lasers, 810-nm diode lasers and 940 nm lasers. But these lasers are rarely used. Why is this so?

First, let's look at 755-nm long-pulsed alexandrite laser. The melanin–Hb absorption coefficient ratio is 0.7 for 595 nm, 5.5 for 755 nm, and 3.2 for 1064 nm [14], i.e., the melanin–Hb absorption coefficient ratio of alexandrite laser is higher than that of the Nd:YAG laser. Thus, alexandrite lasers can be used safely and effectively only in Caucasians. Nevertheless, the epidermis must be cooled. Also, the high melanin–Hb absorption coefficient ratio makes the laser difficult to be applied to small blood vessels with TRTs similar to the epidermal layer. Thus, by applying thermal kinetic selectivity, the laser can be applied to large, blueish vessels that cool down slowly. Also since large vessels have higher deoxyHb than HbO_2, 755-nm alexandrite lasers with a high absorption coefficient for dexoxy-HbO_2 are effective. Thus, alexandrite lasers are not suitable for treating diffuse facial redness on the face. Long-pulsed alexandrite laser is mainly used for laser hair removal and pigmentation treatment.

Second, 810-nm diode lasers have very low power and cannot produce short pulse durations. Therefore, only thick blood vessels of 2–4 mm can be treated [13]. Since blood vessels on the face are usually less than 1 mm, 800-nm lasers are also rarely used for vascular treatment.

Finally, the long-pulsed Nd:YAG laser is a typical NIR laser. The melanin–Hb absorption coefficient ratio is higher than that of 595-nm laser, but when metHb is generated and the absorption coefficient is increased, it is possible to lower the melanin–Hb absorption coefficient ratio. The laser also penetrates deeply and can treat thick blood vessels. Then what are the disadvantages of long-pulsed Nd:YAG lasers? First, since the absorption coefficient of Hb is lower than that of the 500–600 nm wavelength lasers, it must have a high power to be effective, but there is a limit to the power. Therefore, it is difficult to make a short pulse duration. In addition, since the laser uses metHb, it takes time for metHb to be produced. Since metHb starts being produced at more than 4 ms and is most often produced at 10 ms, it is difficult to treat thin blood vessels with TRTs of 4–5 ms or less. TRTs of 5 ms are a 0.1-mm thick blood vessel, which corresponds to the minimum blood vessel thickness that can be observed with the eye (Fig. 6.8). In other words, blood vessels less than 0.1 mm correspond to invisible erythema. Therefore, long-pulsed Nd:YAG lasers cannot cure erythema. Second, although the long-pulsed Nd:YAG laser has a higher absorption coefficient of metHb than other chromophores, it is also absorbed by melanin and

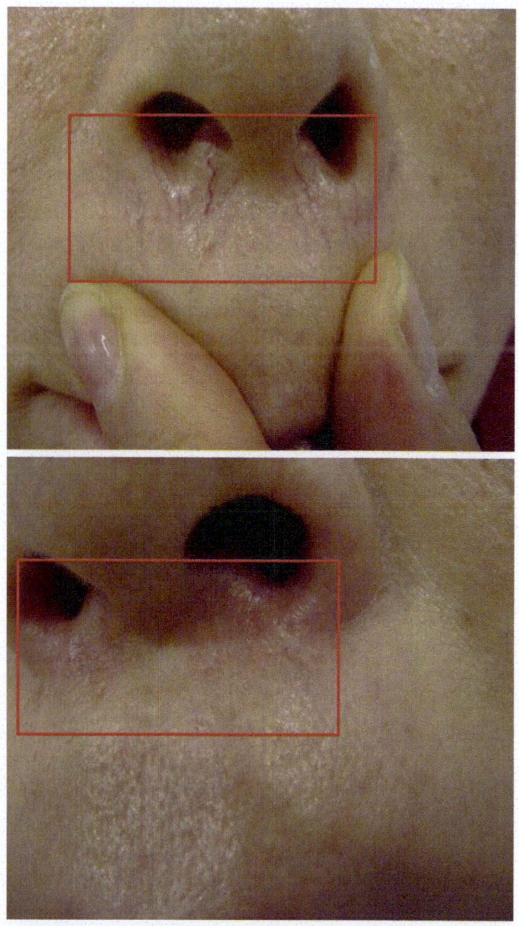

Fig. 6.8 Photos before and after visible blood vessel treatment with 1064 nm long-pulsed Nd:YAG laser. The parameters are spot size 2 mm, pulse duration 8 ms, and fluence 125 J/cm^2

water, so there is a risk of blister and burn. In addition, long-pulsed Nd:YAG laser has a deep OPD. Therefore, when a burn occurs, the deep dermis is damaged resulting in a severe burn. Therefore, epidermal cooling is also important in long-pulsed Nd:YAG lasers and fluence should be adjusted carefully.

Based on these findings, in a paper by Ross et al. the following was proposed for treating facial blood vessels [14]. First, when the skin color is bright or epidermal cooling is sufficient, the wavelength of 532–595 nm is recommended for treating blood vessels of 0.1–0.5 mm. Second, in patients with Fitzpatrick skin types I and II, and when the epidermal cooling is sufficient, 755-nm wavelength is recommended for blood vessels of 0.4–1.6 mm because it is less painful. Third, 940 nm, 980 nm, and 1064 nm lasers are recommended for the treatment of patients with darker skin or blood vessels of 0.7–1.6 mm, if small spot sizes and the lowest possible fluence for blood vessel contraction are used. The wavelength of 755 nm is not suitable for Koreans because there are more Fitzpatrick skin types III, IV, and V than Fitzpatrick skin types I and II. Therefore, when treating Koreans, first, 532–595-nm vascular laser can be selected on the premise of sufficient epidermal cooling. The disadvantage is that only blood vessels of 0.1–0.5-mm thickness can be treated and blood vessels thicker are difficult to treat. Second, 940, 980, and 1064-nm wavelengths are recommended because they are safe in darker skin. However, because there are few lasers currently on the market that have wavelengths of 940 or 980 nm, 1064 nm wavelength seems appropriate.

6.2.3 Types of Vascular Laser by Pulse Duration

This time, let's look at pulse duration without considering the wavelength. TRT of 30–100 μm blood vessels is 0.4–4.5 ms and they can be treated with 585 nm PDL with a 450 μs pulse duration (Table 6.1). On the other hand, the pulse duration of 585 nm PDL is too short to treat a thicker vessel with a TRT of 4.5 ms or more. In addition, blood vessels thicker than 0.1 mm have a TRT of 4.5 ms or more and can be treated with 595 nm long-pulsed PDL with a pulse duration of 1.5 ms or more, but thin blood vessels with TRTs of 1.5 ms or less cannot be treated.

Considering only the pulse duration, it is not possible to treat blood vessels of every size with only one vascular laser. Currently, 595-nm long-pulsed PDL is developed to produce a range of pulse durations from 0.45 to 40 ms, which can cure many blood vessels. However, as mentioned earlier, no matter how long the pulse duration, there is a wavelength limitation, so large blood vessels cannot be treated. Therefore, at least two or more vascular lasers are needed to treat blood vessels of every size.

Then which laser should we buy? I recommend buying the 1064-nm long-pulsed Nd:YAG laser first and later, the 595 nm PDL. The reason for this is as follows. First, the cost of purchasing the long-pulsed Nd:YAG laser is lower. Second, as explained above, NIR lasers can treat both thin and thick blood vessels and thus can treat many blood vessels. Third, due to epidermal bypass effect, NIR lasers have fewer epidermal side effects than 500–600 nm wavelength

Table 6.1 Types of vascular lasers and TRT. (Modified from [15])

Type of laser	Wavelength (nm)	Pulse duration	TRT	Target
Pulsed dye laser	585	450 μs	0.4–4.5 ms	Blood vessels (30–100 μm)
Long-pulsed dye laser	595	1.5 ms (0.45–40 ms)	> 4.5 ms	Blood vessels (> 0.1 mm)
KTP	532	1–100 ms	< 446.4 ms	Blood vessels (up to 1 mm)
Long-pulsed Nd:YAG	1064	5–300 ms		
IPL	500–12,000	2–200 ms		
Copper bromide	577, 511	10–1000 ms, quasi-continuous wave		

lasers. However, long-pulsed Nd:YAG lasers cannot treat erythema, blood vessels corresponding to TRT of less than 5 ms. In this case, using the genesis technique of the long-pulsed Nd:YAG laser first improves erythema to some extent.

Of course, most of the blood vessels on the face are not thick blood vessels. Recently released PDLs have less purpura and fewer side effects than 1064-nm long-pulsed Nd:YAG lasers. So if we need to choose just one vascular laser, we should buy a 595-nm PDL. In many laser texts, the golden standard for facial vascular lasers is known as the 595-nm long-pulsed PDL. However, the problems are the high purchase cost and maintenance cost. I recommend purchasing 1064-nm long-pulsed Nd:YAG laser first or if you want to put the effect first, regardless of cost, I recommend buying a 595 nm long-pulsed PDL.

For reference, what is the range of TRT that can be effective for a specific pulse duration? The pulse duration should be less than or equal to TRT. If the pulse duration is equal to TRT, there would be no problem, but if the pulse duration is small, how small can the pulse duration be, so that it is still effective? Although there is nothing known about this, but based on the fact that the pulse duration of 450 μs is effective up to 4.5 ms TRT (Table 6.1), I think that it may be effective up to about ten times the TRT of the pulse duration, and may not be effective at more than ten times the TRT.

6.2.4 Vascular Laser for Koreans

Now let's look at the specifics of the pros and cons of each vascular laser and what problems they have when applied to Koreans.

The 532-nm KTP laser has the same blood absorption coefficient as the 585-nm PDL [2], while the pulse duration varies from 1 to 100 ms [15] enabling treatment of variety of blood vessels, and because it has a true long pulse, purpura rarely occurs. However, 532-nm KTP laser does not have deeper OPD than 585 nm and has a high absorption coefficient for Hb, so it cannot treat large blood vessels and has a high absorption coefficient for melanin, so it is not suitable for Asians and darker skin [2].

577-nm copper vapor laser has the highest Hb absorption coefficient, but like 532-nm KTP, the laser still has a high melanin absorption coefficient, which makes it inadequate for darker skin, especially Fitzpatrick skin type V [16]. Also, since the laser has a quasi-continuous wave and a pulse duration of 10 ms or more, it cannot treat small blood vessels corresponding to TRT 10 ms or less (Table 6.1).

When Fitzpatrick skin types IV and V were treated with 585-nm PDL for port-wine stain (PWS), treatment progress was slower than Caucasians, multiple treatment sessions were required, and the treatment efficacy was reported to be lower. However, it is known that the treatment effect of telangiectasia with 585-nm PDL does not differ according to ethnicity [16]. Therefore, it is not necessary to completely exclude 585-nm PDL from the vascular treatment of Asians due to the fact that several treatments are required for the treatment of PWS and the therapeutic effect is somewhat inferior [2]. Disadvantages of 585-nm PDL are that there is a downtime in which purpura occurs and that blood vessels larger than 0.1 mm cannot be treated.

595-nm long-pulsed PDL adopts the 595-nm wavelength with a lower melanin absorption coefficient and a deeper OPD to improve the shortcomings of 585-nm PDL (Fig. 6.9). The laser has been improved for use in treating blood vessels of various sizes by increasing the pulse duration and reducing side effects through epidermal cooling. Thus, the laser is currently the most optimal laser for PWS in Asians and also purpura rarely occurs [2]. However, since the absorption coefficient of Hb is lower than that of 585-nm PDL, the power must be increased, resulting in high costs in purchasing and maintenance.

IPL is also known as an effective method for treating PWS, but it is known that it should be performed only by those with much experience [2]. 1064 nm long-pulsed Nd:YAG laser can be used to treat blood vessels not only on the face but also on every part of the body. It is known that the pigmentation side effects such as

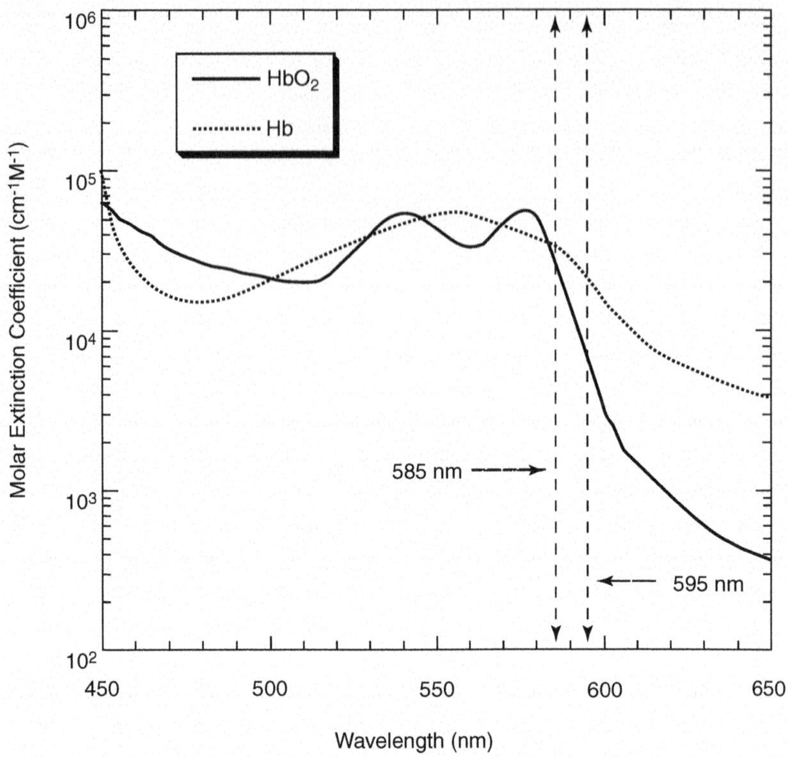

Fig. 6.9 Absorption spectra of Hb and HbO_2 in the region 450–650 nm. Reproduced from [17]

hypopigmentation do not occur. It is the most suitable laser for darkly pigmented skin. However, erythema cannot be cured with this laser [2].

6.3 Determination of Pulse Duration

TRTs of blood vessels vary greatly depending on the size of blood vessel (Table 6.2). From barely visible blood vessels (100 μm) to largest vessel visible on the face (1 mm), there is a 100-fold difference of TRT from 4.8 to 446.4 ms. It seems very difficult to determine the pulse duration for such a wide TRT range. Is it really?

There are three ways to calculate the TRT of blood vessels. First follows the theory of selective photothermolysis, in which the heat of the blood is transferred to the blood vessel wall and is coagulated. In this case, TRT can be calculated by considering only the blood inside the blood vessel wall as the target tissue [TRT]. Second,

Table 6.2 Thermal relaxation time (TRT) of blood vessels [2, 18].

Size (μm)	TRT (ms)	Depth (μm)	Comments
10	0.048	100	Uniform pink color
20	0.19		
50	1.2		
100	4.8		Smallest size of blood vessels visible
200	19.0	250	
300	42.6		
400	80		
800	300		
1000	446.4		

also follows the theory of the photothermolysis, in which the blood vessel is the target tissue. In this case, TRT can be calculated by calculating the TRT of the blood vessel itself. This is the TRT we are currently using (Table 1.13). We will define this as TRT' in this book. Third, TRT may be calculated using thermal damage time (TDT), which is the time when the heat of the blood vessel reaches the blood vessel wall by the extended theory of selective photothermolysis [TDT] [19]. Comparing these three, the TRT of the blood inside the blood vessel is the shortest, the TDT reaching the vessel wall by the extended theory is the longest, and TRT′ calculated by considering the blood vessel as the target tissue is in between (TRT < TRT'< TDT).

Christiansen et al. measured the vessel diameter and wall thickness of the blood vessels and studied the appropriate pulse duration according to the thickness of the blood vessels when using long-pulsed Nd:YAG lasers [19]. Measurements of the vessel diameter and wall thickness of the blood vessels revealed interesting facts. The blood vessels of 0.25 mm or less had the similar thickness of vessel diameter and wall thickness. For blood vessels of 0.25 mm or more, although the vessel diameter increased, wall thickness did not increase as much, so the blood vessel wall becomes relatively thin compared to the thickness of the entire blood vessel (Table 6.3).

TRT blood lumen was calculated by the theory of selective photothermolysis and TRT blood vein is the TRT′ calculated by considering the blood vessel itself as the target tissue and TDT blood vein is the TDT calculated by the extended theory (TRT blood lumen < TRT blood vein < TDT blood vein, Fig. 6.10). When applying the extended theory, the pulse duration should be equal to or shorter than the TDT blood vein and longer than the TRT blood lumen (TDT ≥ PD > TRT).

Vascular therapy mainly uses coagulation that occurs at temperatures below 100 °C, so the Arrhenius equation applied to temperatures

Table 6.3 TRT and TDT according to Altshuler et al. [20] for rectangular Nd:YAG (1064 nm) light pulse treatment of telangiectasias. Reproduced from [19]

Vessel diameter d mm	Wall thickness t_w mm	Blood lumen diameter d_i mm	TRT Blood lumen (ms)	TRT Blood vein (ms)	TDT Blood vein (ms)
0.1	0.035	0.03	0.4	5	140
0.25	0.08	0.09	3.9	30	610
0.5	0.12	0.27	32.5	120	1200
1.0	0.15	0.7	236	480	2400

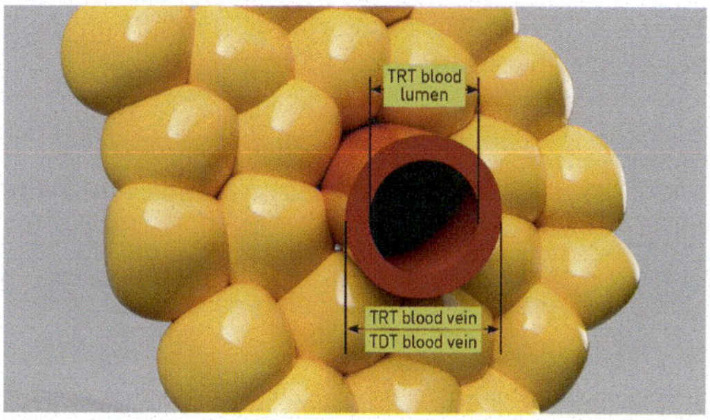

Fig. 6.10 TRT blood lumen, TRT blood vein, TDT blood vein. Published with kind permission of © Jin Kwon Cho 2019. All rights reserved

below 100 °C is applied (see Sect. 3.6.3 in "Chap. 3"). Therefore, any pulse duration longer than TRT and equal to or less than TDT produces the same effect. However, the longer the pulse duration, the fewer side effects (method B in nonablative rejuvenation), so based on TRT blood vein (TRT′), the pulse duration should be equal to or shorter than TDT blood vein and longer than TRT blood vein (TDT ≥ PD > TRT′). On the other hand, the longer the pulse duration, the worse the pain. In particular, 1064 nm has a high absorption of water, which causes considerable pain during long pulse duration. Considering these two points, let's think about the pulse duration of two blood vessels.

First, the pulse duration of blood vessels smaller than 0.25 mm should be in between TRT blood vein and TDT blood vein and close to TRT blood vein (TRT′ < PD ≤ TDT). Second, in blood vessels larger than 0.25 mm, since the pulse duration is quite long and vessel wall is relatively thin compared to vessel, by ignoring the vessel wall and applying the theory of selective photothermolysis, it is possible to set the pulse duration equal to or less than the TRT blood lumen (PD ≤ TRT).

Through these hypotheses, Christiansen et al. found that for blood vessels smaller than 0.25 mm, pulse durations slightly exceeding TRT blood vein are appropriate. And for blood vessels larger than 0.25 mm, pulse durations shorter than or equal to TRT blood lumen are appropriate.

The actual effective pulse duration according to the size of the blood vessel (Table 6.4) shows

Table 6.4 Theoretical and previously clinically proven Nd:YAG parameters used as settings in the FF (fixed fluence)-treated side. Reproduced from [19]

	Blue vessels			Red vessels		
Vessel size mm	Pulse duration (ms)	Spot size (mm)	Fluence J/cm^2	Pulse duration (ms)	Spot size (mm)	Fluence J/cm^2
<0.3	25	1.5	210	12	1.5	210
0.3–0.5	32	3	250	16	3	250
0.5–1.0	45	3	285	25	3	285
1.0–2.5	64	5	200	–	–	–

that the pulse duration of small blood vessels less than 0.3 mm is 12–25 ms, which is larger than TRT blood vein (5 ms) and much smaller than TDT blood vein (140 ms). Pulse duration of large blood vessels of 0.5–1.0 mm is 25–45 ms, similar to or shorter than TRT blood lumen (32.5–236 ms). Therefore, in order to treat blood vessels of 0.1 to 1 mm using a long-pulsed Nd:YAG laser, only pulse duration of 12–45 ms should be selected instead of 4.5–446.4 ms.

In one laser text, it was revealed that a pulse duration of 0.5 ms (or 0.45 ms) for a thickness of 60–100 μm (erythema) and a pulse duration of 10 ms for a thickness of 150–300 μm is ideal. In the case of multiplex lasers that simultaneously irradiate 595 nm and 1064 nm, it is stated that 150–400-μm blood vessels were most effectively treated by 10-ms pulse duration and 400–1000 μm blood vessels at 40-ms pulse duration [7]. Therefore, when treating blood vessels of the face, only four pulse durations (0.45, 5, 10, and 40 ms) need to be used. According to the thermal kinetic selectivity, treatment may be performed sequentially from large pulse duration to small pulse durations of 40, 10, 5, and 0.45 ms. Since most of telangiectasia occurring on the face are thin blood vessels less than 200 μm, I rarely use the pulse duration of 40 ms, but mainly use 10, 5, and 0.45 ms.

In addition, when considering the pulse duration, two lasers, a 1064 nm long-pulsed Nd:YAG laser having a pulse duration of 5 ms or more and a 595 nm PDL having a pulse duration of 0.45–40 ms, could be purchased.

6.4 Spot Size

Blood vessels are located at various depths in the dermis. Therefore, lasers with deeper OPD are recommended. If so, it would be better to increase the spot size so that the OPD becomes deeper. Even with the same fluence, larger spot sizes require more photons to be irradiated, so higher power is required. Long-pulsed Nd:YAG lasers also require higher power to increase spot size. The long-pulsed Nd:YAG laser has already increased the power due to their low absorption of Hb and it is difficult to increase the power further. What shall we do?

There are three factors involved in OPD: Spot size, wavelength, and power density. Which of these factors is the most important for OPD? The most important factor is the wavelength. Christiansen et al. stated that because 532-nm KTP or 575–595 nm PDL has a large scattering coefficient (30–35 mm^{-1}), OPD is limited to 2 mm or less even if the spot size was increased to 6–8 mm [19]. However, the scattering coefficient of 1064 nm Nd:YAG laser is 12 mm^{-1}, which is only 1/3 of the 500–600 nm wavelength lasers and OPD is 2.5 mm or more even when the spot size is reduced to 1.5–3 mm. Thus, Christiansen et al. described that 1064 nm Nd:YAG lasers penetrate deeper than 500–600-nm wavelength lasers.

Therefore, long-pulsed Nd:YAG lasers have a deep OPD without increasing the spot size. Rather, Nd:YAG lasers have the advantage of using small spot sizes. First, even if side effects occur, the range of side effects is small. Second, small spot sizes require higher energy than large spot sizes, but because the total amount of energy is small, small spot sizes cause less pain than large spot sizes. Therefore, it is safer to use small spot sizes when treating blood vessels with long-pulsed Nd:YAG lasers. The disadvantage is that because the spot size is small, the procedure time is long when the entire face is treated.

Ross et al. proposed matching the spot size to the blood vessel thickness for deeply penetrating wavelengths [6]. In other words, treatment of 2-mm thick blood vessel is sufficient for a 2-mm spot size. Usually, blood vessels larger than 1 mm are not common on the face. In addition, in the case of a 2–3 mm punch biopsy, it is known that even if the wound is left without suture, the wound regeneration time may be slow but cosmetically there is no problem [21]. Therefore, I use a spot size of less than 3 mm when treating blood vessels with a long-pulsed Nd:YAG laser.

6.5 Clinical End Point

Wanner et al. suggested various clinical end points of vascular therapy for each vascular lesions [22]. In port-wine stain (PWS) the suggested clinical end point for PDL was purpura limited to spot size, while the suggested clinical end point for both 755-nm long-pulsed alexandrite laser and 1064-nm long-pulsed Nd:YAG laser was the transition to purple blue in color. In infantile hemangioma, the suggested clinical end point was a temporary subtle purpura or a slight blackening of a lesion within 1 min. In telangiectasia, immediate vessel darkening or immediate vessel disappearance was suggested as the clinical end point. In senile hemangioma, purpura without petechiae was suggested as the clinical end point, and in the case of venous lake, vessel darkening or disappearance was suggested as the clinical end point.

Let's consider in detail the clinical end point of telangiectasia. Why do blood vessels darken or disappear? And what happens if higher energy is given?

Suthamjariya et al. used 532-nm and 1064-nm long-pulsed Nd:YAG lasers to irradiate small vessels in a hamster's cheeks with various energy and captured changes in the vessels with a high-speed camera [23].

The results show a series of various changes as the energy increases. In order of low to high fluence, based on the threshold for blood coagulation and threshold for cavitation, no changes in blood vessels or occasionally temporary vasodilatation are observed below blood coagulation threshold. In the coagulation threshold, coagulum appears in the blood vessels, sometimes flowing along the bloodstream, but most adhere to blood vessel walls. Above blood coagulation threshold, blood vessels contract, and coagulum elongates, resulting in thread-like appearance or vessel disappearance (Fig. 6.11).

In the threshold for cavitation, intravascular cavitation occurs and the cavitation push out the coagulum blocking blood flow resulting in vessel disappearance or vessel wall rupture (Fig. 6.12). At higher fluences, extravascular cavitation occurs and vacuoles grow up to 20 times the thickness of vessels at very high energy. This results in vessel wall rupture and hemorrhage, perivascular tissue shrinkage, and damage to surrounding tissue (Fig. 6.13).

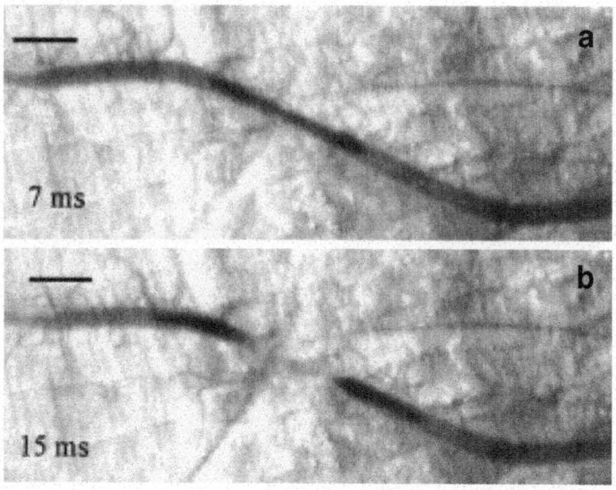

Fig. 6.11 Irradiated with 532 nm, 25 ms, 220 J/cm^2. Coagulum elongates (a) and separates the center of the irradiated area (b) resulting in immediate vessel disappearance. (Modified from [23])

I summarized the above into six phenomena (Table 6.5). The above phenomena are a description through microscopic observation. How do these phenomena look clinically to the laser physician's eyes and which is the most ideal vascular treatment?

First, blood coagulation is not an appropriate phenomenon for vascular treatment. If only coagulum occurs and the blood vessels are not blocked, the coagulum will someday fall off and the blood vessels will remain unchanged. Second, in vasoconstriction and thread-like appearance, blood vessels may disappear after blockage of blood vessels or blood vessels may regenerate due to recanalization. So vasoconstriction and thread-like appearance may or may not be what we desire. However, side effects from vasoconstriction and thread-like appearance will not occur. Clinically, darkening of blood vessels is observed. However, very small blood vessels are difficult to distinguish due to insignificant color change and it is also difficult to distinguish from blood coagulation. Third, the authors of the paper consider vessel disappearance as the appropriate response. Clinically, there is a distinct reaction in which blood vessels disappear. Fourth, intravascular cavitation is more likely to cause blood vessels to disappear because it acts to further block the blood vessels by pushing the coagulum in the vessels. However, sometimes hemorrhage occurs, and clinically, blood vessels disappear, but purpura may occur. Although this may be an appropriate response to vascular therapy, there may be some downtime. Fifth, extravascular cavitation breaks blood vessels, resulting in disappearance of blood vessels. Clinically purpura that lasts up to 10–14 days occurs. This cannot be covered by makeup, making normal

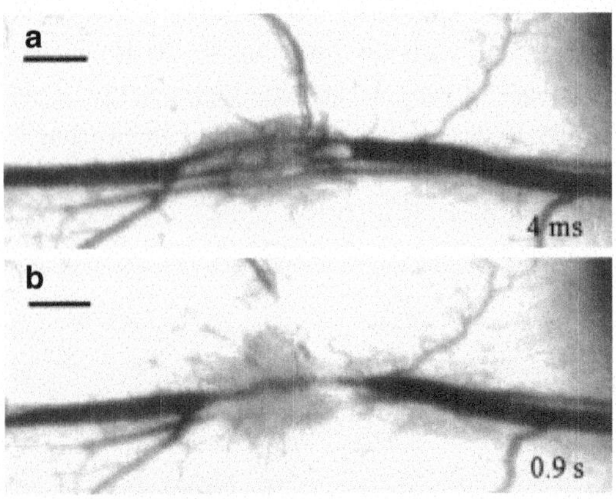

Fig. 6.12 Irradiated with 1064 nm, 25 ms, 400 J/cm^2. Cavitation in vessels destroy the vessel walls (**a**) resulting in hemorrhage (**b**). Modified from [23]

Table 6.5 Summary of vessel changes with energy

Microscopic findings	Thresholds and clinical end points
Blood coagulation	Threshold for blood coagulation. Darkening
Vasoconstriction, thread-like appearance	Darkening
Vessel disappearance	A useful clinical end point associated with good results. Disappearance
Intravascular cavitation	Threshold for cavitation. Disappearance, little purpura
Extravascular cavitation (bubble formation), vessel wall rupture and hemorrhage	Purpura (~10–14 days)
Shrinkage of perivascular tissue	Gray and white discoloration

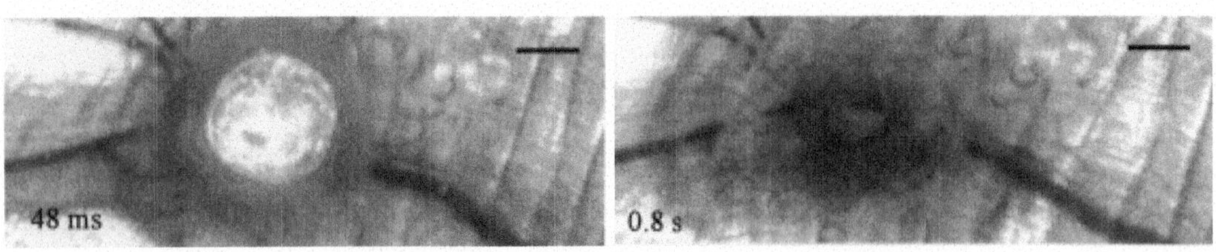

Fig. 6.13 Irradiated with 532 nm, 50 ms, 160 J/cm^2. Huge bubbles develop, causing significant hemorrhage and perivascular tissue damage. Modified from [23]

social life difficult for patients. Thus, although this may be one method of vascular therapy, it is not an appropriate method. In addition, blood vessels may regenerate and recur. Sixth, shrinkage of perivascular tissue occurs due to extravascular cavitation that does not end with purpura but damages the tissue around the blood vessels. This phenomenon has a high risk of scarring. Clinically, gray and white discoloration can be seen.

Of the six phenomena, I think that the second (vasoconstriction, thread-like appearance) and the third (vessel disappearance) phenomena are the most appropriate for vascular therapy. The disappearance or darkening of blood vessels is considered as the clinical end point. Of course, the second phenomenon may recur later, but I think it is better to relapse than to have side effects. If it recurs, it can be treated again.

The fourth phenomenon (intravascular cavitation) also results in vessel disappearance, but I think there is a high chance of side effects. In order for intravascular cavitation to occur, vaporization of blood must occur. At this time, I do not think that only vaporization occurs. When the temperature rises, the damage threshold of protein degeneration and the survival threshold of tissue necrosis occurs before vaporization (see Sect. 9.2.4 in "Chap. 9"). Thus, vaporization means that tissue necrosis has already occurred. In other words, scarring may occur later. For the same reason, I think that the extravascular cavitation of 585–595-nm PDL laser and long-pulsed laser is different. In both lasers, blood vessels are ruptured and purpura occurs at temperatures above vaporization. However, when using PDL lasers, the power density is increased in a short time, so the mechanical damage is greater than that of thermal damage, such as Q-switched lasers or Er:YAG lasers. Conversely, when using long-pulsed lasers, there is a high possibility of scarring due to high thermal damage like CO_2 lasers. Therefore, in extravascular cavitation caused by PDL, purpura may occur, but scarring is unlikely. Long-pulsed lasers, on the other hand, are more likely to cause scarring later as well as purpura.

6.5.1 Disadvantages of Long-Pulsed Nd:YAG Lasers

Wang et al. investigated 61 patients with flat port-wine stain (PWS) on face that had never been treated [24]. One side of the lesion was irradiated with 595-nm PDL and the other half with multiplex laser with 595 nm and 1064 nm wavelengths. The results showed no difference in effect between the PDL only side and the multiplex laser side. However, crusting or blistering occurred in two patients (3%) in the PDL-only side and 19 patients (31%) in the multiplex laser side. Scarring occurred in three patients in the multiplex laser side.

This paper compares the effects and side effects of 595-nm PDL and multiplex laser (595-nm PDL is irradiated first, and after an interval of 1 s, 1064-nm Nd:YAG is irradiated). Although the multiplex laser irradiates 595-nm PDL, the effect is similar to that of using the long-pulsed Nd:YAG laser alone, because first, the metHb is made from PDL and the 1064-nm long-pulsed Nd:YAG laser raises the temperature of metHb as chromophore. The results show that long-pulsed Nd:YAG lasers have higher side effects, as explained previously about the difference in side effects between the PDL and the long-pulsed lasers.

Yang et al. treated port-wine stains (PWS) in 17 patients. The lesion was divided into four areas [25]. One area was treated with 595-nm PDL (Scleroplus; Candela Corp, Wayland, MA) and the parameters were 8 J/cm^2, 7 mm, 1.5 ms. The other three areas were treated with 1064-nm Nd:YAG laser (Modified Coolglide; Altus Medical, Inc., Brisbane, CA) with fluences of 1.0, 0.8, and 0.6 times the minimum purpura dose (MPD). MPD was defined as fluence with a slightly blackening reaction (purpura) that lasted at least 15 min after at least two to three trials. The results show that, first, the MPD of long-pulsed Nd:YAG laser varied greatly from 40 to 250 J/cm^2 when measured by fluence. Second, the objective improvement between PDL and long-pulsed Nd:YAG laser (MPD 1.0) was 50–75%, i.e., there was no difference. Third, patient satisfaction measured by VAS (visual analog scale) was 4.85 and 5.84, respectively. Long-pulsed Nd:YAG laser showed higher satisfaction ($p < 0.05$). Purpuras in long-pulsed Nd:YAG lasers lasted 3 days, while purpuras in PDLs lasted for 7–10 days. In other words, the recovery period of patients with long-pulsed Nd:YAG laser was short. Fourth, at the beginning of the study, long-pulsed Nd:YAG laser, like PDL, was performed with defined parameters. But after scarring occurred in the first patient, the study was conducted after defining the MPD. The energy of the patient with scarring was 1.2 times and 1.7 times the MPD.

As can be seen in this paper, both PDL and long-pulsed Nd:YAG lasers have the same effect if they have the same energy levels that cause the same response to tissue. However, even if long-pulsed Nd:YAG laser has only 1.2 times the MPD, side effects such as scarring may occur. On the other hand, PDL is known to be safe even when irradiated with two times the MPD without epidermal cooling. In other words, long-pulsed Nd:YAG laser has a narrower therapeutic window than PDL. In addition, MPD in long-pulsed Nd:YAG laser varies from 40 to 250 J/cm^2 when measured by fluence. Thus the fluence is difficult to adjust and scarring may occur during testing. However, because the duration of purpura was short, the satisfaction of long-pulsed Nd:YAG laser was higher than that of PDL, but if PDL also has the technology to reduce energy and minimize purpura, I think patient satisfaction will be similar (This will be explained again in "ideal macropulse").

Why do long-pulsed Nd:YAG lasers have narrow therapeutic window and various MPDs? First, when 1064 nm long-pulsed Nd:YAG laser is irradiated, the absorption coefficient increases three times due to metHb production. In addition, coagulum occurs and the loss of water increases the concentration of chromophores. Therefore, Nd:YAG laser has a long pulse duration and as a result, temperature rises rapidly. Second, percentage of dermal blood vessels is 0.05 in pink PWS and 0.25 in dark purple and hypertrophic PWS. Bulk dermal heating is proportional to the total energy per unit volume. The total energy is related not only to temperature but also to the proportion of blood vessels. Therefore, MPD is different for each lesion and the treatment range is narrowed because Nd:YAG laser penetrates deeper than PDL and consequently increases the ratio of blood vessels [25].

On the other hand, why is PDL safe? Next, we will look at macropulse used in long-pulsed PDL.

6.6 Pulsed Dye Laser

6.6.1 Macropulse

Macropulse is a method of irradiating several small pulses (subpulse) in succession to make the pulse duration longer than the pulse duration of small pulses [2]. It is also called "Train pulse," because the connection of the pulses is similar to that of train. Macropulse's typical laser is the PDL.

If the original pulse duration is 1.5 ms, the laser should be continuously irradiated for 1.5 ms (Figure 6.14a) and the irradiation must be completed after 1.5 ms. This is called the "true long pulse" [16]. However, the actual PDL we use, V-beam, cannot produce a long pulse duration of 1.5 ms, but only 0.45 ms. So 0.45 ms is irradiated three times consecutively to increase the temperature for 1.5 ms, similar to a true long pulse.

The reason for creating macropulse was as follows. In order to produce a true long pulse, high power was required, but it was difficult to produce high power when long-pulsed laser was being developed. At this time, it was found that irradiating one time and irradiating multiple times could get the same result. Thus, a long-pulsed laser was created using macropulses that continuously collect and irradiate low-energy subpulses (Fig. 6.15).

Macropulse is applied to various lasers. As seen earlier, PDL and Er:YAG lasers also use macropulses. I also think that the PTP mode of 1064-nm Q-switched Nd:YAG laser and the low-power multipass type diode laser (e.g., Soprano laser in hair removal) also applied the concept of macropulse.

Then what is the difference between macropulse and true long pulse? First, the main differ-

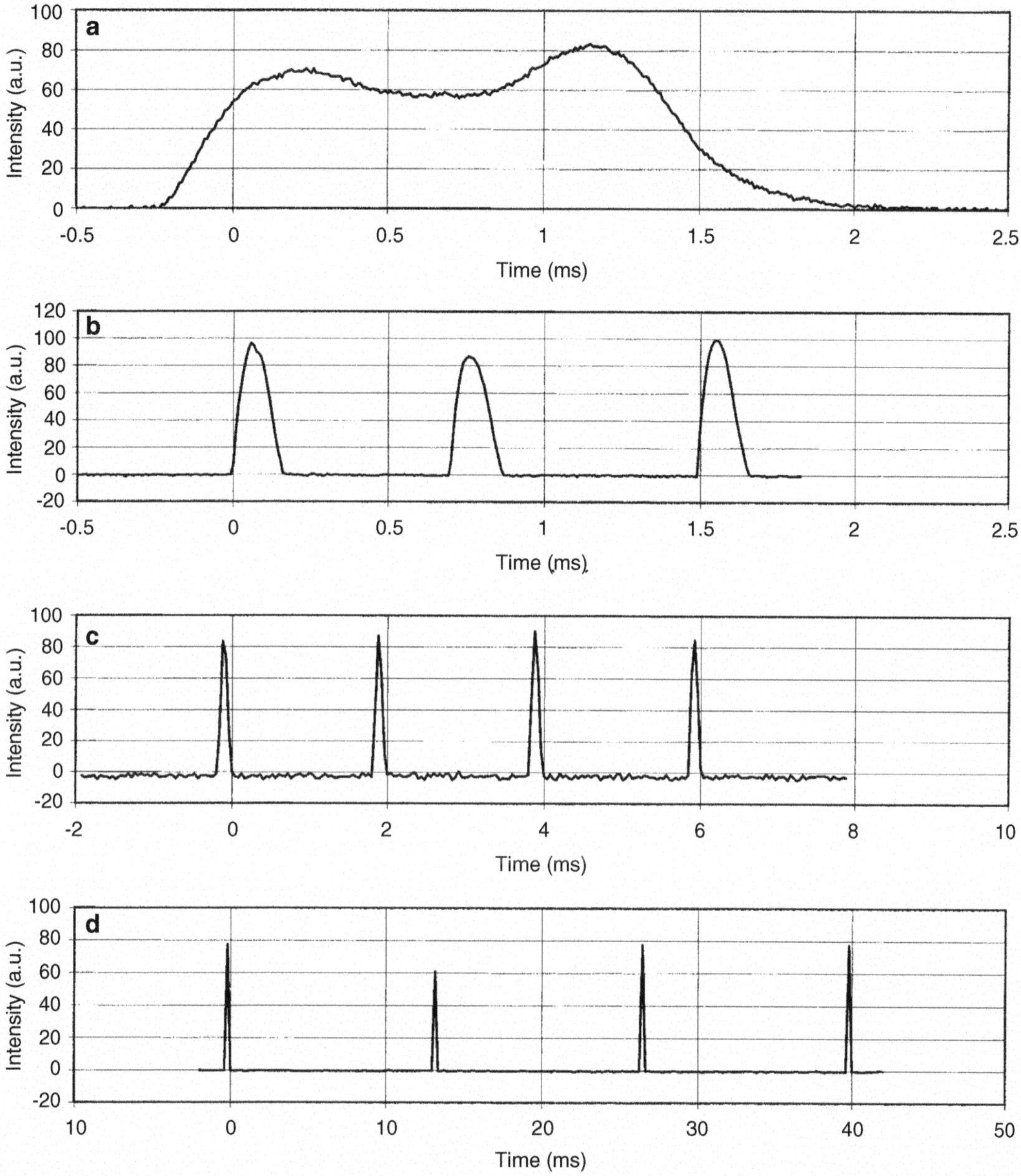

Fig. 6.14 Contour of laser pulses (**a**): ScleroPlus 1.5 ms, (**b**) V-bem 1.5 ms, (**c**) V-beam 6 ms, and (**d**) V-bem 40 ms. (Reproduced from [17])

ence is that it is difficult for macropulses to produce higher temperatures than true long pulses. During the break between subpulses, the temperature drops, resulting in a lower temperature than the true long pulse. However, this can act as an advantage because of the lower temperature there are fewer side effects (see "True long pulse vs false long pulse (macropulse)").

Second, the characteristics of the subpulse remain [2]. For example, in the case of PDL, when a long pulse duration in milliseconds is made with macropulse, purpura should not occur due to photothermal effect. However, the characteristics of the subpulse of 0.45 ms remain and purpura occur by photomechanical effect.

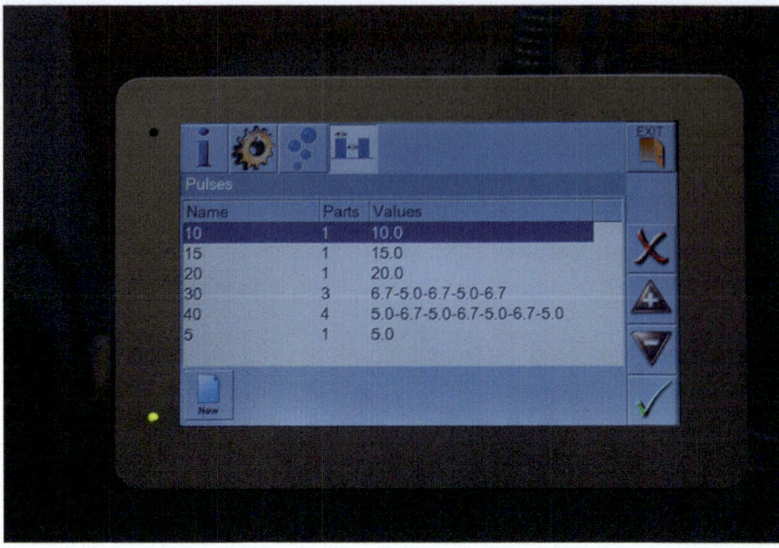

Fig. 6.15 Pulse duration of a 1064-nm long-pulsed Nd:YAG laser. 20 ms or less is a true long pulse but 30 ms or more is macropulse

Third, even with the same type of laser, response and actual fluence of each lasers may vary even if the same pulse duration and fluence are used. This is because the pulse duration and shape of the subpulse, fluence, and number of subpulse shots vary from manufacturer to manufacturer.

6.6.2 Are Laser Parameters Interchangeable?

It is often thought that even lasers of the same wavelength cannot share laser parameters because of the difference of actual energy. Is this true? A laser machine is a machine that converts light energy of weak power into laser of high power. Different flash lamps use different amounts of photons but produce photons of the same wavelength. Also, if the same photon quantity is measured when the output is measured, the energy will be the same even if the manufacturers are different. Therefore, even if the manufacturers are different, laser parameters can be shared if measured output values are the same.

But macropulse is an exception. Macropulse cannot share laser parameters because different manufacturers have different pulse duration and shape of the subpulse, fluence, and number of subpulse shots [19]. In other words, if it is a true pulse laser, even lasers manufactured by other manufacturers can share parameters. In particular, Q-switched lasers are true pulses, allowing us to share parameters. Therefore, the same result can be obtained if the parameters are the same even if a laser different from the one presented in the paper is used.

However, it is difficult to share 100% of all parameters between lasers. Besides the pulse structure such as macropulse, handpiece specifications (beam type and quality) and cooling devices are different from manufacturer to manufacturer. In addition, as the laser is used, the output of the lamp is reduced, so the actual fluence is reduced compared to the fluence displayed on the instrument panel. Thus, energy parameters may be different between lasers of the same manufacturer.

Then, on what basis can we compare the results with each other and choose parameters based on the results in the paper? What we can set as a reference is the clinical end point [7]. In other words, the energy level can be estimated through the tissue reaction caused by the laser. For example, if lentigo darkens at 16 J/cm^2 with manufacturer A's 755-nm long-pulsed alexandrite laser and darkens at 20 J/cm^2 with manufacturer B's, we can conclude that even though the fluences are different, energy levels are similar. Of course, it is not possible to compare the exact energy level with the clinical end point. There are observational errors, severe deviations, and above all, in some cases, clinical end points do not occur.

6.6.3 True Long Pulse Versus False Long Pulse (Macropulse)

In particular, we must note the first difference between macropulse and true long pulse. As opposed to true long pulses, marcopulse is also called false long pulse. When comparing IPL, a typical example of true long pulse and PDL, a typical example of false long pulse, some say IPL is better. Is it better just because it is named "true?" What is the specific difference between a true long pulse and a false long pulse (macropulse)?

What we eventually want is to raise the temperature to the threshold where blood vessels coagulate and contract. However, not only temperature but also time plays an important role in thermal changes below 100 °C. In other words, it is subject to the Arrhenius equation (see Sect. 9.2.3 in "Chap. 9"). There are two possible treatment methods according to the Arrhenius equation. First, a method of raising a high temperature in a short time (method A), and second, a method of raising a low temperature in a long time (method B). Both methods have the same effect. However, plan B has fewer side effects and a wider therapeutic window (see Sect. 9.2.6 in "Chap. 9").

In IPL, the temperature is raised in a short time as light is continuously irradiated during the pulse duration. On the other hand, in PDL, the temperature raises during subpulse, but the temperature drops while cooling at the delay time. The second subpulse is irradiated without falling to the original temperature, so the temperature is higher than the temperature generated during the first subpulse. Repeatedly, the temperature rises slowly for a long time. This corresponds to method B in Arrhenius equation. Therefore, I believe that both IPL and PDL have the same effect if an appropriate pulse duration and an appropriate fluence are selected, but PDL is safer than IPL.

Let's look at why the Arrhenius equation applies to vascular laser therapy rather than the theory of selective photothermolysis.

6.6.4 Arrhenius Equation

The three phases of optical thermal model are optical phase, thermal phase, and tissue denaturation process (see Sect. 3.7.1 in "Chap. 3"). First, in optical phase, the wavelength and depth of target tissue are considered. Second, thermal phase is the thermodynamic heating process. This is a process in which the theory of selective photothermolysis and the extended theory of selective photothermolysis are applied as a process of locally increasing temperature. Therefore, pulse duration should be considered. Third, tissue denaturation process is a chemical process. Just because the only temperature rises locally by the thermal phase, the tissue is not denatured. In order for the tissue denaturation to occur in the photothermal effect below 100 °C, sufficient time is required in addition to the temperature (Arrhenius equation).

Based on this concept, Murphy et al. defined various times during laser irradiation process (Fig. 6.16) [26].

First, pulse duration (pulse width, t_p). Pulse duration determines the total energy entering the tissue. Second, total denaturation time (t_{tden}). This is the time lasting over 43 °C in tissue. The minimum temperature at which tissue denaturation occurs is known to be above 5 °C of body temperature. Murphy et al. considered this temperature to be 43 °C. Third, effective denaturation time (t_{eden}). This is the time when 99% of actual tissues are denatured. The temperature at this time can be defined as effective (or threshold) temperature (T_{eden}). Therefore, the effective denaturation time is less than or equal to the total denaturation time ($t_{eden} \leq t_{tden}$). Fourth is TRT (t_{TRT}) defined by the theory of selective photothermolysis and the extended theory of selective photothemolysis.

The important fact here is that there is no link between the desired effective denaturation time (t_{eden}) and TRT (t_{TRT}) which is the

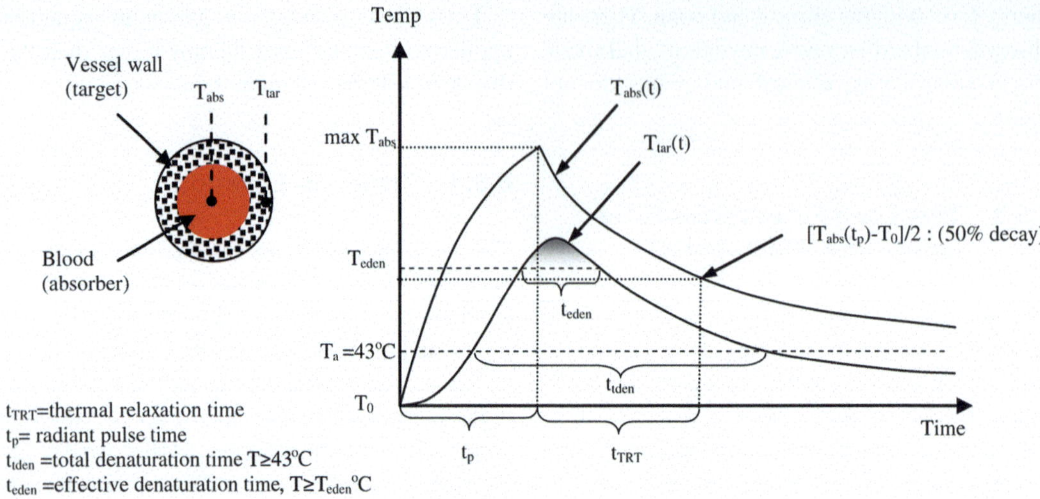

Fig. 6.16 Once $T \geq 43$ °C in the target tissue, the denaturation process starts up slowly and continues for the total denaturation time t_{tden}. However, the denaturation process accelerates exponentially with increasing temperature, and, therefore, it is useful to introduce the "effective" denaturation temperature, T_{eden}, and corresponding time t_{eden} over which most of the denaturation takes place. Reproduced from [26]

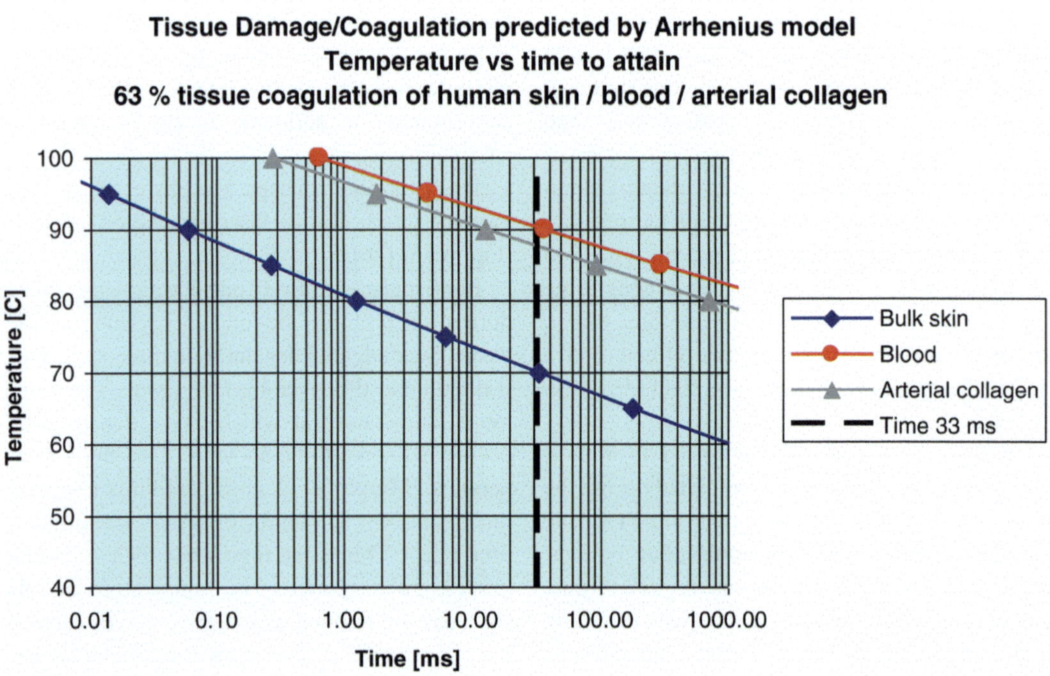

Fig. 6.17 Tissue denaturation temperature dependency versus time predicted by the Arrhenius model for bulk skin, blood, and arterial collagen (Reproduced from [26])

basis of pulse duration in laser treatment in transient heating process.

Now let's review vascular treatment based on Arrhenius equation (Fig. 6.17). Based on 33 ms, the coagulation temperatures for blood, arterial collagen, and bulk skin are 90.4, 88, and 70 °C, respectively. Therefore, according to the Arrhenius equation, if the temperature of the entire skin rises, the arterial collagen or bulk skin will denaturate before the blood coagulates, which will cause side effects. One way to overcome this is by the theory of selective photothermolysis or the extended theory of selective photothermolysis. That is why TRT (or TDT) is of primary importance. Ultimately, however, tissue denaturation is based on Arrhenius equation. In this case, the important time is T_{eden}, not TRT.

Phenomenon that was not treated by actual TRT was observed in vascular treatment. The blood vessel thickness of PWS is 10–300 μm and the corresponding TRT is 0.057–51 ms. Pulse durations of 0.0003–0.36 ms was used in PDL, according to the TRT, but treatment-resistant vessels were found. Why does this phenomenon occur? The arterial collagen should be above 99.4 °C and the blood vessel should be above 101 °C for collagen denaturation to occur below 0.36 ms. Therefore, intravascular cavitation occurs and the blood vessel wall is destroyed, resulting in purpura [26]. This is not the desired outcome because blood vessels with destroyed walls can be regenerated.

Conversely, let's look at the blood vessels of the minimum thickness that can be treated according to the Arrhenius equation (Fig. 6.17). Arterial collagen should be at least 100 °C. At this time, the time corresponding to the Arrhenius model is 0.296 ms. The vessel thickness corresponding to 0.296 ms TRT is 25.5 μm. Therefore, no matter how short the pulse duration of PDL laser, it is impossible to treat blood vessels of 25.5 μm or less by photothermal effect alone. Erythema appears different in color depending on the thickness of blood vessels. Ten to twenty micrometer blood vessels appear as diffuse pink lesions and 50 μm relatively large blood vessels appear as purple lesions [7]. Therefore, PDL cannot treat pink erythema.

This time, let's look at the blood vessels of the maximum thickness that can be treated. For example, assuming that there is a PDL laser having a pulse duration of 1.5–10 ms, the collagen temperature of the artery corresponding to the pulse duration is 95.7 and 90.7 °C, respectively, and the temperature of the blood does not exceed 100 °C. If the irradiation method is continuous irradiation, i.e., true long pulse, it is possible to treat blood vessels up to 150 μm thick corresponding to 10 ms TRT. Therefore, PDL lasers with a maximum pulse duration of 10 ms cannot treat blood vessels larger than 150 μm [26].

Based on the above, let's see why macropulse is used in PDL laser. For example, let's consider a PDL with a true pulse of 0.45 ms pulse duration. The pulse duration of 0.45 ms can treat blood vessels corresponding to a thickness of 30–100 μm. If the laser is irradiated with the pulse duration of 0.45 ms with true pulse, blood vessels can be treated without purpura. However, considering the Arrhenius formula, the method of using high energy in a short pulse duration (method A) has a narrow therapeutic window. In addition, as the blood vessel bursts in temperatures over 100 °C, purpura may occur, resulting in blood vessel recurrence. On the other hand, in the method of using low energy in a long pulse duration (method B), due to the long pulse duration (e.g., 4.5 ms), 30–100 μm blood vessels corresponding to pulse duration of 0.45 ms are spared and cannot be treated due to thermal kinetic selectivity (TRT < PD) in the thermal phase of the optical thermal model. In summary, method B cannot treat blood vessels because of thermal kinetic selectivity (TKS). To overcome this, macropulse is used. When using a macropulse that irradiates low-energy subpulses (0.45 ms) multiple times, photons are selectively absorbed in blood vessels of 30–100 μm (TRT ≥ PD), and because the subpulse is repeated and has a long pulse duration, blood vessels do not burst and the range of treatment can be broadened.

Macropulse can also be used to treat thick blood vessels. For example, if the minimum maintenance temperature generated by the subpulse is about 88 °C and is maintained for a period of 40 ms, blood vessels with a thickness of up to 300 μm can be treated.

6.6.5 Regeneration and Recurrence of Blood Vessels

The paper mentioned earlier by Murphy et al. is based on the premise that the temperature of blood should not be above 100 °C because purpura should not occur. Why should there be no purpura during PDL?

After vascular laser treatment, the blood vessels regenerate and symptoms recur. Neovascularization occurs even after sclerotherapy for the treatment of varicose veins as well as after vascular lasers [2]. This is very confusing, but there is still little research on this phenomenon.

The mechanism of occurrence is assumed as follows. In the wound-healing process, tissue is regenerated as the damaged tissue is replaced with new blood vessels. Vascular lasers also damage the skin and new blood vessels regenerate and recur. It is believed that inflammatory cells generated during wound-healing process secrete various cytokines, especially cytokines that increase angiogenic factors.

Prevention methods are as follows. First, we can try Rapamune (Pfizer Inc. New York, NY, USA), a drug to prevent long-term rejection reaction in kidney transplant patients. Rapamune is known to inhibit cytokine production and there are some reports that it is effective for revascularization after laser treatment. Second, imiquimod is an immunomodulator which was used to prevent recurrence after laser on PWS, but the results were poor.

Considering the mechanisms of blood vessel regeneration and recurrence, I believe that shrinking blood vessels or creating intravascular coagulation to block blood vessels is a way to reduce blood vessel regeneration and recurrence, rather than rupturing blood vessels and developing inflammation. So how do we keep the minimum maintenance temperature for blood vessel coagulation while the subpulse temperature does not exceed 100 °C?

6.6.6 Ideal Macropulse

Figure 6.18 shows the fluence in which purpura occurs according to pulse duration and the number of subpulses. This figure shows that purpura threshold increases as subpulse increases. What does the fact that "purpura threshold increases as subpulse increases" mean?

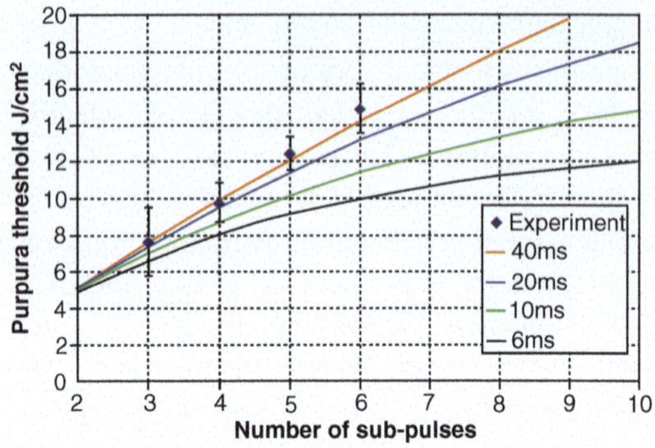

Fig. 6.18 Purpura threshold versus number of subpulses. Experimental data are for a 595-nm dye laser, 40-ms pulse duration published in [27]. Modeling calculations (*solid lines*) for 40, 20, 10, and 6 ms based on Mirkov et al. [10]. An increased number of subpulses have a larger effect, increasing the purpura threshold for the longer pulses. (Reproduced from [7])

The thing to note here is that the fluence of the y-axis is only the sum of the fluences of the subpulse. For example, when irradiating four subpulses at a pulse duration of 40 ms, the energy of subpulse where purpura starts to occur is 2.5 J/cm^2. There are four 2.5 J/cm^2 beams, so the instrument panel displays 10 J/cm^2. To make it easier to understand, I drew a pulse profile of a subpulse in which purpura occurs at 10 ms pulse duration (Fig. 6.19).

In Fig. 6.19, when the number of subpulses are 3, 6, and 8, the fluence of each subpulse is 2.3, 1.9, and 1.6 J/cm^2, respectively. As the number of subpulses increase, the fluence of each subpulse is decreased. In other words, rather than thinking that "purpura threshold increases as subpulse increases" it is better to think that "each subpulse energy decreases as subpulse increases."

Then what is the difference between a small number of subpulses and a large number of subpulses?

Earlier, it was revealed that minimum maintenance temperature of the subpulse should be maintained at, for example, 88 °C without exceeding 100 °C. The temperature change of the macropulse rises to a high temperature when the subpulse is irradiated, and then the temperature drops during the delay time when there is no irradiation. The lowest temperature should be

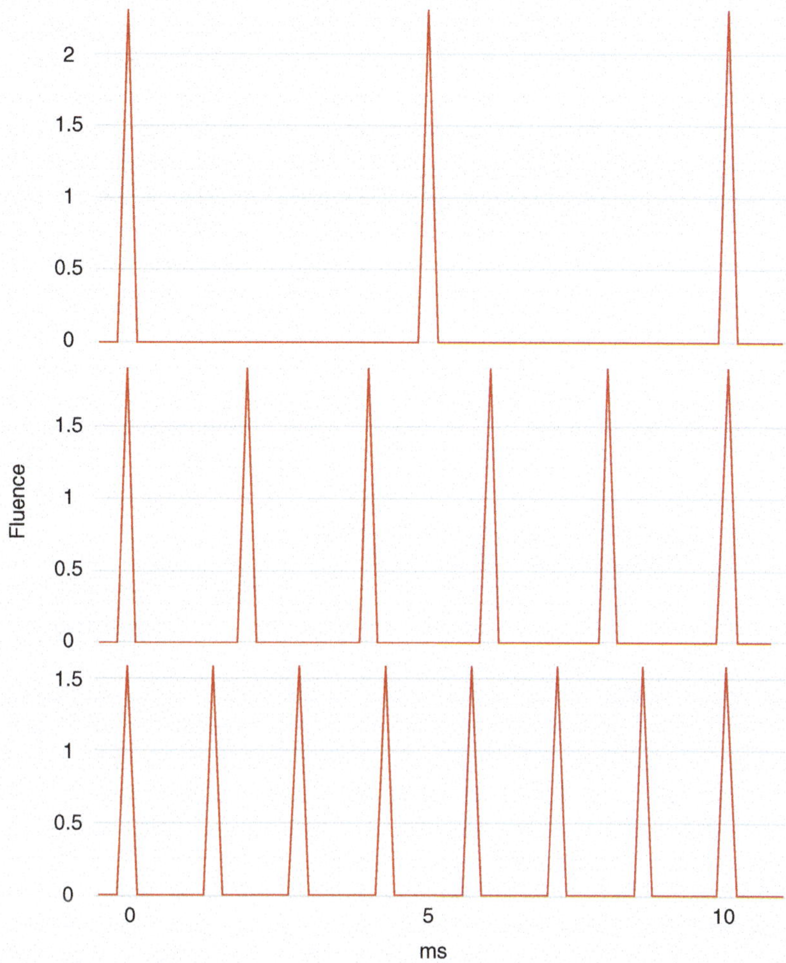

Fig. 6.19 Figure showing subpulse corresponding to purpura threshold at 10 ms pulse duration. The number of subpulses are 3, 6, 8 from top to bottom. Published with kind permission of © Jin Kwon Cho 2019. All rights reserved

above 88 °C, the minimum maintenance temperature. The higher the temperature of subpulse, the higher the minimum temperature at delay time. However, when the temperature of subpulse is too high that it exceeds 100 °C, purpura occurs. In particular, purpura will occur if chromophore concentration is high even though the energy of subpulse is the same. In addition, even if the temperature generated by subpulse does not exceed 100 °C, if high temperature is repeated, it is likely that purpura will occur because it eventually exceeds 100 °C. So how can the subpulse maintain the minimum maintenance temperature above 88 °C without exceeding 100 °C? This is done by increasing the number of subpulses. If the subpulse is irradiated before the temperature drops sufficiently in the delay time after the subpulse, the minimum maintenance temperature can be increased, while the subpulse temperature may be lowered. Therefore, it was reported that PDL with eight subpulses, compared to PDL with four subpulses in the past, reduced the energy of the subpulse, so there was no immediate or delayed purpura so that vascular treatment could be performed without downtime [28].

For reference, the shorter the pulse duration, the lower the energy of subpulse. For example, in Fig. 6.18, it can be seen that as the number of subpulses increases at pulse duration 6 ms, the increase of purpura threshold is small. This is because the energy of each subpulse decreases rapidly because there is not enough time for cooling between the subpulses.

Then what is the appropriate fluence in macropulse? Let's look again at Fig. 6.18 again. The graph in this figure depicts the fluence representing purpura threshold. The desired reaction is vessel contraction or vessel blockage due to intravascular coagulation without purpura. Therefore, energy that is lower than the purpura threshold should be irradiated. For example, the purpura threshold of PDL with eight subpulses at 20 ms is 16 J/cm^2. There are reports that PDL with eight subpulse at 20 ms treated successfully blood vessels below 600 μm without downtime only with fluence of 9–10 J/cm^2.

6.7 Parameters of Vascular Laser Therapy

Based on the above, let's summarize the laser parameters for vascular therapy.

First, depending on the wavelength, there are 500–600 nm wavelength lasers (532-nm long-pulsed laser, 585-nm PDL, 595-nm long-pulsed PDL, and IPL), 1064-nm long-pulsed Nd:YAG lasers and multiplex lasers that irradiated both 595 and 1064 nm. Among these, long-pulsed Nd:YAG lasers are cheaper to purchase or maintain. Since few Asians have erythema as the main symptom, the first laser I recommend is the 1064-nm long-pulsed Nd:YAG laser. Telangiectasia could be treated with Nd:YAG laser and erythema treatment may be first attempted with the Genesis technique. For treatment of unresolved erythema, an additional purchase of 595 nm long-pulsed PDL that is expensive but safe and effective may be needed. Second, pulse duration should start with 30–40 ms considering vascular thickness and thermal kinetic selectivity, and then reduced to 10 ms, 5 ms, 1.5 ms, or 450 μs sequentially while checking clinical end points. Third, Large spot sizes are good for deep penetration, but small spot sizes are better for long-pulsed Nd:YAG lasers. Fourth, fluence is determined by observing at clinical end points. The best clinical end point is vessel disappearance. Darkening is not the best clinical end point, but is considered as a good clinical end point. The rupture of blood vessels and the development of purpura may be considered as a clinical end point, but due to frequent recurrence and long downtime, I do not recommend this clinical endpoint. However when using long-pulsed Nd:YAG lasers, purpura should never occur. Therefore, energy that is equal to or lower than the fluence that causes vessel disappearance should be used. Fifth, fluence should be lower than purpura threshold, when using macropulse of PDL or multipulse of IPL. Stacking PDL or IPL is effective without any significant side effects, but long-pulsed Nd:YAG laser should never be stacked. Excessive residual heat may be generated and there is a high possibility of scarring. Sixth, epidermal cooling is essential for vascular treatment.

6.8 Side Effects of Vascular Laser Therapy

The use of vascular lasers may cause a variety of side effects. There may be pain. In PDL, there may be snapping and burning sensation. Topical anesthesia may be used to reduce pain. When using vascular laser, it is better to use topical anesthesia without vasoconstriction (tetracine, Ametop®) than topical anesthesia with vasoconstriction (lidocaine and prilocaine, Emla®) [1]. Also, after applying topical anesthesia, erythema sometimes appears, which can hinder treatment. In addition, it may be better not to apply topical anesthesia when treating blood vessels because the pain, which is a marker of possible side effects, may be eliminated and serious side effects may not be noticed.

Purpura (bruising) may occur, especially during PDL treatment, usually lasting 7–10 days, up to 15 days. Purpura cannot be covered by makeup, so sufficient consultation with the patient is required prior to treatment. Discoloration, blisters, or scabs are rare, but they can be caused by excessive treatment or energy. In these cases, the epidermis becomes gray or pale white after treatment. The patient should be advised to visit the hospital immediately if these phenomena occur and active treatment is required. Infections and herpes may occur, but this is not common. Hyperpigmentation or hypopigmentation may appear but this is also not common. Excessive energy may cause skin texture changes or scarring. Scars, in particular, are rare in PDL, but caution should be exercised in long-pulsed Nd:YAG lasers, have a high incidence and can be severe. The last side effect is lesion persistence (nonresponders), i.e., lesions that remain despite laser treatment.

6.9 Non-laser Treatments for Vascular and Erythema Treatment

So far, we have reviewed lasers for the treatment of blood vessels and erythema. However, vascular lasers, especially PDLs, are expensive to purchase and maintain. Is there a way to treat blood vessels and erythema without great cost? I suggest the following four methods.

First, a 1064-nm long-pulsed Nd:YAG laser may be used to perform the so-called Genesis technique. Schmults et al. performed Genesis technique on nine patients using a long-pulsed Nd:YAG laser and found that the thickness of collagen fibers decreased, skin quality improved, and erythema improved [29].

Second, CO_2 lasers can be used to treat blood vessels. Chung et al. used pinhole technique with 1 mm spot, 1 W, continuous mode using a CO_2 laser [30]. Papillary dermis was irradiated at intervals of 3 mm. A case of improved facial telangiectasia was reported. Of course, CO_2 laser pinhole therapy may have side effects such as PIH or blood vessel regeneration and recurrence. However, for a small number of telangiectasia, senile hemangioma, and spider hemangioma, CO_2 laser pinhole therapy may be used.

Third, botulinum toxin can be used. Bloom et al. mixed 300 units of botulinum toxin (Dysport) with 3 mL of normal saline and used a total of 15–45 units (average 25 units) to inject the skin of nose, cheeks, forehead, and chin resulting in erythema improvement [31]. Bloom et al. speculated that acetylcholine plays an important role in vasodilatation and that erythema improves because botulinum toxin inhibits acetylcholine. Kim et al. compared and observed 12-week progression of 24 mild-to-moderate erythematotelangiectatic type rosacea by subcutaneously injecting botulinum toxin into one cheek and normal saline in the other cheek [32]. The botulinum toxin (prabotulinum toxin A; NABOTA, Daewoong Pharmaceutical, Seoul, Korea) was mixed with normal saline to a very low concentration of 1 U per 0.1 mL. A total of 15 U was injected intradermally into 30 points with 0.05 mL at each point with intervals of 1 cm. The results showed that erythema improved from 4 to 8 weeks. In addition to erythema, increased skin elasticity and skin hydration were statistically significant.

Fourth, medication is possible. Although it is important to treat the blood vessels or the erythema itself, it is more important to know why they developed in the first place (Table 6.6). There are various causes of facial flushing or erythema, all of which can make the face to appear red. Therefore, detailed examination and accurate diagnosis should be made before laser treatment. If appropriate diagnosis is made, drug treatment alone may be sufficient. For example, acne should be treated with retinoids (isotretinoin) or antibiotics (doxycycline) before laser treatment. For atopic dermatitis, topical pimecrolimus (Elidel cream 1%) or tacrolimus cream may be administered. Mild steroid lotion or topical ketoconazole may be effective for seborrheic dermatitis on the face. For perioral dermatitis,

Table 6.6 Acute and chronic causes of a "red face" [33]

Acute	Chronic
Erysipelas Acute flare of eczema: • Atopic • Allergic contact or irritant Polymorphic light eruption Phototoxic eruptions	Acne vulgaris Acne fulminans Rosacea Pyoderma faciale Seborrheic eczema Perioral/orbital dermatitis Psoriasis Discoid lupus erythemtosus/ systmemic erythematosus Gram-negative folliculitis Drug induced: • Steroid • Immunomodulators • Epidermal growth factor receptor (EGFR) inhibitors

doxycycline for 6–12 weeks may have dramatic effects on erythema [33].

In particular, rosacea is one of the most common causes of erythema, so detailed examination and diagnosis are necessary. For the treatment of rosacea, topical metronidazole (MetroGel) can be used once a day and 20% azelaic acid can be used once or twice a day. Oral doxycycline 100–200 mg/day may be used. Isotretinoin 0.5 mg/kg/day for 20 weeks may be used as well. For flushing and erythema caused by rosacea, topical brimonidine gel 0.33% (Mirvaso gel) may be used as alpha2-adrenergic agonist. Even with a dose of a sweet pea, once a day may be effective. For flushing and erythema caused by rosacea, oral nonselective beta-adrenergic blocker carvedilol 3.125–6.25 mg can be gradually increased by two to three times a day to 31.25 mg. Significant improvement can be seen within 3 weeks [21].

Since perioral dermatitis or rosacea is a disease that is not cured and recurs continuously, accurate diagnosis, and sufficient explanation to the patient are important before starting treatment.

6.10 Treatment of Ecchymoses by Vascular Laser and IPL

Recently, as botulinum toxin or filler procedures have increased, interest in preventing and treating bruising caused by the procedure has increased. In particular, many studies have been conducted to quickly remove bruises by vascular laser or IPL.

First, let's summarize various terms for bruises [34]. Ecchymoses refers to the phenomenon of extravasation of blood out of ruptured blood vessels, causing the skin to turn red or blue. It is usually a patch of 1 cm or more, with broad and ambiguous boundaries. Ecchymosis is not telangiectasia, so does not disappear by diascopy. Causes include both traumatic and nontraumatic causes. Bruises, on the other hand, are ecchymoses caused by damage. Therefore, the phenomenon that occurs after botulinum toxin or filler procedure is a bruise, which belongs to ecchymoses.

Purpura has a clear border with dark purple spots or patches that are 4–10 mm in size. Purpura is closer to rash than bruise. Diascopy test is needed for differential diagnosis with telangiectasia. Unlike ecchymoses, purpura is not caused by damage, but rather by infection, medication, and blood clotting disorders. Petechiae have the same cause and symptoms as purpura, but is smaller than 4 mm, which results from capillaries bursting.

Ecchymoses are usually accompanied by pain and inflammation of surrounding tissues and the color of the skin changes sequentially as oxyHb degrades. In the clinical course of ecchymoses, red blood cells (RBCs) leaking out of blood vessels are first broken down and Hb is released, turning the skin red. Within 1–2 days, the red iron in the blood changes and the skin turns from red to blue or purple. At 6 days, the skin turns green and at 9 days, heme breaks down into biliverdin (green) and bilirubin (yellow), turning the skin yellowish-brown. Most ecchymoses recover within 2–3 weeks and return to normal skin color.

The most common areas of bruise after filler procedures are perioral and periorbital areas and in the skin layer, it occurs just below the skin, in superficial dermal and immediate subdermal planes. Deeper injections are known to reduce bruises and fanning or threading techniques are known to increase the possibility of bruises. In particular, less bruise occurs with the use of deeper bolus injection technique on pre-periosteal level. Among patients, middle-aged and old-age patients are more prone to bruises due to thin skin and subcutaneous fat layer and reduced blood clotting function.

Preventive measures to reduce bruise during filler procedures include first, cessation of anticoagulants such as aspirin or warfarin (aspirin, warfarin, dipyridamole, clopidogrel, nonsteroidal anti-inflammatory drugs (NSAIDs), fish oil, vitamin E supplements, St. John's Wort, garlic tablets, gingko biloba, and ginseng) 10 days prior to procedure. Second, the most thin needle or blunt cannula should be used, injection should be slow, and the number of injection points should be minimized. Third, ice packs or cold compression should be applied for a few minutes immediately after injection. Fourth, patients must be instructed to avoid vigorous exercise during the first 24 h to avoid raising blood pressure.

Traditionally, simple observation has been known as the treatment of choice for treatment of bruises that have already occurred [35]. Cold compression, 15% hydrogen peroxide or OTC (over-the-counter) products such as vitamin K cream have been used, but they have not been very effective.

Recently, many studies have been conducted on the treatment of bruises using vascular lasers such as PDL and IPL [34]. DeFatta RJ et al. irradiated PDL (V-beam, Candela) with 10 mm spot size of 6 J/cm^2 and 10 ms to 20 patients with postoperative ecchymoses. The results showed that ecchymoses decreased in 63% of patients and early PDL-treated patients had better results. Karen et al. irradiated PDL at 7.5 J/cm^2 and 6 ms with a 10 mm spot size to 10 patients. The results showed that the size of the bruises of the PDL-exposed sites was much lower than that of the non-PDL-exposed sites, and that the most effective treatment was when PDL was irradiated 24–48 h after damage, when Hb was the most frequent. Mayo et al. reported that the use of PDL immediately after procedure was more effective than cold compression, hydrogen peroxide, and bruise creams. Alegre-Sánchez et al. observed bruises almost disappeared or improved significantly 24 h after PDL procedure, and observed that bruises that were shallow, darker and had less edema were more susceptible to treatment than bruises that were deep, had less color change and had severe edema. Verner I et al. irradiated IPL (Dye-VL module, Alma Beauty Rejuve, Alma Lasers US, Buffalo Grove, IL) with wavelengths from 500 to 600 nm at 7–10 J/cm^2, 10 ms, 3 cm^2 spot size to 11 patients who had bruises after filler procedure [34]. The results showed that all the bruises improved 48 h after IPL all bruises improved.

The mechanism by which vascular laser improves bruises is not yet accurate, but it is thought that when the laser is irradiated to the Hb of the red blood cells leaking out of the blood vessel, the energy is transferred to the cell membrane and the cell membrane is deformed and cell lysis occurs, improving bruises [36]. Less efficacy in PDL treatment for late bruises, compared to early bruises are thought to be because of bilirubin. Bilirubin has a yellow color and the absorption curve is the highest at 460 nm, which is very far from 585 nm or 595 nm used in PDL lasers, so it is difficult to treat bilirubin with PDL because its absorption is low. Yellow bruises are a late phenomenon, so PDL should be used early. For the same reason, it is thought that bruises that are deep, have less color change and have severe edema are less susceptible to treatment because there is less Hb, the chromophore and the laser is at a depth difficult to penetrate.

Alegre-Sánchez A et al. irradiated PDL using 10 mm spot size at various pulse durations (0.5 vs. 6 ms) and various energies (5 J/cm^2 vs. 8 J/cm^2) [36]. As a result, it was found that the method of using high energy (8 J/cm^2) at short pulse durations (0.5 ms) was the most effective. However, high-energy parameters at short pulse durations may cause patient discomfort and side effects such as scabs, blisters, temporary pigmentation changes, and even aggravation of bruises. Therefore, in bruises after cosmetic procedures such as fillers, low energy at long pulse duration is recommended.

References

1. Allemann IB, Goldberg DJ (2011) Basics in dermatological laser applications. Karger Medical and Scientific Publishers
2. Goldman MP (2006) Cutaneous and cosmetic laser surgery. Mosby Elsevier, Philadelphia, PA
3. Nouri K (2018) Lasers in dermatology and medicine: dermatologic applications. Springer International Publishing
4. Park SH, Yeo WC, Koh WS, Park JW, Noh NK, Yoon CS (2014) Laser dermatology plastic surgery, 2nd edn. (Korean). Koonja, Seoul
5. Anderson RR, Parrish JA (1983) Selective photothermolysis: precise microsurgery by selective absorption of pulsed radiation. Science 220(4596): 524–527
6. Ross EV, Domankevitz Y (2005) Laser treatment of leg veins: physical mechanisms and theoretical considerations. Lasers Surg Med 36(2):105–116
7. Raulin C, Karsai S (2011) Laser and IPL technology in dermatology and aesthetic medicine. Heidelberg: New York

8. Keyvan N (2012) Lasers in dermatology and medicine. Springer-Verlag, London
9. Welch AJ, Gemert MJCV (2011) Optical-thermal response of laser-irradiated tissue. Dordrecht: London
10. Mirkov M, Sherr EA, Sierra RA, Lloyd JR, Tanghetti E (2006) Analytical modeling of laser pulse heating of embedded biological targets: an application to cutaneous vascular lesions. J Appl Phys 99(11):114701
11. Issa MCA, Tamura B (2018) Lasers, lights and other technologies. Springer
12. (2000) Appendix. Laryngoscope 110(S95):31–37
13. Ross EV, Smirnov M, Pankratov M, Altshuler G (2005) Intense pulsed light and laser treatment of facial telangiectasias and dyspigmentation: some theoretical and practical comparisons. Dermatol Surg 31(9 Pt 2):1188–1198
14. Ross EV, Meehan KJ, Domankevitz Y, Trafeli JP, Annandono J, Jacoby M (2010) Use of a variable long-pulse alexandrite laser in the treatment of facial telangiectasia. Dermatol Surg 36(4):470–474
15. Stratigos A, Dover JS (2000) Overview of lasers and their properties. Dermatol Ther 13(1):2–16
16. Kauvar A, Hruza G (2005) Principles and practices in cutaneous laser surgery. CRC Press
17. Kimel S, Svaasand LO, Cao D, Hammer-Wilson MJ, Nelson JS (2002) Vascular response to laser photothermolysis as a function of pulse duration, vessel type, and diameter: implications for port wine stain laser therapy. Lasers Surg Med 30(2):160–169
18. Lee W (2008) Principles of IPL and its uses (Korean). MDworld, Seoul
19. Christiansen K, Drosner M, Bjerring P (2015) Optimized settings for Nd:YAG laser treatments of leg telangiectasias. J Cosmet Laser Ther 17(2):69–76
20. Altshuler GB, Anderson RR, Manstein D, Zenzie HH, Smirnov MZ (2001) Extended theory of selective photothermolysis. Lasers Surg Med 29(5):416–432
21. Habif TP (2015) Clinical dermatology. Elsevier, St. Louis, MO
22. Wanner M, Sakamoto FH, Avram MM, Chan HH, Alam M, Tannous Z et al (2016) Immediate skin responses to laser and light treatments: therapeutic endpoints: how to obtain efficacy. J Am Acad Dermatol 74(5):821–833. quiz 34, 33
23. Suthamjariya K, Farinelli WA, Koh W, Anderson RR (2004) Mechanisms of microvascular response to laser pulses. J Invest Dermatol 122(2):518–525
24. Wang T, Chen D, Yang J, Ma G, Yu W, Lin X (2018) Safety and efficacy of dual-wavelength laser (1064 + 595 nm) for treatment of non-treated port-wine stains. J Eur Acad Dermatol Venereol 32(2):260–264
25. Yang MU, Yaroslavsky AN, Farinelli WA, Flotte TJ, Rius-Diaz F, Tsao SS et al (2005) Long-pulsed neodymium:yttrium-aluminum-garnet laser treatment for port-wine stains. J Am Acad Dermatol 52(3 Pt 1):480–490
26. Murphy MJ, Torstensson PA (2014) Thermal relaxation times: an outdated concept in photothermal treatments. Lasers Med Sci 29(3):973–978
27. Tanghetti E (2003) Extended pulse format dye laser and its effects on therapeutic efficacy. Lasers Surg Med 15:29
28. Ross EV, Uebelhoer NS, Domankevitz Y (2007) Use of a novel pulse dye laser for rapid single-pass purpura-free treatment of telangiectases. Dermatol Surg 33(12):1466–1469
29. Schmults CD, Phelps R, Goldberg DJ (2004) Nonablative facial remodeling: erythema reduction and histologic evidence of new collagen formation using a 300-microsecond 1064-nm Nd:YAG laser. Arch Dermatol 140(11):1373–1376
30. Chung BY, Han SS, Moon HR, Lee MW, Chang SE (2014) Treatment with the pinhole technique using erbium-doped yttrium aluminium garnet laser for a cafe au lait macule and carbon dioxide laser for facial telangiectasia. Ann Dermatol 26(5):657–659
31. Bloom BS, Payongayong L, Mourin A, Goldberg DJ (2015) Impact of intradermal abobotulinumtoxinA on facial erythema of rosacea. Dermatol Surg 41(Suppl 1):S9–S16
32. Kim MJ, Kim JH, Cheon HI, Hur MS, Han SH, Lee YW et al (2019) Assessment of skin physiology change and safety after intradermal injections with botulinum toxin: a randomized, double-blind, placebo-controlled, split-face pilot study in rosacea patients with facial erythema. Dermatol Surg 45(9):1155–1162
33. Layton AM (2009) Dermatological causes of a 'red face'. Medicine 37(5):249–254
34. Verner I, Prag Naveh H, Bertossi D (2019) Treatment of injection-induced ecchymoses with light/laser-assisted technology. Dermatol Ther 32(3):e12861
35. Jeong GJ, Kwon HJ, Park KY, Kim BJ (2018) Pulsed-dye laser as a novel therapeutic approach for post-filler bruises. Dermatol Ther 31(6):e12721
36. Alegre-Sanchez A, Saceda-Corralo D, Segurado-Miravalles G, de Perosanz-Lobo D, Fonda-Pascual P, Moreno-Arrones OM et al (2018) Pulsed dye laser on ecchymoses: clinical and histological assessment. Lasers Med Sci 33(3):683–688

7 Pigment Lasers

7.1 Pigmented Lesions in Darker Skin

Darker skin, unlike Caucasians, has the following characteristics of pigmented lesions [1]. First, pigmentary changes such as lentigines and seborrheic keratosis are major features of photoaging in darker skin, while wrinkling is a major feature of photoaging in Caucasians. Second, women of darker skin are susceptible to melasma and acquired bilateral nevus of Ota-like macules (ABNOM). Third, the main goal of pigmentation treatment of darker skin is postinflammatory hyperpigmentation (PIH). Fourth, people with darker skin are less likely to have melanoma, and therefore, when removing congenital melanin lesions such as the nevus of Ota or congenital melanocytic nevi (CMN), there is less concern for skin cancer.

Pigmented lesions are in demand in darker skin, and even though the risk of skin cancer is low, due to side effects such as PIH, this is not an area that can be easily treated with lasers.

7.2 Mechanism of Pigment Removal

7.2.1 Types of Pigment Lasers

Pigment lasers can be classified into Q-switched lasers, long-pulsed lasers, ablative lasers, and fractional lasers according to their mechanisms (Table 7.1) [1]. There are currently three Q-switched lasers: 694-nm ruby laser, 755-nm alexandrite laser, and Nd:YAG laser that produces two wavelengths of 1064 and 532 nm. There are two long-pulsed lasers: 532-nm long-pulsed KTP lasers and 755-nm long-pulsed alexandrite lasers.

One type of long-pulsed laser is the 1064-nm long-pulsed Nd:YAG laser. However, this laser is not used for pigment treatment. The reason why the long-pulsed Nd:YAG laser is not used for pigment treatment is as follows. First, in the treatment of epidermal pigmentations, the 1064-nm wavelength has low epidermis absorption due to the epidermal bypass effect. Increasing the flu-

Table 7.1 Types of pigment lasers by mechanism

Mechanisms	Types of pigment laser
Pigment-selective Q-switched lasers	Q-switched ruby laser (694 nm, 25 ns) Q-switched alexandrite laser (755 nm, 50–100 ns) Q-switched Nd:YAG laser (1064 nm, 532 nm, 5–15 ns)
Less-selective long-pulsed lasers	Long-pulsed laser (532 nm, 755 nm) IPL
Non-pigment-specific ablative lasers	CO_2 laser Er:YAG laser
Non-pigment-specific fractional lasers	1550-nm Er:Glass laser (Fraxel®) CO_2 pinhole method

J. D. Lee et al., *Principles and Choice of Laser Treatment in Dermatology*,
https://doi.org/10.1007/978-981-15-6556-4_7

ence to compensate for the low absorption coefficient increases the risk of burns in the dermis. Second, in the treatment of dermal pigmentations, long-pulsed lasers cannot be used for treatment if cells are scattered independently, such as nevus of Ota or ABNOM (thermal kinetic selectivity, TKS). Third, melanocytic nevi can be cured, but the therapeutic window is very narrow due to bulk heating, as explained in Sect. 6.5.1 in "Chap. 6."

IPL is not a laser but can be included as a long-pulsed laser of the pigment laser because it exhibits a photothermal effect like a long-pulsed laser with a millisecond pulse duration. Ablative lasers are CO_2 lasers and Er:YAG lasers. Some may not consider fractional lasers as pigment lasers, but I included them in pigment lasers because of the melanin shuttle phenomenon.

7.2.2 Melanin Shuttle

Fractional lasers do not irradiate the entire skin, but instead irradiates parts of the skin, leaving normal tissue between the beams, so that the regeneration of the tissue from the normal tissues is faster, reducing side effects (fractional photothermolysis). The area irradiated with a fractional laser beam is called the microscopic treatment zone (MTZ), and the tissue that is irradiated, necrotized, and is pushed out of the skin is called microscopic epidermal necrotic debris (MEND) (Fig. 7.1). Since MEND contains not only epidermal keratinocytes but also melanin in keratinocytes, laser texts often refer to them as "melanin shuttle." Although the term MEND includes "epidermal," it also includes dermal tissue because fractional laser beam reaches the dermal layer and may also include dermal melanin pigmentations. Therefore, a fractional laser can theoretically be applied to both epidermal and dermal pigmentation treatments.

7.2.3 Mechanism of Pigment Removal

How is melanin pigment removed? Let's think about the epidermis and the dermis separately. First, let's look at the pigment removal process of the epidermis.

Kawada et al. performed biopsies over time after the treatment of lentigines with IPL (Fig. 7.2) [2]. The results show that 30 min after the IPL procedure, a subepidermal cleft begins to form under the epidermis. After 24 h, epidermis

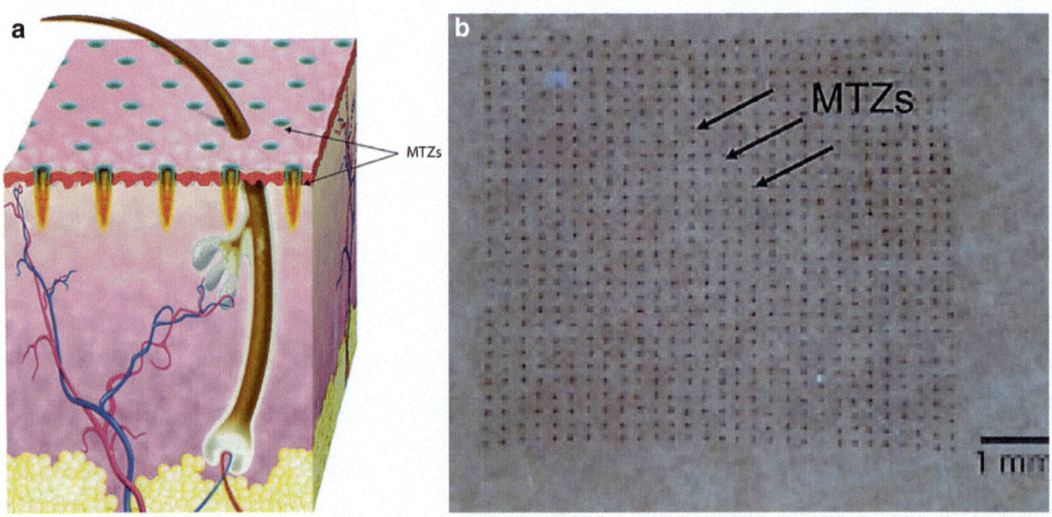

Fig. 7.1 (**a**) Schematic picture of FP (fractional photothermolysis) depicting MTZs (microscopic treatment zones) surrounded by unharmed tissue. (**b**) Clinical picture depicting MTZs surrounded by unharmed tissue. (Reproduced from [1])

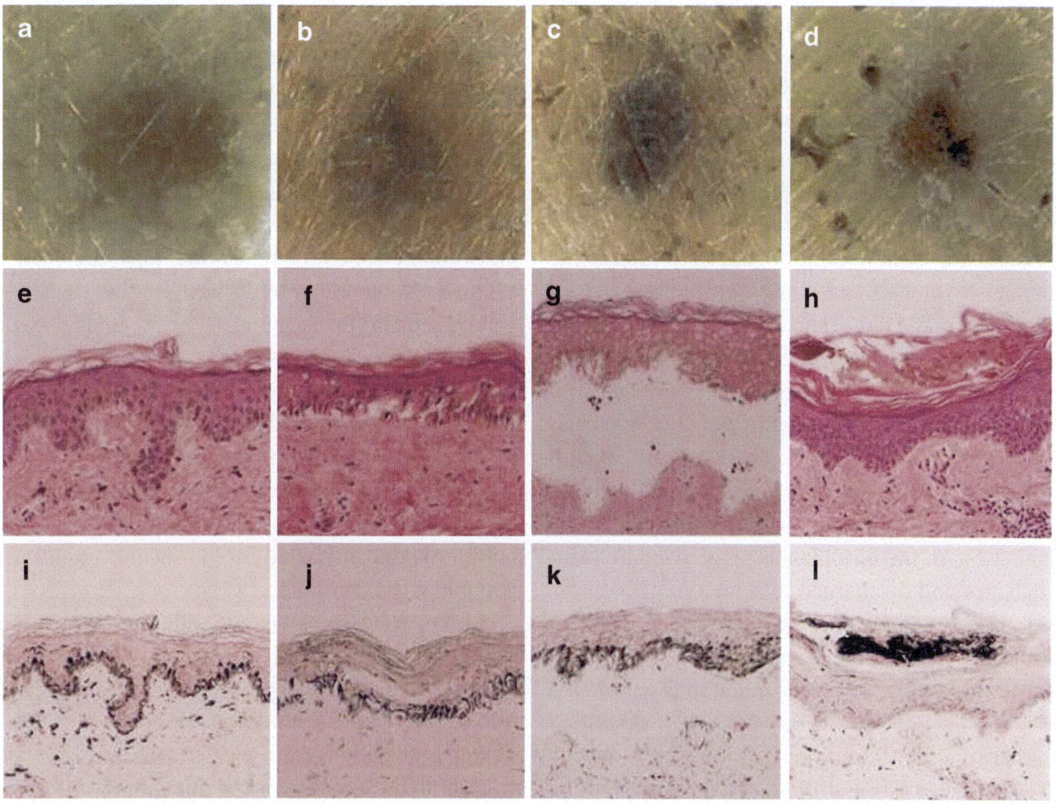

Fig. 7.2 Sequential videoscopic (**a**–**d**) and histopathological findings (**e**–**l**) of pigment spots of solar lentigines. Pigment spots at pre-irradiation (**a**, **e**, **i**), 30 min (**b**, **f**, **j**), 24 h (**c**, **g**, **k**), and 7 days (**d**, **h**, **l**) after irradiation of intense pulsed light were shown (**e**–**h**, hematoxylin-eosin staining; **i**–**l**, Masson–Fontana staining; ×200). (Reproduced from [2])

degeneration and worsening of cracks are observed. A week later, crust removal and regeneration of a new layer of the epidermis were observed.

In other words, the mechanism of epidermal pigment removal using IPL is as follows. The epidermal pigment coagulates and the rapid differentiation of pigmented keratinocytes are induced by thermal heating, and new keratinocyte and new epidermal layers are formed (epidermal turnover), resulting in pushing out the coagulated epidermal pigment.

Therefore, pigments are removed from the epidermis in two ways (Table 7.2). First, Q-switched lasers or long-pulsed lasers coagulate and crust epidermal tissues, accelerate epidermal turnover, regenerate new epidermal layers, and eject crusts out of the epidermis. Second, the pigment can be removed by ablating the skin tissue with ablative lasers such as the CO_2 laser.

Table 7.2 Mechanism of pigment removal by pigment location [3].

Pigment location	Mechanisms of pigment removal
Epidermis	1. Epidermal turnover within the crust 2. Ablation
Dermis	1. Epidermal turnover within the crust 2. Transported lymphatically 3. Rephagocytosis by local macrophages 4. MEND—"Melanin shuttle"

In the dermis, pigments are removed in four ways. Consider the process of removing tattoo pigment with a Q-switched laser [1]. Fibroblasts contain tattoo ink. Shooting a Q-switched laser explodes the tattoo ink and breaks the fibroblast. Histologically, a "ring cell" is created in which a cavity is formed in the fibroblast and the tattoo ink is dispersed around the cell. Visually, it appears as a whitening phenomenon. At this time, the tattoo pigment is removed in three ways. First, some exploded tattoo ink may escape the dermal layer and reach the epidermal layer or may even come out of the epidermal layer. Tattoo ink that reaches the epidermal layer is removed through epidermal turnover, one of the mechanisms of epidermal pigment removal. However, this is not a common case, and only occurs with very high energy, and is not recommended due to side effects. Second, a portion of tattoo ink that comes out of the fibroblast is phagotized by macrophages and discharged into the lymphatic vessel. Third, some tattoo inks are phagotized by fibroblasts and remain trapped around blood vessels. And last, the dermal pigment is also removed through the MEND of fractional laser described earlier (melanin shuttle).

Then what is the difference between pigment removal of the epidermis and the dermis?

First, long-pulsed lasers cannot be used to treat dermal pigments. Except for tattoos, TRTs of dermal pigmented lesions such as ABNOM, nevus of Ota, and dermal melasma, have TRTs of cell units, 1–30 μs. This is because the cells are separated from each other and exist as independent cells. Therefore, the treatment of dermal pigmented lesions has no effect when irradiated with millisecond long-pulsed laser due to thermal kinetic selectivity (TKS). However, tattoo and congenital nevi have a high risk of scarring even with a little high energy [1]. This is because when the temperature is higher than coagulation, there is no problem in the epidermal layer but burns and scarring may occur in the dermal layer.

Second, if the dermal pigment is removed with an ablative laser, there is a high risk of scarring. For example, the CO_2 laser may be used to cut the epidermis and the dermis to remove the pigments from the dermis, but there is a high probability of scarring due to poor skin regeneration. At this point, we will review wound healing.

Wound healing can be divided into primary, secondary, and third intention (wound closure), depending on how the wound is closed [4]. First, the primary intention is the closure of wounds immediately after injuries. Examples are surgical wounds and clean lacerations. Scars are less likely to occur because of the approximation of the wound edge by a thread, glue, tape, mechanical devices, or skin graft or flap. Second, the secondary intention is how open wounds heal. Granulation tissue formation and epithelialization take place. Myofibroblasts appear on the third day of the wound to enhance skin barrier function recovery, resulting in wound contracture. Third, the tertiary intention is a method in which the wound is closed by the first intention, but the wound is healed by the second intention due to wound dehiscence.

There are two ways of epithelialization in secondary intention. First, epithelialization proceeds as keratinocytes proliferate and migrate in the normal epidermal basal layer around the wound. Second, keratinocytes differentiate and epithelialize from epidermal appendages of epidermal origin, such as the eccrine gland, apocrine gland, hair, and nails [5]. Therefore, if the epidermis and only part of the dermis are damaged (split-thickness wound), the epithelialization is good with the help of both methods, and the skin barrier function is well restored without granuloma. But if the epidermis and the deep dermis is damaged (full-thickness wound), there is no epidermal appendage, so the epithelialization occurs by the keratinocytes from the normal epidermal basal layer around the wound, delaying the recovery of skin barrier function resulting in granuloma formation and eventually scarring (Fig. 7.3) [6].

This method of removing pigmentation by burning the epidermal and dermal layers with a CO_2 laser is likely to cause side effects, so dermal pigmentations should not be treated with ablative lasers. However, if the range is very narrow, even full-thickness wounds may not be a problem for regeneration. When a 2–3 mm punch biopsy is performed for tissue biopsy and the wound is left without suture, it is known that there is no problem cosmetically despite the slow regeneration

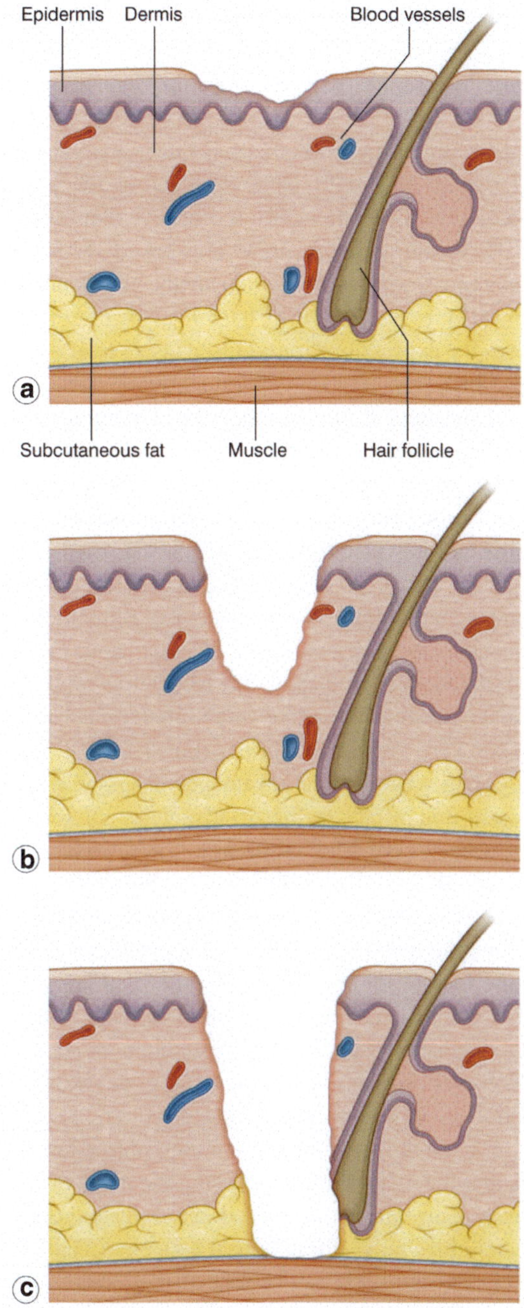

Fig. 7.3 Comparison of erosion, partial-thickness, and full-thickness wounds. (**a**) Erosion: only the epidermis is lost. (**b**) Partial-thickness wound: the epidermis and part of the dermis are missing but some adnexal structures remain. (**c**) Full-thickness wound: all of the epidermis and dermis along with adnexal structures are missing. The full-thickness skin loss involves the subcutaneous fat tissue and may extend down to, but not through, the underlying fascia. (Reproduced from [7])

Table 7.3 Type of pigment laser by location

Epidermal melanin lesions	Dermal melanin lesions
1. Q-switched laser (532 nm, 694 nm, 755 nm) 2. Long-pulsed laser (532 nm, 755 nm), IPL 3. Ablative laser (CO_2, Er:YAG laser) 4. Fractional laser, pinhole method	1. Q-switched laser (694 nm, 755 nm, 1064 nm) 2. Fractional laser, pinhole method

time [6]. Therefore, treatment with very thin beams such as fractional lasers or pinhole therapy with CO_2 lasers can be used to treat dermal pigmentations by reducing side effects.

7.2.4 Types of Pigment Lasers by Location

Considering the mechanism of pigmentation removal as described earlier, pigment lasers of the epidermal layer and dermal layer can be classified as follows (Table 7.3). Epidermal pigmented lesions can be treated with Q-switched lasers, long-pulsed lasers, ablative lasers, fractional lasers, or pinhole methods. Dermal pigmented lesions can only be cured with Q-switched lasers and fractional laser or pinhole methods. Let's remember that only two lasers can be used, especially for dermal pigmented lesions.

7.2.5 Photothermal Versus Photomechanical Effect

What specific changes do photothermal and photomechanical effects cause in the skin? Also, what is the difference between long-pulsed lasers that mainly produce a photothermal effect and Q-switched lasers that mainly produce a photomechanical effect, and which laser is more effective for pigment treatment and has fewer side effects?

Lee et al. analyzed why more PIH occurs in ABNOM and less PIH occur in Ota nevus when treated with Q-switched lasers by comparing biopsy results [8]. The results of the biopsy are as follows. In the case of ABNOM and Nevus of Ota, melanocytes are distributed in the dermal layer, but ABNOM is mainly distributed in the upper dermis with many blood vessels, and Nevus of Ota is distributed throughout the dermis.

The melanocytes of ABNOM are close to the epidermis and are mainly distributed in the upper dermis with many blood vessels. Why does this cause more PIH? Treatment of ABNOM with a Q-switched laser breaks the melanosomes of melanocytes in upper dermis due to shock wave of photomechanical effect. I think the expression 'explosion' is more correct. The exploded melanosomes and shock waves can damage the nuclei of melanocytes and destroy melanocyte walls. Furthermore, the surrounding blood vessels and epidermal cells can burst. When blood vessels burst, the purpura may form, and PIH is generated by nitric oxide (NO) in the blood vessels. In addition, epidermal cell damage results in the release of cytokines such as prostaglandin (PG) and leukotriene (LT). On the other hand, nevus of Ota has relatively little damage to surrounding blood vessels or epidermal cells, resulting in less PIH. In other words, Q-switched lasers using photomechanical effects damage not only melanosomes or melanocytes that we want but also the surrounding normal tissue. Therefore, side effects such as PIH appear.

What about long-pulsed lasers that mainly generates a photothermal effect? In the treatment of lentigines, the use of a long-pulsed laser first raises the temperature of melanosomes, which in turn increases the temperature of melanocytes or keratinocytes containing melanosomes. Adjusting the pulse duration will raise the temperature of the basal layer that consists of melanocytes and keratinocytes. For example, if the temperature rises to the point where coagulation occurs (typically about 70 °C), basal layer coagulates and degenerates, eventually falling out of the epidermal layer. What about the other tissues next to the basal layer? As the heat transfers from the basal layer, the temperature of other tissues will increase, but not as high as 70 °C but around 65 °C, and the temperature of the tissue next to it will be lower around 60 °C. In conclusion, the basal layer coagulates and the temperature of surrounding tissues also rise, but no degeneration occurs.

Treatment by photothermal effect coagulates (I call it "baking") without affecting the surrounding tissues. In addition, I believe that fewer PIHs occur because they are baked without breaking the cell walls, which are the main causes of PIH (see Sect. 4.7 in "Chap. 4"). One laser text uses the expression "long-pulsed lasers treat gently" [9].

Yamashita et al. examined the change of lentigines after irradiating IPL and 694-nm Q-switched ruby laser. After irradiating Q-switched ruby laser, crusts were observed by transmission electron microscope (TEM) [11]. Broken melanosomes, denatured melanosomes, and vacuole after the disappearance of the melanosomes were observed. On the other hand, TEM observed that even after the irradiation of IPL, intact melanosomes like intact epidermal basal layer were found in the crusts (Fig. 7.4) [10].

Then what are the advantages of Q-switched lasers and what are the disadvantages of long-pulsed lasers? The advantages of Q-switched lasers are as follows. Despite the possibility of PIH with increased energy, it can completely eliminate melanocytes or keratinocytes that contain melanosomes. Thus, perfect treatment is possible. So, in Caucasians with low risk of PIH, Q-switched laser is the best pigment laser. However, Koreans have a high risk of developing PIH, making Q-switched lasers unsuitable [12].

One of the disadvantages of long-pulsed lasers is that there is a limit in reducing the pulse duration. Currently, long-pulsed alexandrite lasers can reduce pulse duration to 0.1–0.3 ms. That is, only the cell layer can be treated. Since melanocyte TRT is 1–30 μs, cells themselves cannot be cured [13]. But on the contrary, this might be an advantage. For example, if there are lentigines in the epidermis and ABNOM in the dermis, treatment with a long-pulsed alexandrite laser will treat the lentigines in the epidermis, and the ABNOM in the dermis will be spared due to thermal kinetic selectivity [9]. Thus, ABNOM is not affected. In other words, when melanocytes such

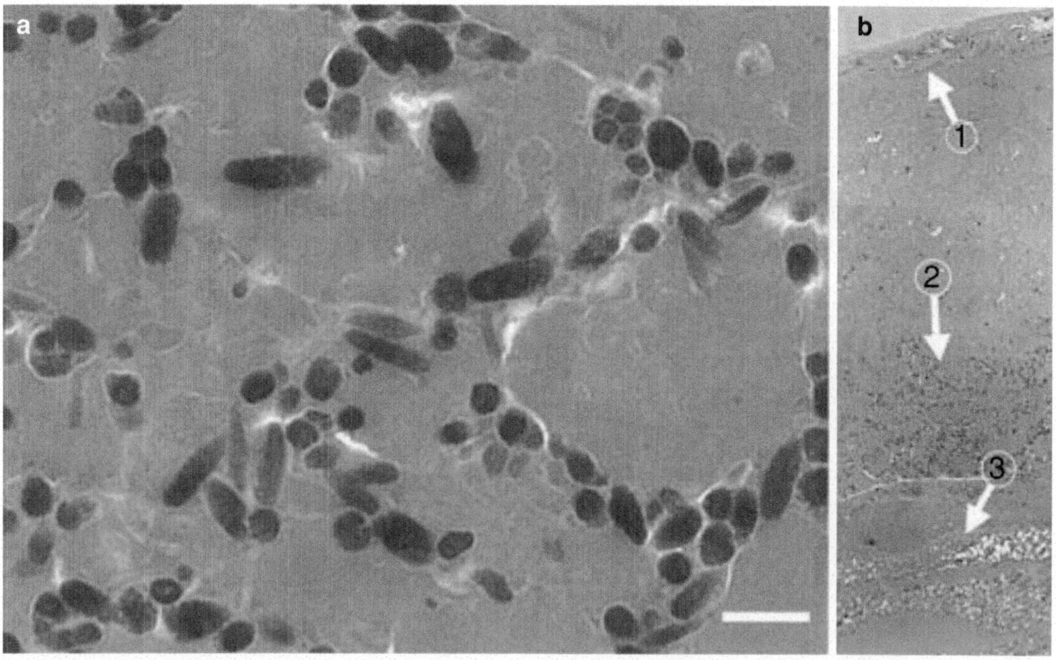

Fig. 7.4 Microscopic structure of microcrust imaged by TEM (transmission electron microscopy). Many melanosomes are observed in the microcrust that sloughed off the skin surface of a pigmented spot. (**a**) Melanosomes in the microcrust. (**b**) The vertical block image of the microcrust constructed by TEM images. Arrows 1–3 show: the stratum corneum, melanosomes, and a part of the newly synthesized stratum corneum, respectively. Bar = 500 nm. (Reproduced from [10])

as ABNOM, nevus of Ota, and dermal melasma are sparsely distributed in the dermal layer, the treatment of epidermis with long-pulsed laser does not affect the dermis. After the epidermis is treated, melanocytes in the dermal layer can be treated with a Q-switched laser. However, side effects may occur in the case of nevus consisting of a cell layer or a cell nest or in tattoos in which particles are aggregated [9]. Therefore, when using long-pulsed lasers, caution should be taken in areas with nevus or tattoo.

In laser texts, it was described that when epidermal pigmented lesions were treated with CO_2, Q-switched, and long-pulsed lasers, 50%, 10%, 1% PIH occurred, respectively [1, 14]. Long-pulsed laser has the fewest side effects, but they have to be repeated several times. Chan et al. found that when treating lentigines 532-nm Q-switched and 532-nm long-pulsed lasers were equally effective. But 532-nm Q-switched lasers had a higher risk, and when Q-switched alexandrite lasers and long-pulsed alexandrite lasers were compared, the results showed that both had the same effect, but the Q-switched laser had 22% PIH and long-pulsed lasers 6%. Finally, they concluded that long-pulsed alexandrite lasers are safe [12].

In theory and papers, we can see that long-pulsed lasers are safer than Q-switched lasers. However, there are some things to watch out for in long-pulsed lasers. Pulse stacking is possible for Q-switched lasers, but long-pulsed lasers have a high risk of side effects after pulse stacking (Fig. 7.5). For example, even though the first and second irradiations may be OK, the third irradiation may cause skin blanching or white discoloration due to residual heat accumulation. Skin blanching or white discoloration suggests a sign of necrosis [9]. Therefore, long-pulsed lasers need to be treated with one shot, then cooled for a sufficient time and then re-irradiated, or post cooling should be used for pulse stacking. For example, when treating certain lentigines with a long-pulsed laser, a desired clinical endpoint

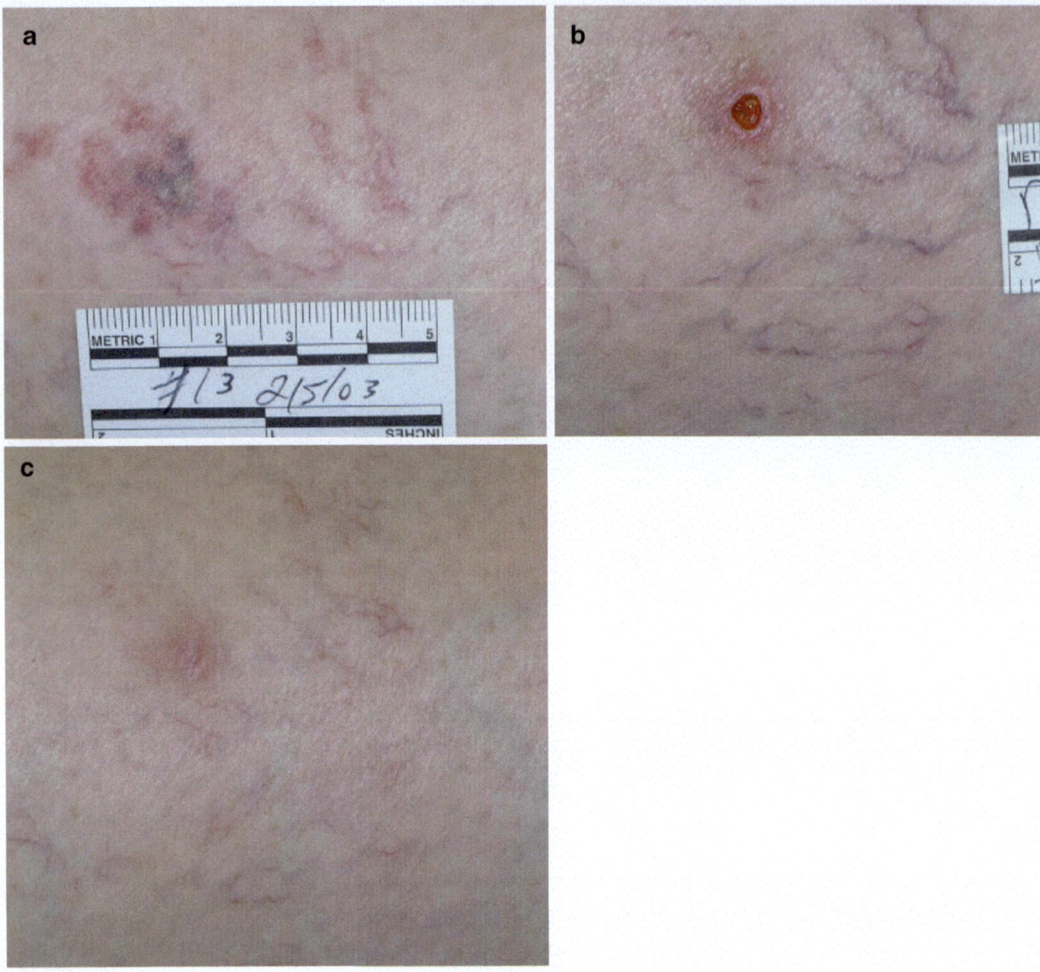

Fig. 7.5 It shows ulceration and healing after inadvertent stacking at one site: 1064-nm pulse, 6-mm spot, 200 J/cm^2, convective cold air chilling, 2 pulses at 1 Hz. (**a**) One day after treatment—note white color is the harbinger of necrosis. (**b**) Three weeks later, ulceration has occurred. (**c**) After 4 months, the ulcer has healed with a small scar. (Reproduced from [15])

does not occur after one shot, immediately re-irradiating may cause burns.

Therefore, I first irradiate the lentigines in the entire face with one pass with the same fluence with a long-pulsed alexandrite laser. During the second pass, only the lentigines without clinical end points (in the case of lentigines, darkening, and perilesional erythema) are re-irradiated. At this time, the lentigines first irradiated were sufficiently cooled before the second pass. Another method is to irradiate the lentigines and then cool it by an ice cube, or in urgent cases, I use my finger to absorb heat and re-irradiate.

7.3 Wavelength

7.3.1 Pigment Laser for Koreans

Then what kind of pigment laser should I buy?

As explained in "Chap. 2," theoretically, the photothermal effect is safer than photoacoustic effect, and as described earlier, when treating epidermal pigmented lesions, the incidence of PIH was said to be high in the order of long-pulsed lasers, Q-switch lasers, and ablative lasers. On the contrary, which laser has the most obvious effect? Theoretically, Q-switched lasers break cells, so pigment can be removed with just one procedure, hence, Q-switched lasers can be considered the most effective. However, Q-switched lasers can eliminate melanocytes with dark melanosomes, but they can't get rid of melanocytes with light melanosomes. On the other hand, the most effective laser is the ablative laser because, despite PIH, ablative laser burns not only pigments but also the surrounding tissue. Therefore, in order of effectiveness (the opposite of the order of safety), the three lasers are ablative lasers, Q-switched lasers, and long-pulsed lasers.

Specific wavelengths are as follows (Table 7.4): Due to epidermal bypass effect, in order to treat epidermal pigmentations, wavelengths below 800 nm should be selected, and the closer to 800 nm, the safer. There are only two long-pulsed lasers below 800 nm, 532-nm long-pulsed KTP lasers, and 755-nm long-pulsed alexandrite lasers. 755-nm long-pulsed alexandrite lasers are safer than 532-nm long-pulsed KTP lasers. Also, in the case of Q-switched lasers, in order of safety: 755-nm Q-switched alexandrite lasers, 694-nm Q-switched ruby lasers, and 532-nm Q-switched Nd:YAG lasers. There are two types of ablative lasers, CO_2 laser and Er:YAG laser. As explained in "Chap. 10," Er:YAG laser ablates thinly and has low residual thermal damage (RTD) so there are fewer side effects. Therefore, Er:YAG laser is safer than the CO_2 laser.

There are so many lasers that can be used to treat epidermal pigments. Which laser should we buy first? I think it is best to buy the cheapest and most effective laser first. Next, buy the safest laser. I think lasers in between are ambiguous. They do not have a definite effect and are not without side effects. Therefore, when buying an epidermal pigment laser, you must first buy the most effective and inexpensive CO_2 laser. After using the CO_2 laser as much as possible, and when you feel the limitations of a CO_2 laser, then buy the safest long-pulsed alexandrite laser. Similarly, if you want to buy a Q-switched laser, first buy a 532-nm Q-switched Nd:YAG laser, then buy a 755-nm Q-switched alexandrite laser.

Dermal pigment lasers are Q-switched laser and fractional laser or pinhole therapy. According to the epidermal bypass effect, the dermal layer must be irradiated with a wavelength of 800 nm or more, and the only possible Q-switched laser is 1064-nm Q-switched Nd:YAG laser. Therefore, only Q-switched Nd:YAG lasers are needed to treat dermal pigments. Fortunately, the cost of purchase is also lower than other Q-switched lasers. For fractional lasers or pinhole therapy, first, purchase a low-cost CO_2 laser to try pinhole therapy, and if you feel the limitations, then consider purchasing a 1550- nm fractional Er:Glass laser.

Table 7.4 Choice of pigment laser

For epidermal pigment	
1. Long-pulsed laser	755 nm > 532 nm
2. Q-switched laser	755 nm > 694 nm > 532 nm
3. Ablative laser	Er:YAG > CO_2
For dermal pigment	
Q-switched laser	1064 nm
Fractional laser	Er:Glass, CO_2 pinhole method

7.3.2 Q-Switched Laser Selection

There are three types of Q-switched lasers: ruby lasers, alexandrite lasers, and Nd:YAG lasers. Which of these three Q-switched lasers is best for treating dermal pigmentations in Koreans?

In "Chap. 5" we reviewed that due to the epidermal bypass effect, lasers with melanin longer wavelength and low absorption coefficient for melanin are safer. We also reviewed that lasers with a wavelength above 800 nm are also appropriate lasers for the treatment of dermal pigmentations (epidermal bypass). Therefore, when treating dermal pigmentations, 1064-nm Q-switched Nd:YAG laser is the safest and the most suitable laser for Koreans. But other than the advantage of epidermal bypass effect is there any other advantages of Q-switched Nd:YAG lasers?

Table 7.5 shows some of the advantages of Nd:YAG lasers.

First, Nd:YAG laser has the deepest light penetration depth. For example, consider tattoo removal. When removing a tattoo, you must con-

Table 7.5 Melanin-specific lasers (Q-switched lasers). (Modified from [16])

Type	Ruby	Alexandrite	Nd:YAG
Wavelengths (nm)	694	755	1064
Penetration depth	Deep	Deeper	Deepest
Absorption by melanin	Good	Good	Bad
Pulse duration (ns)	20–40	50 or 100	5–10
TRT of melanosom	TRT > PD	TRT ≥ PD	TRT > PD
Photoacoustic effect	Moderate	Mild	Severe

sider the location of the tattoo particles. Tattoo particles are located at various positions in the dermal layer. Thus, because Nd:YAG laser penetrates the deepest of the three Q-switched lasers, it can eliminate even the deepest tattoo particles [9].

Second, Nd:YAG laser has the shortest pulse duration. Tattoo particles vary in size from 30 nm to 5 μm. TRT of tattoo particles ranges from 10 to 1000 ns. Thus, ruby lasers of 20–40 ns cannot treat tattoo particles of 20 ns or less in TRT, and alexandrite lasers of 50 to 100 ns cannot treat tattoo particles of 50 ns or less. Thus, Nd:YAG lasers can treat tattoo particles of various sizes. In addition, the treatment mechanism of Q-switched lasers is the photomechanical effect, so the shorter the irradiation time, the higher the power density and the greater the photomechanical effect. In other words, the explosive force is greater. Therefore, Q-switched Nd:YAG lasers, which have the shortest pulse duration will break tattoo particles better, resulting in better tattoo removal.

However, if you think of melanosomes, not tattoo pigments, the greater photomechanical effect is not always good. For example, breaking melanosomes of melasma with high explosive power can result in the aggravation of melasma. In this case, a Q-switched alexandrite laser with the longest pulse duration and the weakest explosive power may be a good choice. This is why some laser physicians claim that Q-switched alexandrite lasers are better than Q-switched Nd:YAG lasers for laser toning.

7.4 Pulse Duration

The pulse duration is fixed in Q-switched lasers, and it does not need to be adjusted. However, in the long-pulsed lasers or IPL, the determination of pulse duration is important. In "Chap. 3" we reviewed that due to thermal kinetic selectivity (TKS) when determining pulse duration, long to short pulse duration should be applied. So specifically, how should we set pulse duration when treating lentigines with long-pulsed lasers?

7.4.1 Simple Rule of Thumb

$$\mathrm{TRT} \fallingdotseq d^2 / gk.$$

When calculating TRT, it is necessary to accurately calculate geometric factor g and the constant k by inserting specific values. However, it can be calculated simply by the rule of thumb [9]. That is, most TRTs are similar to the square of target tissue diameter.

$$\mathrm{TRT}(\mathrm{second}) \fallingdotseq \mathrm{diameter}^2(\mathrm{mm}).$$

For example, a 0.5 μm melanosome is 5×10^{-4} mm in terms of mm and its square is 25×10^{-8} s. That is, 250 ns. The square of 0.1 mm, the vessel thickness of port wine stain (PWS), is 1×10^{-2} s and 10 ms in terms of a millisecond. In other words, it is the same as TRT we knew before.

7.4.2 Pulse Duration Selection in Long-Pulsed Lasers

We will calculate this simple rule of thumb by inserting specific values for lentigines. Since lentigines are confined to the epidermis, thus the thickness is less than that of the epidermis which is less than 100 μm, so the TRT of lentigines will be less than 10 ms.

As shown in Table 7.6, when the size of lentigines decreases to integers of 10 μm, such as 100, 90, 80, 70, and 60 μm, the TRT decreases to

Table 7.6 Thermal relaxation time calculated with the simple rule of thumb

Target size (μm)	Target size (mm)	TRT (s)	TRT (ms)
150	0.15	0.025	22.5
100	0.10	0.0100	10.0
90	0.09	0.0081	8.1
80	0.08	0.0064	6.4
70	0.07	0.0049	4.9
60	0.06	0.0036	3.6
50	0.05	0.0025	2.5
40	0.04	0.0016	1.6
30	0.03	0.0009	0.9
20	0.02	0.0004	0.4
10	0.01	0.0001	0.1

10, 8.1, 6.4, 4.9, and 3.6 ms. TRT decreases by root or power root in relation to the diameter. Therefore, the pulse duration should not be decreased integrally by 2 ms such as 10, 8, 6 ms, but it should be decreased according to the TRT for each size. For example, if you want to sequentially treat thin lentigines by 20 μm, such as 100, 80, 60, and 40 μm you should sequentially irradiate with pulse durations of 10, 6, 3, and 1 ms according to the TRT for each size. If you want to sequentially treat by 30 μm, such as 100, 70, 40, and 10 μm you should sequentially irradiate with pulse durations of 10, 5, 1, and 0.1 ms.

Specifically, when I treat lentigines with 755-nm long-pulsed alexandrite laser, I first use a pulse duration of 6 ms and start from one side of the face, eventually irradiating the whole face. Then I return to the first lentigines irradiated and observe the response. The reason for irradiating all the lentigines without checking the clinical endpoint immediately is as follows. This is because the clinical endpoint of long-pulsed lasers in the treatment of lentigines is "delayed" darkening and perilesional erythema. Responsive lentigines are not treated further and the pulse duration is reduced to 3 ms to re-irradiate only the unresponsive lentigines. Afterward, the pulse duration is sequentially reduced to 1 and 0.3 ms.

Usually, the TRT of the lentigines is about 0.35 ms, so I rarely use the pulse duration of 6 ms. I frequently use 3, 1, and 0.3 ms, and for lentigines that are hard to remove, pulse durations of 0.1–0.2 ms are used sequentially.

7.5 Spot Size

In the Sect. 3.5 of "Chap. 3" we reviewed that when treating the dermis, large spot sizes are useful because the larger the spot size, the deeper the optical penetration depth. How should spot size be adjusted when treating epidermal layers, especially epidermal pigmentations?

Since the epidermal layer is very thin and not where the scattering occurs, the spot size and optical penetration depth are not related. On the other hand, the larger the spot size, the faster the procedure. Thus, I believe that larger spots are still beneficial when treating the epidermal layer.

However, if the skin tone is very dark, the spot size should be adjusted slightly larger than the size of the target tissue to be treated. The main strategy for the treatment of epidermal layers is to use selective photothermolysis to take advantage of absorption coefficient differences. However, there is a problem when there is little difference in the absorption coefficient. For example, if lentigines are too light and the skin tone is light as well, the treatment may not be effective but the spot size does not matter. However, if the skin tone is dark and there is not much difference of absorption coefficient between lentigines and skin tone, hypopigmentation may occur in response to melanin pigmentation in normal skin as well as the lentigines. (see Sect. 5.1.3 in "Chap. 5"). Smaller hypopigmentation is less noticeable. The reasons why tiger print (footprint) by IPL is more noticeable are because it is artificially looking (rectangular) and large in size [17] (Fig. 7.6). Therefore, if the skin tone is dark, it is safe to make the spot size as small as possible, slightly larger than the size of the target tissue.

7.6 Fluence

7.6.1 Tissue Degeneration Process

What changes occur in the tissue degeneration process when treating pigmented lesions by lasers? What happens to pigmented lesions when pulse stacking as in vascular therapy? There is no

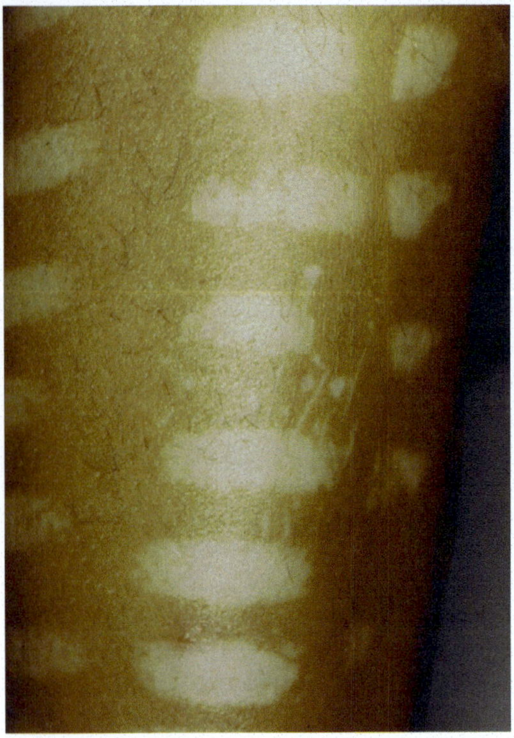

Fig. 7.6 Hypopigmentation by IPL after a vacation in the sun. (Reproduced from [18])

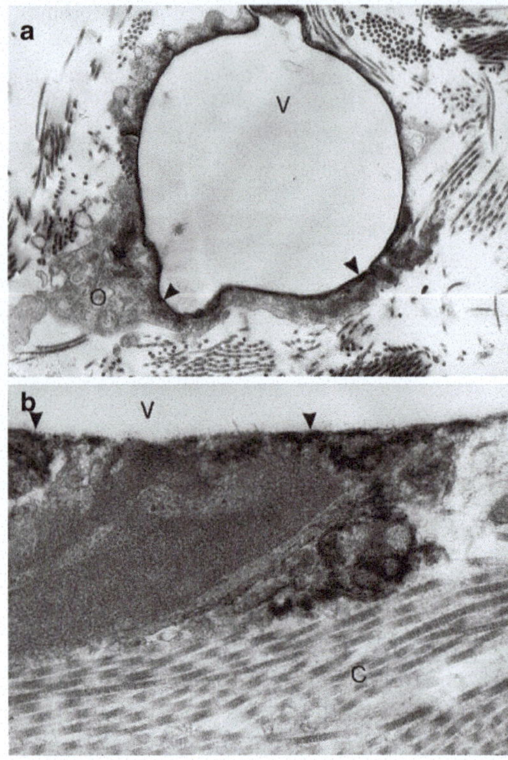

Fig. 7.7 (**a**) Electron microscopy immediately after laser treatment. A large intracellular vacuole (V) is a line with residual pigment and compressed cellular components (arrows). Other cytoplasmic organelles (O) appear intact. (Uranyl acetate and lead citrate, ×11,000). (**b**) Residual pigment (arrows) along the edge of a vacuole (V). Chromatin within the nucleus appears undamaged. Collagen fibers (C) adjacent to the vacuole show normal banding and structure. (Uranyl acetate and lead citrate, ×38,000). (Reproduced from [19])

detailed explanation about specific changes and treatments in laser texts, but I believe that the following two phenomena occur:

First, above the coagulation temperature, melanocytes and keratinocytes containing melanin will be coagulated. If the tissue becomes darker as the coagulation occurs, the absorption coefficient increases, so the temperature may increase rapidly after pulse stacking. In other words, unlike stable changes in temperature by pulse stacking of 500–600 nm wavelength vascular lasers, pulse stacking of pigmented lesions has a high risk of side effects due to rapid temperature rise as with 1064-nm wavelength lasers in vascular lesions.

Secondly, increasing energy with Q-switched laser causes whitening. Whitening is a phenomenon in which vacuoles appear in cells histologically and appear white clinically (Fig. 7.7). Once whitening occurs, pulse stacking does not have any effect because all the photons will be scattered. But what happens to pulse stacking 20 min later, after whitening disappears?

Using these two phenomena, let's review in detail how to treat pigmentations.

7.6.2 Repeat Pulse Method

A laser text describes pulse stacking by the following sentence [20]: "With pigment lesions, repeated laser pulses delivered over short periods (0.25–1 s) intervals results in progressive graying or darkening of the lesions." After reading this sentence, I decided to name the method of pulse stacking as "repeat pulse method."

Then what is the specific parameter of the repeat pulse method for pigmentation treatment? In "Chap. 3," we reviewed that in the repeat pulse method we should adjust the frequency, pulse count, and fluence. Because there are three variables, various parameters can exist. I chose to fix two variables, frequency and pulse count and decided to adjust fluence only.

I mainly use the repeat pulse method to treat epidermal pigmentations. The parameters are as follows: In 532-nm Q-switched Nd:YAG laser, 5 mm spot size with a frequency of 4 Hz, and a pulse count of four shots. Fluence starts at 0.3 J/cm^2. The clinical endpoint is moderate darkening and delayed perilesional erythema. Fluence is increased by 0.1 J/cm^2 if there is no change. Specifically, four shots are irradiated at 0.3 J/cm^2 and, if there is no change, four shots are irradiated again at 0.4 J/cm^2 after at least 10 s interval to rule out heat accumulation effect. Usually, fluence does not exceed 0.4 J/cm^2. In the case of very light lentigines, the fluence may be increased. Conversely, if 0.3 J/cm^2 is used and immediate whitening is produced, it can be lowered to 0.2 J/cm^2.

How can we fine-tune the repeat pulse method? For example, if the response is too strong at 0.3 J/cm^2 and the reaction is too weak at 0.2 J/cm^2, how should we fine-tune the parameters? Nothing is fixed, but in my case, I fine-tune in order of fluence, pulse count, and frequency. For example, if the reaction is too strong at 0.3 J/cm^2, 4 Hz, four shots, and it is too weak at 0.2 J/cm^2, I try three shots at 0.3 J/cm^2. If it is still too strong, frequency is lowered to 3 Hz and only three shots are irradiated.

The advantages of the repeat pulse method for epidermal pigmentation treatment are as follows. First, low-cost 532-nm Q-switched Nd:YAG lasers are economical because it can produce photothermal effects like long-pulsed lasers. Second, it is effective in light lentigines, which are difficult to treat with long-pulsed lasers, by repeat pulse method. However, the disadvantage is that the tissue degeneration step of the pigmented lesion increases the absorption coefficient rapidly at a temperature higher than the coagulation, so pulse stacking after darkening state may result in a high risk of side effects due to rapid temperature rise. Therefore, after darkening additional irradiation must be avoided. This is why the repeat pulse method for pigmentation treatment is very difficult and should be used with caution.

The reason why 5 mm spot is used in the repeat pulse method using 532-nm Q-switched Nd:YAG lasers is because the beam quality is decreased at the spot size less than 4 mm and the fluence is higher than that of the instrument panel. I think this is because when the Q-switched Nd:YAG converts the 1064-nm wavelength to 532 nm using KTP, a flat top mode is not executed at small spot sizes and it is difficult to maintain low fluence.

7.7 Reducing Optical Penetration Depth

7.7.1 R20 Method

Kossida et al. compared the results of single shot irradiation and R20 method for tattoo treatment using Q-switched alexandrite laser [21]. In the R20 method, a single shot with the same parameters as conventional tattoo treatment is irradiated, and after a 20-min interval, the shot is repeated for a total of four shots. Therefore, the total procedure takes about 1 h excluding anesthesia. The results showed that 61% of tattoos were completely removed after only one R20 method. The averages of expert-made tattoos were 88% brighter, and the amateur tattoos were 84% brighter.

However, most of the photographs in this paper were based on blurry tattoos, which made it difficult for me to trust them. So, I tried the R20 method on dark tattoos myself. Figure 7.8 shows the result after two sessions of a conventional single shot and CO_2 fractional laser. The tattoo pigment did not become much brighter (B). However, the R20 method was used only once, and the tattoo pigment became much brighter (C). In addition, two more R20 trials resulted in nearly 90% of tattoo removal (D).

The principle of the R20 method is as follows: The tattoo pigments in the dermal layer exist in various locations (figure 7.9d). If we consider the dermal layer divided into upper and lower parts and we shoot a single shot with a Q-switched laser, the photons will progress from the epider-

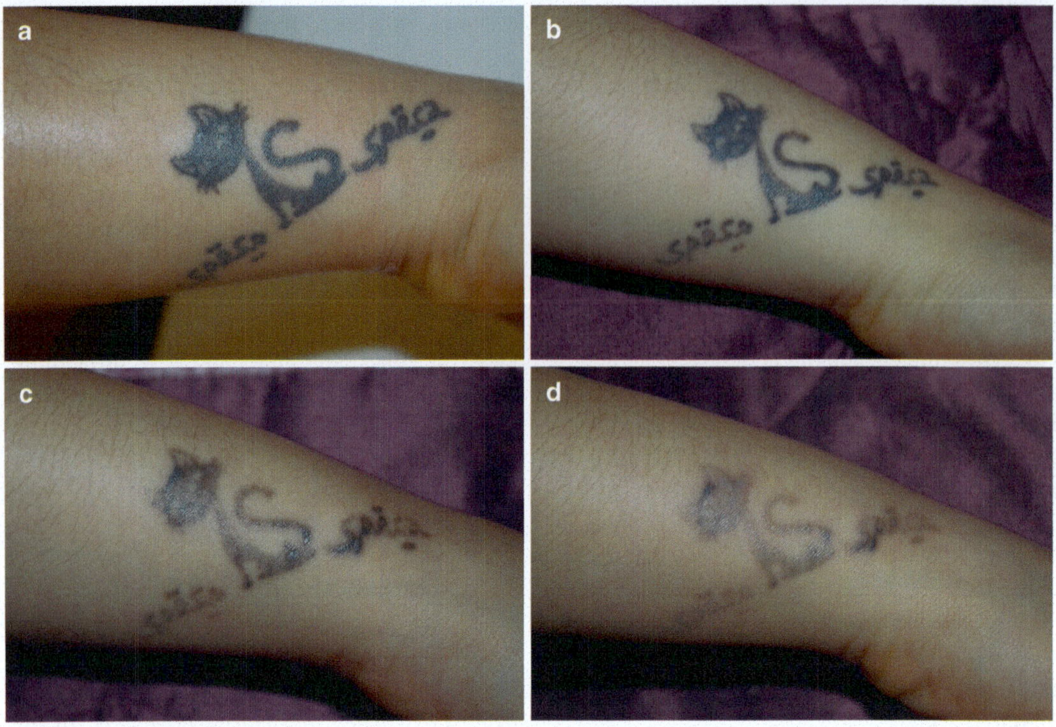

Fig. 7.8 (**a**) Tattoo before treatment (**b**) Results after two tattoo removals using conventional methods. (**c**, **d**) Results after one and three trials with R20 method

mal layer to the upper and lower parts of the dermal layer. The photons will be absorbed mostly by the tattoo pigment in the upper part of the dermal layer where they first meet, and the cells will be broken to form vacuoles. The lower part of the dermis will not have many photons, no vacuoles and the tattoo pigment will remain. Repeated laser irradiation after 20 min will cause the vacuole on the upper part of the dermal layer to disappear, and the tattoo pigment will be broken into smaller pieces, resulting in less absorption and scattering, resulting in more photons reaching the lower part of the dermal layer. Therefore, it is possible to break the tattoo pigment at the lower part of the dermal layer.

In other words, the R20 method removes even deeper tattoo pigments with one procedure in a day. To remove tattoos satisfyingly with existing Q-switch lasers, it is known that amateur tattoos take five times and professional tattoos take 10–15 times at intervals of 1–3 months. However, the R20 method is a new way to reduce the number of procedures.

7.7.2 Kono Technique

Kono technique is the so-called window technique used in private practice. To treat congenital nevus, Kono et al. first irradiated a 694-nm normal mode (meaning a long pulse duration like a long-pulsed laser) ruby laser to coagulate the upper portion of the congenital nevus and then pushed and peeled off the coagulated skin with wet gauze, and then irradiated the lower portion of the congenital nevus by 694-nm Q-switched ruby laser (Fig. 7.10) [22].

Kono technique is similar to the R20 method, but it not only removes the pigment at the top but also physically removes the skin itself to deepen the optical penetration depth.

When can the Kono technique be used? It can be used to treat deep tissue. It can be used to remove congenital nevus, tattoos, or melanocytic nevus. I use a CO_2 or Er:YAG laser instead of a long-pulsed laser to physically get rid of the top of the skin itself. For example, when removing nevus,

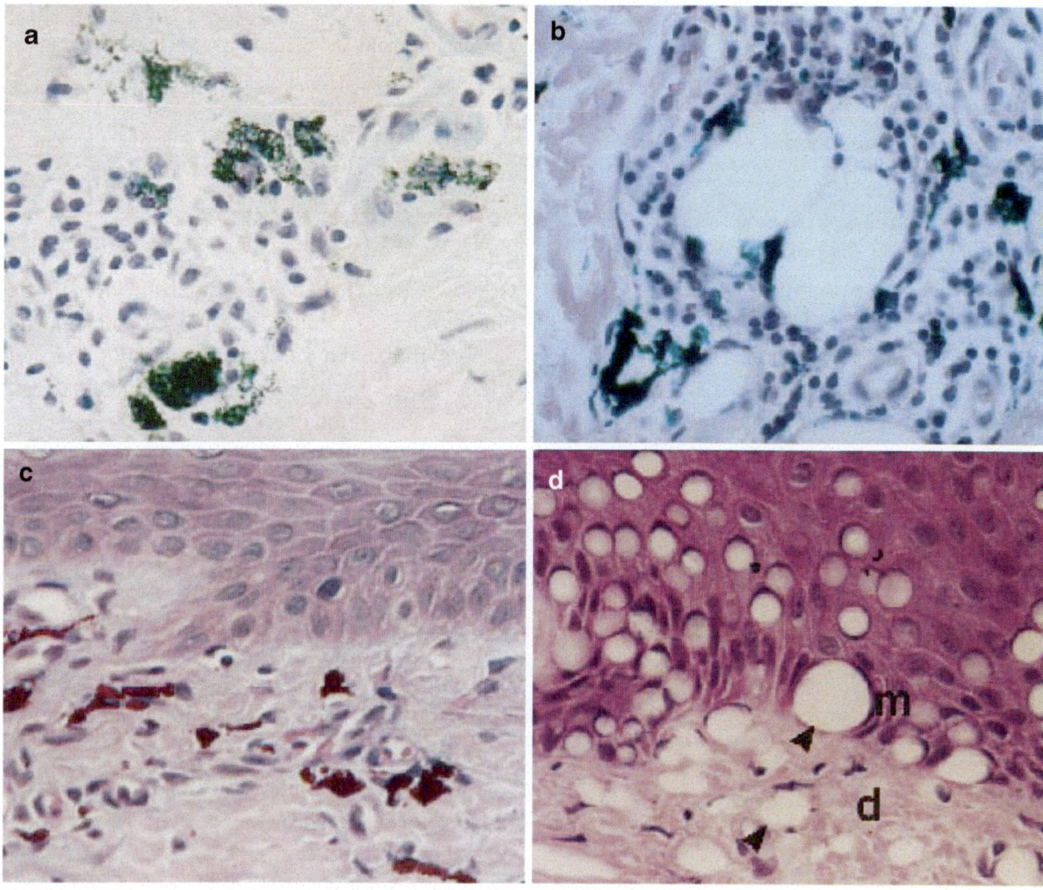

Fig. 7.9 Professional tattoos (all stained with H&E). (**a**) Green tattoo comprising green and black pigment particles within dermal mononuclear cells (×240); (**b**) vacuolation of a black but not green tattoo at 1064 nm (×240); (**c**) red tattoo containing red particles (×240); (**d**) vauolation (arrows) of epidermal melanocytes (m) and upper dermis (d) immediately after laser treatment at 532 nm (×240). (Reproduced from [19])

I first use a CO_2 or Er:YAG laser, and then use the Kono technique to process the remaining nevus using a 1064-nm Q-switched Nd:YAG laser. In the case of congenital nevus or tattoo removal, CO_2 fractional laser or pinhole therapy with a CO_2 laser is followed by the Kono technique using a 1064-nm Q-switched Nd:YAG laser.

7.8 Strategy for Pigment Treatment

According to the strategy mentioned in "Chap. 3" we will examine specific strategies for epidermal pigmented lesions and dermal pigmented lesions (Table 7.7).

7.8.1 Strategy for Epidermal Pigment Treatment

If we first think of epidermal pigmented lesions according to strategies, the competitive tissue of epidermal pigmented lesions is normal epidermis tissue (Table 7.8).

First, selective photothermolysis is the main strategy because the target and competitive tissue are horizontal. An important parameter of selective photothermolysis theory is the wavelength. Due to epidermal bypass effect, epidermal pigment lasers should use less than 800 nm, and lasers with wavelengths near 800 nm are safer. Therefore, a 755-nm Q-switched alexandrite laser or a 755-nm long-pulsed alexandrite laser

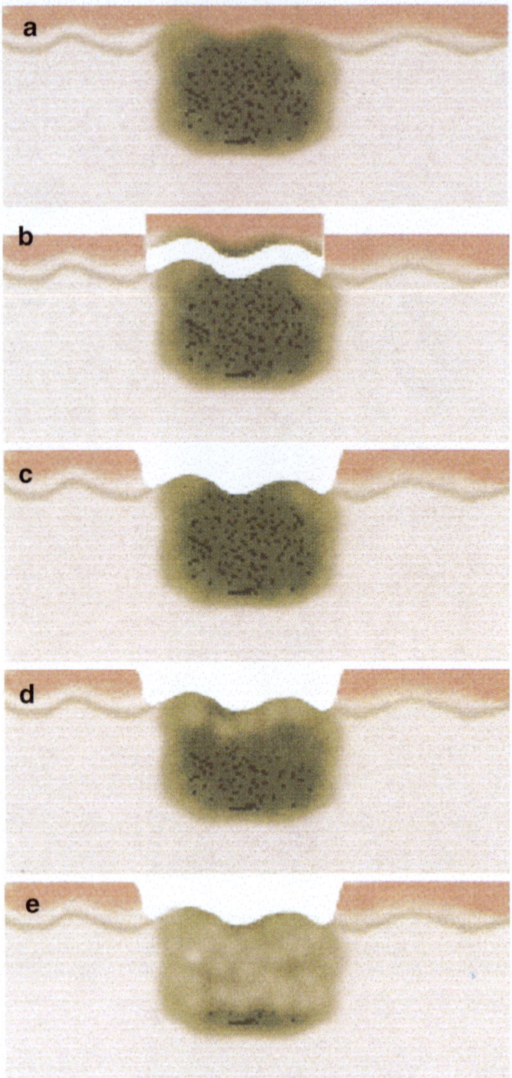

Fig. 7.10 The combination approach: (**a**) before treatment of the pigmented naevus; (**b**) a single pass with the normal-mode ruby laser; (**c**) the epidermis is removed; (**d**) after a single pass with the Q-switched ruby laser; and (**e**) after multiple passes with the Q-switched ruby laser. (Reproduced from [22])

Table 7.7 Laser treatment strategies

Spatially selective temperature elevation
1. Selective photothermolysis
A. Absorption coefficient (wavelengths), concentration of chromophore
B. Pulse duration (thermal kinetic selectivity)
2. Epidermal cooling
3. Fractional photothermolysis

Table 7.8 Target and competitive tissues of epidermal pigmented lesions and dermal pigmented lesions

	Epidermal pigmented lesions	Dermal pigmented lesions
Target tissue	Epidermal pigment	Dermal pigment
Competitive tissue	Surrounding normal epidermis	Epidermis

would be better. When considering laser-tissue interactions, 755-nm long-pulsed alexandrite lasers will be the safest because photothermal effect is safer than photomechanical effect. Because absorption coefficient changes with concentration, "dark lesions should be shot weakly, and light lesions should be shot strongly." Q-switched lasers have a fixed pulse duration, but with long-pulsed lasers, longer pulse durations are used first by thermal kinetic selectivity, and unresponsive lesions should be treated sequentially using shorter pulse durations.

Second, epidermal cooling is not necessary. The reason is explained in detail in the Sect. 3.6.2 in "Chap. 3."

Third, the fractional laser or pinhole method may be meaningful. However, when I tried pinhole therapy with lentigines with a 2 mm spot using Er:YAG laser, PIH could not be completely avoided. I believe that PIH occurs in lentigine treatment with pinhole therapy because the Er:YAG laser or CO_2 laser are both ablative lasers and vaporizes the water of the tissue and the tissue is ablated by the pressure difference between the tissue and water vapor. Thus, I think PIH is inherently unavoidable (see "Chap. 10").

The problem with the strategy using the selective photothermolysis theory occurs when there is no difference in the absorption coefficient between the target tissue and the surrounding tissue. For example, the lentigines may be too bright, or the skin tone itself may be too dark that there is a small difference between the pigmentation and the surrounding normal tissues. How can we effectively treat lentigines if it is bright? Although long-pulsed lasers are safe due to photothermal effects, long-pulsed lasers have no effect on bright lentigines because there is a limit in reducing the pulse duration. Therefore, Q-switched lasers must be used [9]. Because

Q-switched lasers irradiate in nanoseconds, they can destroy cells by exploding melanosomes by photomechanical effects. Therefore, very bright lentigines can be treated. However, side effects should be reduced by increasing the energy little by little. On the contrary, what if the skin tone itself is too dark? Darker skin tones are more likely to cause PIH, so long-pulsed lasers with fewer side effects should be used than Q-switched lasers. Initial energy should be lower than conventional energy. As a side effect, temporary hypopigmentation lasting about a month, such as a tiger print (footprint) that occurs during IPL, may occur in several places. Therefore, patients should be informed in advance of the situation. Using small spots is better, to make them less visible. Without long-pulsed lasers, the 1064-nm Q-switched Nd:YAG laser with the lowest epidermis melanin absorption among Q-switched lasers should be used. As mentioned in "Chap. 3" One-shot toning can be repeated at 4–6 J/cm^2.

7.8.2 When Epidermal Cooling Is Not Effective

There are two cases where epidermis cooling is not effective [9]. The first case is when using ablative lasers with high water absorption, such as CO_2 lasers or Er:YAG lasers. The principle of ablative laser is to vaporize water above 100 °C. However, if the tissue that generates heat with an ablative laser is the same tissue for cooling, then the cooling will reduce the effect of ablation, if the cooling is too strong, below 100 °C. Also, epidermal cooling is meaningless because ablative lasers generate much higher heat than cooling. The second case is because Q-switched lasers only slightly reduce the peak temperature and there is no significant temperature difference, making epidermal cooling meaningless. However, there is an effect of reducing pain.

7.8.3 Strategy for Dermal Pigment Treatment

Considering the strategy of dermal pigment lesions, the competitive tissue of dermal pigment is normal epidermis tissue (Table 7.8). Epidermal cooling maybe most important because it is a vertical relationship, but it is of no use in the treatment of dermal pigmented lesions.

First, wavelengths of 800 nm or more must be used according to the epidermal bypass effect. For pulse duration, Q-switched lasers using nanoseconds should be used according to the theory of selective photothermolysis. Therefore, there is only 1064-nm Q-switched Nd:YAG laser. Since ABNOM, Nevus of Ota, and dermal melasma are present in separate cells, the theory that "dark lesions should be shot weakly and light lesions should be shot strongly" is irrelevant. However, in the case of dermal nevi, the energy needs to be adjusted depending on concentration. Also, in a second camouflage tattoo ("retattoo") over an undesired first tattoo, there may be a lot of tattoo pigments despite the light appearance. Therefore, low energy should be used first to check the reaction.

Second, as mentioned earlier, epidermal cooling is meaningless.

Third, actively use fractional laser or pinhole methods. But, ABNOM or dermal melasma are more likely to develop PIH and melasma may also aggravate by fractional laser or pinhole methods. Therefore, I do not recommend fractional laser or pinhole therapy for ABNOM or dermal melasma. However, in tattoo or congenital nevus fractional laser or pinhole methods should be actively used.

The final strategy is to remove epidermal pigmented lesions first and then perform a stepwise procedure to treat dermal pigmented lesions.

7.9 Treatment of Lentigines

7.9.1 Target Cell and Chromophores of Lentigines

The histological findings of the lentigines are characterized by the proliferation of melanocytes, increased pigmentation around the basal layer, and epidermal growth in which the rete ridges become club shape and are lengthened into the papillary dermis. The mechanism of lentigines is unknown, but histological findings suggest that it is a tumor or hamartoma caused by the proliferation of melanocytes [23]. Therefore, the therapeutic target of laser in lentigines is melanocytes. However, melanocytes do not have enough melanin as the chromophore of lasers. Melanocytes synthesize melanosomes and deliver them to the supranuclear cap of peripheral keratinocytes through dendrites. Melanosomes are divided into four stages (stages I–IV) according to their maturity level [24]. Melanosomes in the first and second stages are "melanin-free" and have "red melanin only," and melanosomes in third and fourth stages are melanosomes that synthesize eumelanin and are commonly found in dendrites.

Hruza et al. irradiated 694-nm Q-switched ruby lasers on normal skin and lentigines [25]. Transmission electron microscopy revealed that the melanosomes in stages 1 and 2 were intact. Therefore, I believe that the irradiation of pigment lasers will not damage melanocytes first, but primarily damages keratinocytes and dendrites of melanocytes, which has the most melanosomes in the third and fourth stages. Yamasita et al. observed lentigines disappearing by the naked eye after irradiation of lentigines with IPL, but melanocytes remained intact on reflection-mode confocal microscopy (RCM) [10]. Melanocytes also remained after the crust of lentigines exfoliated after Q-switch ruby laser irradiation [11]. Mun et al. performed laser toning with a 1064-nm Q-switched Nd:YAG laser observed "dendrectomy" phenomenon in which melanocytes did not disappear but only dendrite disappeared [26].

Target tissue and chromophores are different for lentigines. This makes the treatment of lentigines difficult.

7.9.2 My Treatment of Lentigines

Treatment of epidermal pigments includes long-pulsed lasers including IPL, Q-switched lasers, and ablative lasers. Recently a new laser, picolaser, has been released. I believe that picolasers have similar safety to long-pulsed lasers regarding PIH development (see "Chap. 2"). Another technique is to use the 1064-nm Q-switched Nd:YAG laser with one shot toning at 1–2-week intervals at 4–6 J/cm^2, with the "energy level that does not affect the surrounding cells and only damages the cells."

I think that it is better to repeat the treatment several times starting from the safest treatment. Therefore, I treat lentigines as follows: First, the safest 755-nm long-pulsed alexandrite laser or 755-nm picolaser is irradiated at intervals of 2–4 weeks, and in between, one shot toning at 4–6 J/cm^2 with a 1064-nm Q-switched Nd:YAG laser is performed. If treatment is slow, use a repeat pulse method with a 532-nm Q-switched Nd:YAG laser. This repetition dims lentigines and decreases the size of lentigines. Finally, small lentigines of 1–2 mm size are removed by defocusing with a CO_2 laser.

References

1. Allemann IB, Goldberg DJ (2011) Basics in dermatological laser applications. Karger Medical and Scientific Publishers
2. Kawada A, Asai M, Kameyama H, Sangen Y, Aragane Y, Tezuka T et al (2002) Videomicroscopic and histopathological investigation of intense pulsed light therapy for solar lentigines. J Dermatol Sci 29(2):91–96
3. Raulin C, Karsai S (2011) Laser and IPL technology in dermatology and aesthetic medicine. Heidelberg: New York
4. Bolognia J, Schaffer JV, Cerroni L (2018) Dermatology. Elsevier, Philadelphia, PA
5. Kasai K (2007) Skin spots treatment clinics (Korean edition). Shinheung Med Science, Seoul
6. Habif TP (2015) Clinical dermatology. Elsevier, St. Louis, MO
7. Robinson JK, Hanke CW, Siegel DM, Fratila A, Bhatia AC, Rohrer TE (2014) Surgery of the skin E-book: procedural dermatology. Elsevier Health Sciences
8. Lee B, Kim YC, Kang WH, Lee ES (2004) Comparison of characteristics of acquired bilateral nevus of Ota-like macules and nevus of Ota according to therapeutic outcome. J Korean Med Sci 19(4):554–559
9. Goldman MP (2006) Cutaneous and cosmetic laser surgery. Mosby Elsevier, Philadelphia, PA
10. Yamashita T, Negishi K, Hariya T, Kunizawa N, Ikuta K, Yanai M et al (2006) Intense pulsed light therapy for superficial pigmented lesions evalu-

ated by reflectance-mode confocal microscopy and optical coherence tomography. J Invest Dermatol 126(10):2281–2286
11. Yamashita T, Negishi K, Hariya T, Yanai M, Iikura T, Wakamatsu S (2010) In vivo microscopic approaches for facial melanocytic lesions after quality-switched ruby laser therapy: time-sequential imaging of melanin and melanocytes of solar lentigo in Asian skin. Dermatol Surg 36(7):1138–1147
12. Hruza GJ, Tanzi EL (2018) Lasers and lights. Elsevier, Edinburgh
13. Kang WH (2013) Treatment strateties for pigmentation disorders in skin (Korean). Hansol Medical, Seoul
14. Kauvar A, Hruza G (2005) Principles and practices in cutaneous laser surgery. CRC Press
15. Ross EV, Domankevitz Y (2005) Laser treatment of leg veins: physical mechanisms and theoretical considerations. Lasers Surg Med 36(2):105–116
16. Watanabe S (2008) Basics of laser application to dermatology. Arch Dermatol Res 300(1):21–30
17. Goldman MP, Weiss RA, Weiss MA (2005) Intense pulsed light as a nonablative approach to photoaging. Dermatol Surg 31:1179–1187
18. Stangl S, Hadshiew I, Kimmig W (2008) Side effects and complications using intense pulsed light (IPL) sources. Med Laser Appl 23(1):15–20
19. Ferguson J, Andrew S, Jones C, August P (1997) The Q-switched neodymium: YAG laser and tattoos: a microscopic analysis of laser-tattoo interactions. Br J Dermatol 137(3):405–410
20. Keyvan N (2012) Lasers in dermatology and medicine. [S.I.]. Springer
21. Kossida T, Rigopoulos D, Katsambas A, Anderson RR (2012) Optimal tattoo removal in a single laser session based on the method of repeated exposures. J Am Acad Dermatol 66(2):271–277
22. Kono T, Nozaki M, Chan HH, Sasaki K, Kwon SG (2001) Combined use of normal mode and Q-switched ruby lasers in the treatment of congenital melanocytic naevi. Br J Plast Surg 54(7):640–643
23. Goldsmith LA, Katz SI, Gilchrest BA, Paller AS, Leffell DJ, Wolff K et al (2012) Fitzpatrick's dermatology in general medicine. McGraw-Hill Professional, New York
24. Textbook Compilation Committee in Korean Dermatological Association (2014) Text book of dermatology 6th edition (Korean). Daehanuihak, Seoul
25. Hruza GJ, Dover JS, Flotte TJ, Goetschkes M, Watanabe S, Anderson RR (1991) Q-switched ruby laser irradiation of normal human skin. Histologic and ultrastructural findings. Arch Dermatol 127(12):1799–1805
26. Mun JY, Jeong SY, Kim JH, Han SS, Kim IH (2011) A low fluence Q-switched Nd:YAG laser modifies the 3D structure of melanocyte and ultrastructure of melanosome by subcellular-selective photothermolysis. J Electron Microsc 60(1):11–18

8 Laser Hair Removal

8.1 Introduction

8.1.1 Structure and Function of Hair Follicle

Hair is a cylindrical fiber consisting of tightly adhered, cornified epithelial cells that only mammals have [1]. It is present anywhere on the skin except on palms and soles, distal ends of fingers and toes, boundaries of mucous membranes, and the glans penis.

Hair does not have physiological functions related to life, but hair protects the scalp from sunlight, while eyebrows and eyelashes cover eyes from sunlight and sweat. Also, hair in the nose filters out external stimulus, while the hair in the folds of the skin (armpits, groin) reduces friction.

Hair formation is observed between 9 and 12 weeks of gestation and at about 20 weeks of gestation, hair follicles are completed and hair begins to appear. The number of hair follicles formed at this time does not increase throughout life but decreases with age.

Hair in different parts of the body has different biological and morphological characteristics. In addition, hair receives different effects of hormones on different parts of the body. The hair of the face, body, armpits, and pubic are affected by sex hormones, but eyebrows and eyelashes are not affected by sex hormones.

Hair is divided into lanugo, vellus hair, and terminal hair according to thickness and length. The skin of the fetus is covered with delicate soft pale hair, called lanugo. Lanugo is mostly eliminated before birth. The hair covering most of the young and adult skin is delicate vellus hair (vellus hair) and long, thick terminal hair (terminal hair). Only terminal hairs contain medulla.

Hair thickness is generally determined by the dermal papilla and the hair bulb. In terminal hair, the radius of the hair bulb is 200–300 μm while the thickness of the hair shaft is rather small, 40–120 μm [2]. Vellus hair is less than 40 μm thick and less than 30 mm long [1].

The hair follicle can be divided into three regions: the infundibulum, isthmus, and inferior segments [1]. These regions are divided by the sebaceous gland, and the bulge region, which is where arrector pili muscle attaches to (Fig. 8.1). In the inferior segments, the expanded, bottom part of the hair follicle is the hair bulb. The hair bulb is composed of dermal structures called the dermal papilla and hair follicle structures called the matrix. The infundibulum is the region between the sebaceous gland and the opening of the hair follicle and is an important structure concerning acne [3].

The hair bulb of the terminal hair during anagen period is usually located in the subcutaneous fat layer, and the depth of the hair bulb depends on the thickness of the skin, usually at 2–7 mm

J. D. Lee et al., *Principles and Choice of Laser Treatment in Dermatology*,
https://doi.org/10.1007/978-981-15-6556-4_8

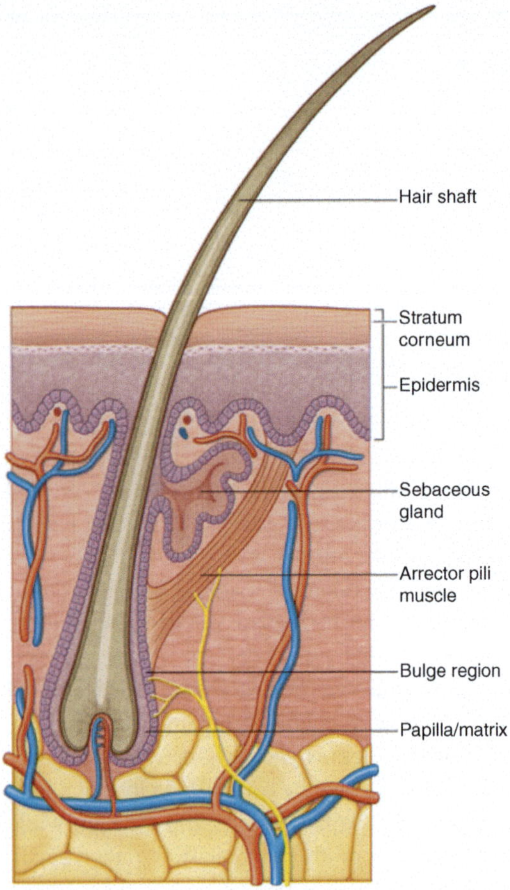

Fig. 8.1 Hair follicle anatomy. (Modified from [4])

depth. The hair bulbs of vellus hair and the thin terminal hair are located in the upper part of the dermis, with a depth of less than 1 mm. The location of hair bulbs varies depending on the hair cycle. In the latter part of the telogen and at the beginning of anagen, the hair bulb is located at the shallowest at 1.5 mm, which is equal to the depth of the bulge region. The bulge region maintains a constant depth regardless of the hair cycle [2].

The inferior segment of the hair follicle consists of five parts: The dermal papilla, the matrix, the hair shaft, the inner root sheath, and the outer root sheath. The hair shaft consists of medulla, cortex, and hair cuticle. The inner root sheath consists of the inner root sheath cuticle, Huxley layer, Henle layer, and companion layer (Fig. 8.2) [1].

Undifferentiated keratinocytes in the hair matrix produce hair shafts and inner root sheaths. As cortex cell grows up in the matrix, it gradually loses its nucleus, and the cytoplasm is filled with keratin fibrils arranged vertically. This keratinization process is different from the epidermal keratinization process after keratohyaline granulation or the inner root sheath keratinization process after trichohyaline granulation. As a result, the epidermis produces soft corneocytes and cortex produces hard corneocytes [1].

The inner root sheath breaks down after reaching the isthmus following complete keratinization. This is why the inner root sheath does not exist on the hair shaft out of the skin surface. It is assumed that the companion layer cells are tightly bound to Henle's layer, but not to the outer root sheath, thus allowing the companion layer to function as a slippage plane between the stationary outer root sheath and the upwards moving inner root sheath. The Huxley layer is thought to play a role in maintaining the shape of the hair shaft.

Melanocytes are between the keratinocytes of the matrix in the hair bulb. The melanin produced by hair follicle melanocytes is phagocytosed by the cells that will later form the hair shaft. The amount of melanin phagocytosed determines the color of hair. The transfer of melanin to keratinocytes in the matrix of hair bulb is similar to the transfer in the epidermis, from melanocytes to keratinocytes. Large melanosomes are found in darker hair and small melanosomes are found in brighter hair. Hair follicle melanocytes produce two kinds of melanin: Eumelanin produces black-brown hair, and pheomelanin produces red-yellow hair.

Melanocytes with melanin are located in the upper part of the hair bulb and the upper outer root sheath of the infundibulum. Amelanotic melanocytes are located in the outer root sheath of the middle and the bottom of the hair follicle and the outer root sheath of the hair bulb. When activated by appropriate stimuli, amelanotic melanocytes produce dendrite, move upward, and produce pigments. Therefore, amelanotic melanocytes play an important role in repigmentation after vitiligo treatment or mechanical ablation [2].

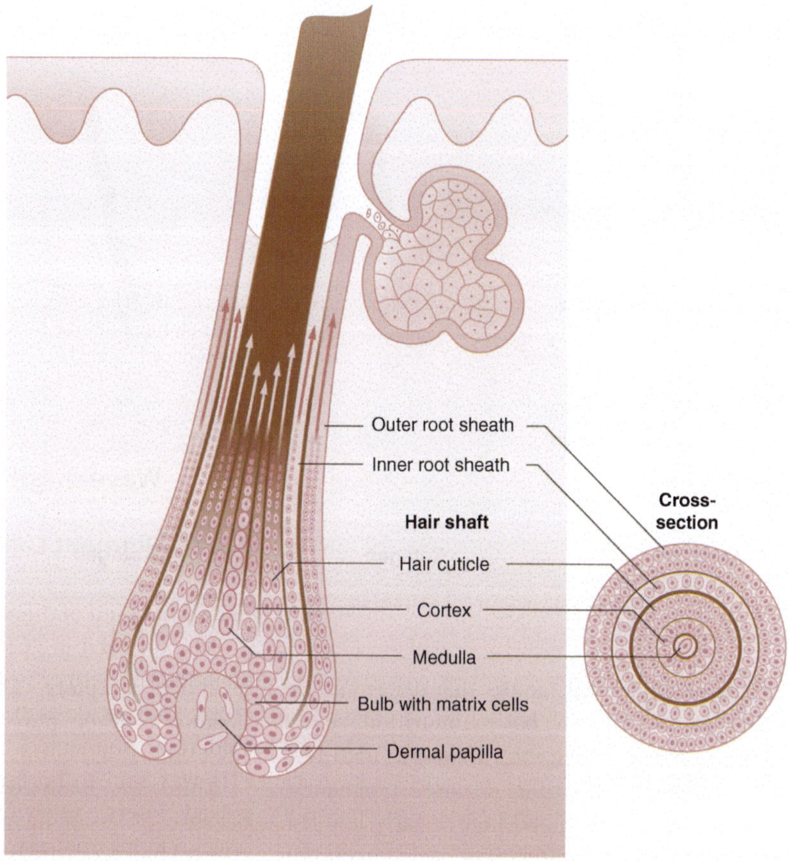

Fig. 8.2 Anatomy of the hair follicle. (Reproduced from [5])

8.1.2 Hair Growth Cycle

Under normal conditions, hair grows, stops growing for a while, falls out and new hair starts to grow again. This is called the hair growth cycle. The hair growth cycle consists of three stages: anagen, catagen, and telogen. If exogen (cycle when hair falls out) is included, it can be seen as four stages [1] (Fig. 8.3).

Adult scalp hair has anagen for 2–8 years, catagen for 2 weeks, and telogen for 1–3 months. At any time, 90–93% of adult scalp hair is the anagen, less than 1% in catagen, and the rest is telogen. The hair growth rate is about 0.3–0.4 mm/day, and each hair follicle repeats 10–20 cycles throughout its life. The number of hairs in telogen is estimated to be 10,000, but 50–100 hairs fall out every day. Human hair growth is periodic, but each hair follicle acts independently. Therefore, shedding, i.e., synchronized fur loss is seen in many animals, does not occur in humans.

During anagen, matrix cells multiply to form hair shafts and inner root sheaths. After anagen, catagen starts, and cell division and melanogenesis stop in the hair bulb, hair bulb contracts, and separates from the dermal papilla. As hair moves up, the inferior segments of the hair follicle are regressed, the growth of inner root sheath stops and the inferior segments of the hair shaft are surrounded by trichilemmal keratin formed in the outer root sheath. This is called club hair. When hair regenerates, a certain signal causes follicular epithelial stem cells to divide and proliferate downward with the dermal papilla to form new hair bulbs, generating new anagen hair, and finally pushing out club hair.

The inferior segments of hair follicles that form the hair according to hair cycle show a lot of histological changes, but the upper hair follicles located above the isthmus are permanent portions with relatively no change.

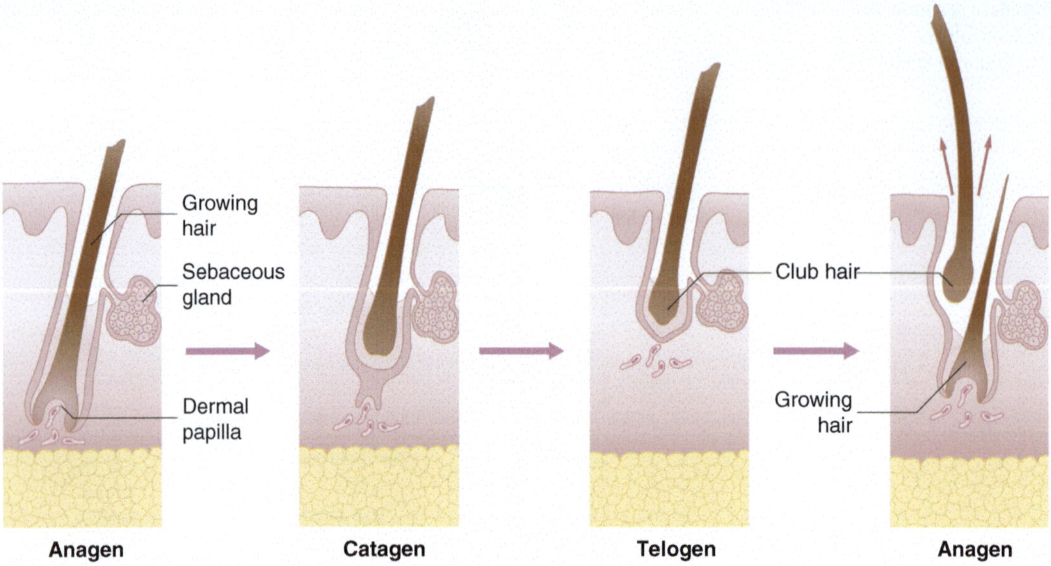

Fig. 8.3 Phases of the growth cycle of hair. (Reproduced from [5])

The physiological factors that determine the hair cycle are unclear, but malnutrition, severe stress (surgery, infection, trauma), and hormonal changes (thyroid disease, pregnancy) may stop hair growth and induce early telogen. Pulling out hair may affect hair cycle but cutting hair does not.

8.1.3 Indications for Hair Removal

There are four main reasons for getting hair removal [6]. First, hypertrichosis. Hypertrichosis refers to the phenomenon of hair growth on parts of the body that are not affected by androgen, regardless of gender. The cause is mostly genetic or ethnic. Also, drugs such as cyclosporine, prednisolone, and phenytoin, diseases such as porphyria, thyroid disease, internal malignancies, malnutrition, or anorexia nervosa may be of cause [7].

Second, hirsutism. Hirsutism is a condition in which women are affected by male hormones and the hairs on the chin, sideburns, chest, inner thighs, back, and abdomen increase. The cause may be idiopathic or maybe because of overproduction of male hormones in ovaries or adrenal glands, increased skin sensitivity to male hormones, or functional differences in male hormone receptors. The most common cause is known to be polycystic ovarian syndrome (PCOS).

Third, the main reason for hair removal is because of cosmetic reasons. Women want to remove hair from areas such as the armpits, philtrum, or calves due to cultural influences, especially gender awareness. Recently, the demand for hair removal is also increasing for men. Men want hair removal for cheeks, neck, sideburns, and calves for cosmetic reasons. In addition, recently many men receive beard hair removal to prevent folliculitis caused by shaving and discomfort caused by frequent shaving.

Fourth, medical reasons. People receive hair removal due to hair-related diseases such as pseudofolliculitis barbae, pilonidal sinus disease, and skin grafts [7]. Pseudofolliculitis barbae (razor humps) is a genetic disease that causes inflammation of the skin due to the curling or spiraling of hair. If the hair is shaved tightly, sharp hair will grow and penetrate the skin. 50–75% occur in blacks and 3–5% in whites. It is most common in cheeks and neck, and can also occur in armpits, pubic areas, and calves [8]. In addition, hair removal may be applied to hirsutism observed in pilonidal sinus disease and hair growth on transplanted flaps after skin transplantation.

8.1.4 Traditional Hair Removal Method

Traditional hair removal methods include shaving, plucking, waxing, and chemical depilatory. However, these methods have the disadvantage of showing only short-term effects. In addition, electrolysis is a method of scorching hair follicles by inserting needles into hair follicles using the Kobayashi insulation needle. However, this method is very inconvenient because the needle has to be inserted into each hair follicle. Thus, application to small areas is possible but it is difficult to apply to large areas [7]. Due to the popularization of hair removal lasers these days, this procedure is not performed anymore.

8.2 Laser Hair Removal

8.2.1 Follicular Stem Cell

The target cell of hair removal laser is hair follicular stem cell that produces hair follicles. However, controversy still exists about the location of hair follicular stem cells [2].

Initially, the growth center of hair was thought to be within the hair matrix. This is because the matrix cells differentiate and form a hair shaft. However, many studies have shown that the matrix is not the only growth center. Surgical removal of the hair follicle containing the matrix did not inhibit new hair follicle regeneration [9]. So, it was thought that the hair matrix and the contiguous dermal papilla interact to form hair follicles. Oliver later studied rat vibrissae and observed that hair follicles regenerated even after removing the dermal papilla and one-third of hair follicle inferior segments. Therefore, hair follicle stem cells were thought to exist in areas other than the hair bulb and the dermal papilla. Cotsarelis et al. specialized slow-cycling cells having the characteristics of hair follicle stem cells in the outer root sheath of the bulge of Wulst in the permanent portion of the hair follicle where arrector pili muscle is attached. Currently, most authors say that hair follicular stem cells exist in the mid-follicular outer root sheath at the insertion of arrector pili muscle within the bulge of Wulst. It is thought that these hair follicle stem cells make the outer root sheath, indirectly form the matrix, and ultimately the hair shaft.

The presence of a hair follicular stem cell in the bulge of Wulst instead of a deeply located hair bulb has several biological advantages. First, hair bulb decays periodically, while the bulge of Wulst is the permanent portion of the hair follicle. It is also in a good position to interact with hair bulbs that come up later in the telogen to make new hair follicles. Second, hair bulbs are easily damaged when plucking, but the bulge of Wulst is safe from damage. Third, the bulge of Wulst is the site where blood vessels develop and provide sufficient nutrients.

The mechanism of the hair cycle, in which hair follicles grow and stop is not yet known. Also, the mechanism by which the hair follicular stem cells of the bulge of Wulst are activated is not yet known. However, recent research suggests a bulge activation hypothesis [9]. The hypothesis of the bulge of Wulst activation is that inactivated stem cells in the bulge of Wulst are activated by dermal papilla-derived diffusible growth factor or direct cell-cell contact when dermal papilla and the bulge of Wulst come closer in telogen late. The bulge of Wulst stem cells is also known to produce sebaceous glands and epidermis, as well as hair follicles and hair shafts. From this, the concept of "pilosebaceous epithelial unit" emerged. Some say that the bulge of Wulst is "housing the ultimate epidermal stem cell."

On the other hand, high-proliferative cells such as hair germ cells, which are different from the bulge of Wulst stem cells, were observed in telogen. Some authors say that these cells are near dermal papilla and play a role in inducing anagen. Dermal papilla is known to determine the size of the hair bulb, the diameter of the hair shaft, and the duration of anagen [9].

8.2.2 Target Cell and Chromophores of Laser Hair Removal

Therefore, the target cells of laser hair removal are considered to be hair follicle stem cells in the bulge region and hair germ cells near dermal

Table 8.1 Target cell and chromophores of laser hair removal

Location	Chromophore	Target cell
Bulge region	Hair shaft	Follicular stem cell
Hair bulb	Hair matrix	Hair germ cell

papilla. The problem is that the bulge region or the dermal papilla are pigment-free sites that do not have chromophores for laser. The pigmented part of the hair follicle is part of the outer root sheath of infundibulum, the hair matrix of the hair bulb, and the hair shaft (Table 8.1). That is, the chromophores of laser hair removal and the target cell are different.

In summary, the mechanism of laser hair removal is as follows. Heat is applied to the chromophores, which are the hair shaft and the hair matrix. The extended theory of selective photothermolysis is then applied to create heat diffusion [10]. As a result, follicular stem cells and hair germ cells, which are target cells, are destroyed. Therefore, when hair is pulled out with tweezers, the chromophore of laser disappears, so there is no hair removal effect.

8.2.3 Optimal Treatment Period

It is hypothesized that there is a suitable hair cycle for laser hair removal because the position and color of chromophores vary depending on the hair cycle [2]. In conclusion, it is known that the hair cycle and laser hair removal effect are not related. So, the following information is for reference only [9].

Melanin density is highest in hair bulbs. When catagen starts, melanin synthesis stops, i.e., the hair bulb in telogen has no pigment. Therefore, the effect of the laser cannot be seen. During initial anagen (early telogen), melanin synthesis is recovered from the hair bulb. In this period, the hair bulb is located near the shallowest bulge region. In addition, the bulge region stem cells of early anagen are active at cell division and are vulnerable to damage. In the second half of anagen, the hair bulb and the dermal papilla are lowered into the dermis, making laser difficult to reach, and stem cells in the bulge region stop dividing, and thus laser hair removal will not have a significant effect. In conclusion, the early anagen (early telogen) is the most effective time to stop hair follicle growth by laser hair removal [2].

The tissue reaction by hair removal laser is thought to occur in three ways. First, hair bulb damage. In the event of damage to the hair bulb, the hair cycle is induced by catagen and telogen, and subsequent hair grows in the same number but becomes thinner and brighter. Second, damage to the bulge. Damage to the bulge region will make hair more compact and permanently turn into hair-like vellus hair. Third, complete degeneration of hair follicle. With high fluence, long wavelengths, and long-pulsed durations of 20–50 ms, hair follicles will denature completely and hair will not grow at all.

If the hair bulb and bulge region are damaged but not fully denatured, there is evidence that the hair cycle is induced to catagen or telogen. Thus, even at low fluences, many hair cycles are synchronized, and when many hairs are subsequently induced to early anagen and laser is irradiated using high fluence and long-pulsed duration, the entire follicle unit will be destroyed and the effect of hair removal will appear. However, if the second laser procedure is initiated too early or too late, then it will not be effective.

The theory of optimal anagen treatment times, however, proved inconsistent with the use of hair removal lasers. Dierickx et al. studied hair removal with a 694-nm ruby laser and 800-nm diode laser. After 9 months, they found that 50% of missing hair was anagen when first treated, but 45% of missing hair was telogen when initially treated. Currently, hair cycles such as anagen or telogen are known to not affect laser hair removal effects [9].

8.2.4 Mechanism and Extended Theory of Selective Photothermolysis in Laser Hair Removal

The mechanism of laser hair removal can be divided into three categories [6]. First, photothermal effect. Using the extended theory, localized heat generated in hair bulb or hair shaft and matrix damages hair follicle stem cells and hair

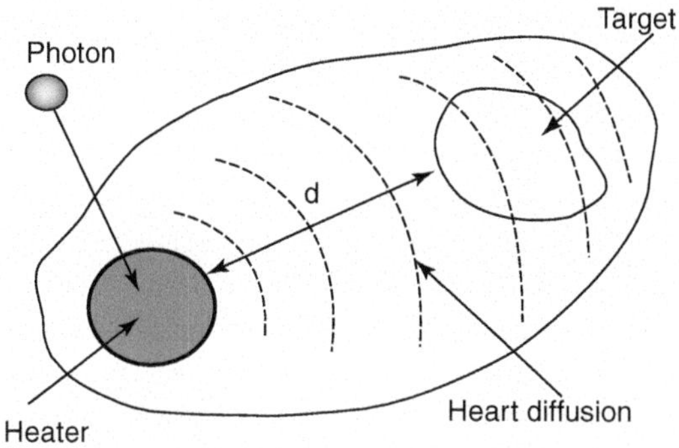

Fig. 8.4 General structure of biological target with space separation between target and absorber (heater). (Reproduced from [11])

germ cells, leading to hair removal (Fig. 8.4). It is the mechanism underlying the hair removal laser currently in use. These lasers include normal mode ruby lasers, long-pulsed alexandrite lasers, 810-nm diode lasers, long-pulsed Nd:YAG lasers, and IPLs. Currently, normal mode ruby lasers are not used for hair removal. Second, photomechanical effect. This mechanism damages hair follicle stem cells and dermal papillae by generating shock waves using nanosecond Q-switched lasers. Q-switched lasers are sometimes irradiated after carbon is applied to the skin. However, this only results in temporary hair loss and is not currently used. After removing eyebrow tattoos, hair growth does not occur for a while, because the photomechanical effect causes temporary hair removal. Third, photochemical effect. By applying the principle of photodynamic therapy (PDT), toxic mediators are made by using photosensitizer, light source, and oxygen, resulting in hair removal. It is theoretically applicable to red hair, yellow hair, and white hair with less black pigment, but more research is needed. Most of the research to date remains at the level of pilot studies.

8.2.5 Hair Growth Cycle and Laser Hair Removal Interval

The hair cycle consists of anagen phase, catagen phase, and telogen phase. Depending on the location of hair, anagen varies. For example, the anagen of eyebrows is 1–2 months, and the anagen of the scalp is 24–72 months. Telogen is relatively constant, ranging from 1 to 6 months, depending on the location of the hair. Therefore, the entire hair cycle, excluding the scalp, is usually about 4–12 months (Table 8.2). For reference, the length of the hair depends on anagen. This is why the hair on the scalp is the longest, and the length of eyebrows and hair on arms are short.

Table 8.2 Hair growth cycle by location

	Duration[a]		
Body area	Anagen	Telogen (months)	% Telogen
Scalp	2–6 years	3–4	10–15
Eyelashes	1–1.5 months		
Eyebrows	1–2 months	3–4	85–94
Moustache	2–5 months	1.5	34
Beard	1 year	2.5	
Chest		2.5	
Axillae			31–79
Arms	1–3 months	2.4	72–86
Thigh	1–2 months	2.3	64–83
Legs	4–6 months	3–6	62–88
Pubic hair			65–81

[a]The means to determine the duration of telogen and anagen were not standardized and vary greatly between authors. (Reproduced from [12])

In animal studies, the change in the destruction of hair follicles according to the hair cycle was observed. In other words, it is known that the laser hair removal effect is best in anagen with strong hair growth and pigmentation, and hair removal effect is poor in telogen or catagen. Therefore, if we ignore catagen, which is a very short period, hair removal interval will have to follow telogen intervals, i.e., telogen should be avoided. In addition, since telogen is slightly different depending on the area of the body, the interval of hair removal procedure should be different according to the area of the body. However, as described earlier, in humans, it is known that the hair cycle does not affect the hair removal effect. Unlike animals, human hair follicles have enough melanin in hair follicles regardless of the hair cycle, so laser hair removal in any hair cycle does not affect hair removal effect.

Then what is the most effective interval for hair removal? Christine Dierickx reported that treatment intervals less than 4 weeks or longer than 8 weeks resulted in decreased efficacy. Navid Bouzari reported that 45-day intervals are more effective than 60- or 90-day intervals for facial and neck hair removal [3].

Clinically, laser hair removal is usually performed at intervals of 4–8 weeks. Hair removal effect is seen in an average of five or more treatments. In general, after three or more treatments, the majority of patients will notice that the number of hairs decreases subjectively and objectively [3].

8.2.6 Permanent Hair Removal or Reduction

Although the term "permanent hair removal" is used in private practice, permanent loss of hair is not possible [7]. To be precise, the term "permanent hair reduction" should be used instead of the term "permanent hair removal."

Permanent hair reduction refers to a long-term, stable reduction of the number of hairs that grow back after a number of laser hair removals. The term "long-term" refers to the time of more than one hair cycle [7]. If hair does not grow during one hair cycle, it is unlikely that it will grow afterward, so permanent hair reduction can be defined as a reduction in the number of hairs that grow again over a period of 4–12 months, for the entire hair cycle except for the scalp (Table 8.2).

The U.S. Food and Drug Administration (FDA) states that permanent hair reduction does not refer to complete hair loss, in which all hair is lost [9]. On the other hand, there are two major factors that affect the subjective satisfaction of patients in the hair removal effect. First, the number and rate of regrowing hairs, and second, the thickness and color of the regrowing hairs [7].

Patients may misunderstand that when they receive laser hair removal, the term "permanency" means that hair will not ever grow again. Fortunately, laser hair removal reduces the number and proportion of hair that grows again, slows hair growth and hair becomes thinner and brighter in color like vellus hair (Fig. 8.5). Most patients are satisfied with the result but a small number of patients may complain that they did not receive "permanent" hair removal (to be exact, complete hair loss). I, therefore, recommend that the pre-procedure explanation to the patient must be explained in more detail. This is how I explain: "Laser hair removal is treated by an indirect method of transferring heat from hair bulb to stem cells. With tweezers, 100 hairs are gradually reduced to 90, 80, and 70 hairs. But this is not so in lasers. 100 stem cells are reduced to 90, 80, and 70 stem cells, resulting in hair becoming thinner and some hair may disappear in this process. However, after five laser hair removals, the number of hairs is significantly reduced and becomes thinner like vellus hair, so most patients are satisfied."

Also, because Beer's law (see "Chap. 1") is applied, it is very difficult for the number of stem cells to become completely zero, resulting in all hair removal. For example, assuming that 50% of all stem cells are destroyed by laser hair removal,

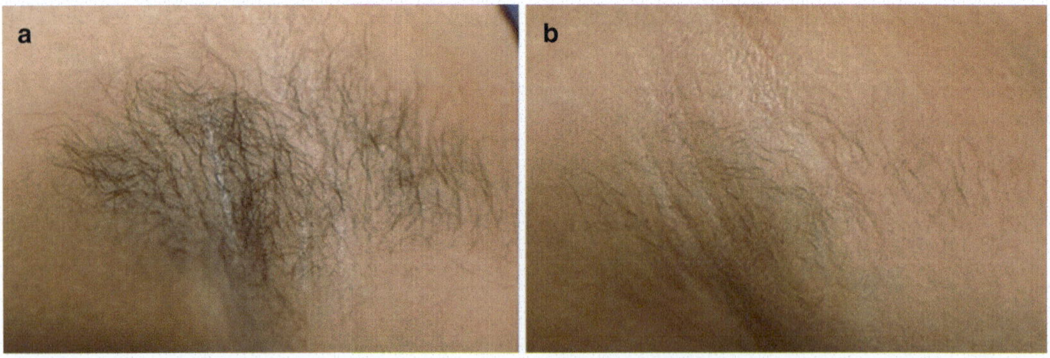

Fig. 8.5 (**a**) Pretreatment of the right axillary area with coarse hair. (**b**) Only fine hair exist after 3 months and five treatment with 1064 Nd:YAG laser. (Reproduced from [13])

100 stem cells are reduced to 50, 25, 12.5, and 6.25 depending on the number of procedures. That is, it is difficult to have zero stem cells, although infinitely increasing the number of procedures may lead to zero.

8.3 Wavelength

8.3.1 Optical Window and Types of Hair Removal Lasers

Looking back at the absorption curves for the three chromophores of skin, the melanin absorption curve continues to decrease from ultraviolet to visible and infrared light, and the water has no absorption curve in visible light, but the curve starts from near-infrared (MIR), gradually increase in the midinfrared (MIR) region. Hemoglobin shows a high absorption curve below 600 nm but shows a low absorption curve after 600 nm. Therefore, below 600 nm, the absorption curve for hemoglobin is high, and above 1200 nm, the absorption curve for water is high.

On the other hand, at 600 nm and 1200 nm, the absorption curves for hemoglobin and water are low or do not exist and only the absorption curves for melanin exist, and scattering is small and optical penetration depth is deep [15]. This area is called the optical window and is suitable for laser hair removal (Fig. 8.6). Scattering is high in wavelengths of less than 600 nm resulting in low penetration depth and can compete with other chromophores such as hemoglobin, causing side effects or diminishing effects. Wavelengths above 1200 nm have low absorption coefficients for melanin, making it difficult to produce high fluence or short pulse durations. Therefore 694-nm ruby lasers, 755-nm alexandrite lasers, 810-nm diode lasers, and 1064-nm Nd:YAG lasers, which have wavelengths corresponding to the optical window, are used as hair removal lasers. And although not a laser, IPL can also be used for laser hair removal because it has a wavelength corresponding to this region. (Table 8.3).

8.3.2 810-Nm Diode Laser

There are two types of 810-nm diode lasers. The first is a high-power single-pass diode laser. An example is the LightSheer™ (Lumenis, Inc., Santa Clara, CA, USA). The power is very high at 1600 W, so one pass alone is effective. But the procedure is painful with potential side effects,

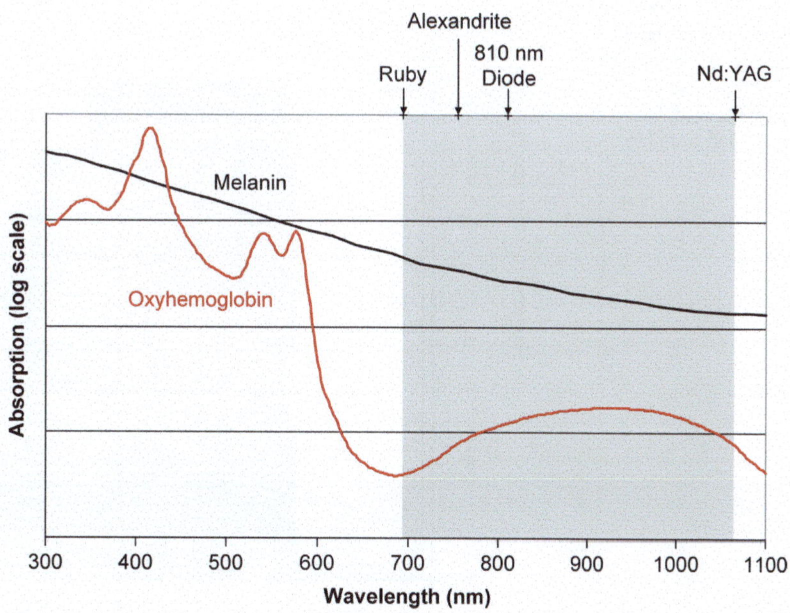

Fig. 8.6 Absorption profile for melanin and oxyhemoglobin. The shaded region identifies the range of wavelengths for lasers commonly used in nonablative dermatological procedures, e.g., tattoo removal, hair epilation. (Reproduced from [14])

and the cost of the laser is expensive. The second is a low-power multipass laser, such as the Soprano® XL (Alma Laser Ltd., Caesarea, Israel). To overcome the low output of 600 W, it works by using the concept of macropulse several times. It is known to have less pain and fewer side effects. Also due to the low output, the cost is cheaper.

Pai et al. compared 42 patients with facial hirsutism with LightSheer™ lasers on half of their faces and Soprano® XL lasers on the other half [16]. The parameters were 25–35 J/cm^2, 2 Hz, 30 ms, and 10 J/cm^2, 10 Hz, 20 ms, respectively. Soprano® XL lasers use lower fluence, with higher repetition. The procedure was performed six times at 4- to 6-week intervals.

The results showed that the overall hair reduction was 85% for LightSheer™ laser and 90.5% for Soprano® XL laser, which was not statistically significant ($p < 0.063$), but Soprano® XL laser was more effective (Fig. 8.7). The thickness of hair was also thinner with Soprano® XL laser (0.02 mm) than LightSheer™ laser (0.05 mm) ($p < 0.0005$) (Fig. 8.8). When the pain was divided into scores from 0 to 10 on the visual analog scale (VAS) (0 = no pain, 10 = unbearable pain), LightSheer™ laser scored 6 points and Soprano® XL laser scored two points, indicating that Soprano® XL laser had less pain (Fig. 8.9).

In conclusion, Soprano® XL laser has similar or better hair removal effects than LightSheer™ laser, while the pain is less. In the past, LightSheer™ laser was known as the golden standard for hair removal lasers. However, with the introduction of Soprano® XL lasers, which were cheaper to purchase and less painful, Soprano® XL lasers became popular in private practice. Currently, low-power multipass diode lasers are still the trend in hair removal lasers.

Then, what is the difference between high-power single pass diode laser and low-power multipass diode laser? The theoretical basis of hair removal laser is the extended theory of selective photothermolysis. Instead of using vaporization, shock waves, or plasma in the target tissue, protein degeneration is used by chang-

Table 8.3 Types of hair removal lasers

Types of hair removal lasers
694-nm normal mode (long-pulsed) ruby laser
755-nm long-pulsed alexandrite laser
810-nm diode laser 1. High-power single pass (e.g., LightSheer™) 2. Low-power multipass (e.g., soprano XL®)
1064-nm long-pulsed Nd:YAG laser
IPL (intense pulsed light)

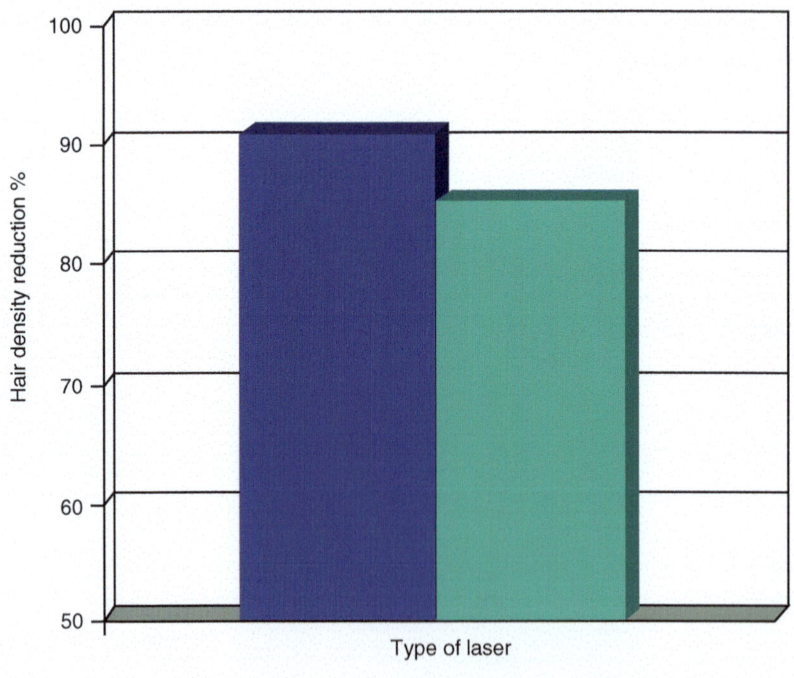

Fig. 8.7 Graph comparing the overall median hair removal percentages for Soprano XL (90.5%) and LightSheer (85%). (Modified from [16])

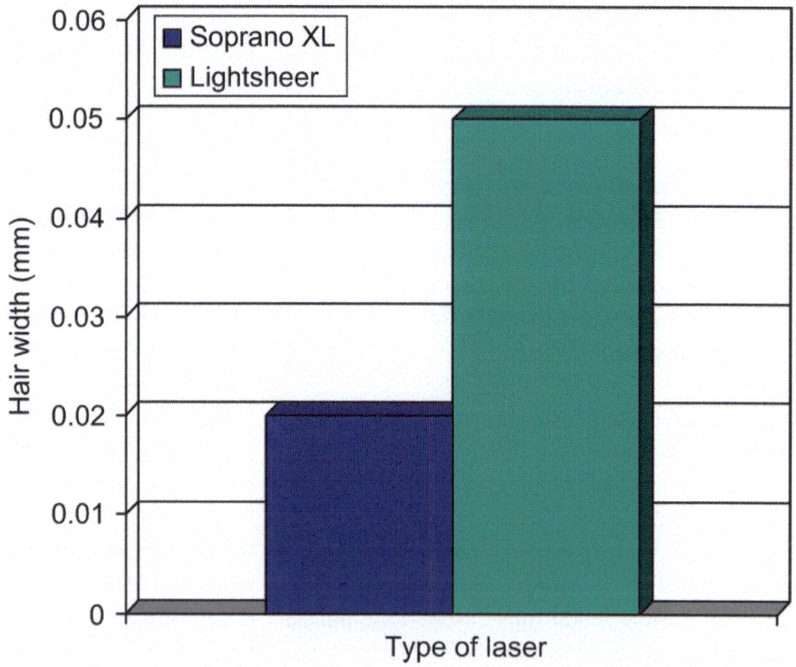

Fig. 8.8 Graph comparing the overall median hair width reduction for Soprano XL (0.02 mm) and LightSheer (0.05 mm). (Reproduced from [16])

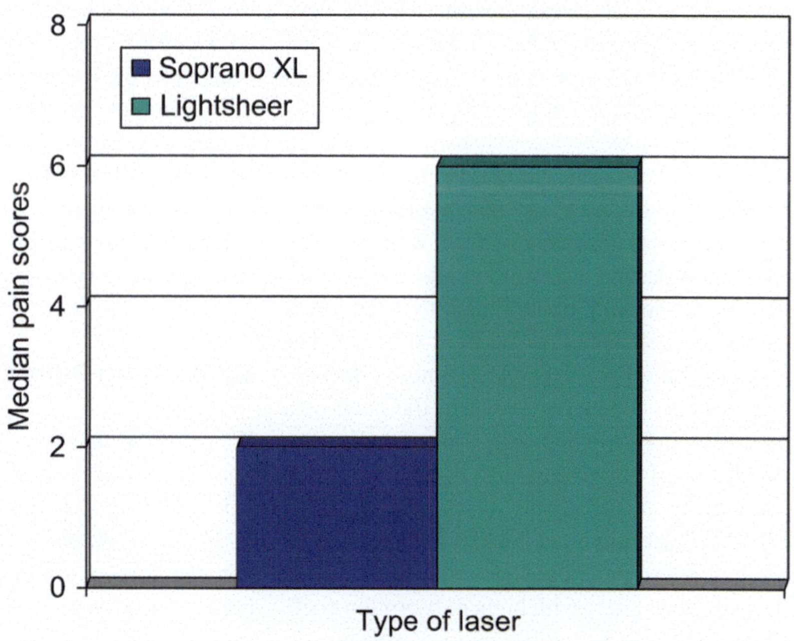

Fig. 8.9 Graph comparing the overall median pain scores for Soprano XL (2) and LightSheer (6). (Reproduced from [16])

ing the temperature to a temperature below 100 °C. Therefore, the Arrhenius formula, which applies to temperatures below 100 °C, is applied (see Sect. 3.6.3 in "Chap. 3"). There are two ways to apply a laser according to the Arrhenius formula. The first is to use a high temperature in a short time (method A), and the second is to use a low temperature in a long time (method B). I think that a high-power single pass diode laser corresponds to method A and a low-power multi-pass diode laser corresponds to method B. So, both lasers will have a similar effect. However, due to the narrow therapeutic window of high-power single pass diode laser, there is a high possibility of side effects and pain. On the other hand, low-power multipass diode lasers can be used safely, but the procedure time is longer than high-power single pass diode lasers.

8.3.3 Problems of Comparative Studies Between Hair Removal Lasers

Since the release of hair removal lasers, many articles have been published comparing the effects of hair removal lasers. In one laser text, 17 randomized clinical trials (RCTs) and 26 nonrandomized controlled clinical trials (CTs) published from 1990 to 2008 were reviewed, and the effect of normal mode ruby lasers, long-pulsed alexandrite lasers, 810-nm diode lasers, long-pulsed Nd:YAG lasers, and IPLs were compared and analyzed [17]. But comparing the effects of wavelengths is meaningless. Theoretically, if the pulse duration is the same and tissue temperature is the same, the result will be the same regardless of wavelength.

Among the papers comparing lasers of two wavelengths for effective hair removal lasers, there are papers comparing effects with the same parameters despite the different absorption coefficients for melanin. In particular, there are often papers that conclude that the laser with a higher melanin absorption coefficient is more effective. For example, for hair removal in the neck of a patient with Fitzpatrick skin type II, a 10 mm spot, 21 ms, 44 J/cm^2 with an 810-nm diode laser was used for one side, and 1064-nm long-pulsed Nd:YAG laser was used for the other side. The result is, not surprisingly, that even with the same fluence, diode lasers with higher absorption coefficients will have better hair removal effects.

Then how should we compare them? For example, the same temperature of the hair bulb should be used as the standard. To compare the temperature equally, the fluence should be increased as the absorption coefficient is lower. Diode laser has a 2.5 times higher absorption coefficient than the long-pulsed Nd:YAG laser. Therefore, the fluence of the long-pulsed Nd:YAG laser should be increased 2.5 times. The long-pulsed Nd:YAG lasers also have an optical penetration depth (OPD) of 3 mm, which is deeper than diode lasers. At this depth, long-pulsed Nd:YAG lasers have 25% more photons than diode lasers. Therefore, increasing the fluence of long-pulsed Nd:YAG laser 2 times (not 2.5 times) will result in the same temperature as diode lasers. Therefore, the fluence of the long-pulsed Nd:YAG lasers should be increased to at least 80 J/cm^2 [15].

Hair removal lasers with longer wavelengths can be thought to be more effective because photons are transferred to deeper hair follicles by longer wavelengths. However, all hair removal lasers that correspond to the optical windows reach the depth of dermis, and OPD (optical penetration depth) does not matter. I think the difference in wavelength in hair removal laser results in the difference in side effects more than the effect. Shorter wavelength hair removal lasers, such as ruby lasers, are suitable for whites because of the higher potential for side effects as many photons are absorbed in the epidermis. In longer wavelength hair removal lasers, such as long-pulsed Nd:YAG lasers, there is less epidermis absorption, so it can be used effectively for blacks, but it can penetrate deeply and cause serious scarring if side effects occur.

8.3.4 Long-Pulsed Nd:YAG Laser

We reviewed that when 44 J/cm^2 is used in 810-nm diode lasers, the fluence of long-pulsed Nd:YAG lasers should be increased to at least 80 J/cm^2, to compare these lasers. The problem is that the fluence of most long-pulsed Nd:YAG lasers cannot be raised to 80 J/cm^2 with a 10 mm spot size due to power limitations. In addition, long-pulsed Nd:YAG lasers have a high risk of burn if multiple pulses are used, such as the low-power multipass method.

Moreover, very short pulse duration is needed to treat thinner and lighter hair. Reducing the spot size significantly allows very short pulse duration, but long-pulsed Nd:YAG lasers do not actually use these parameters because of the high risk of burn and longer procedure time. Therefore, long-pulsed Nd:YAG lasers have less hair removal effect for thin hairs. Long-pulsed Nd:YAG laser is a suitable hair removal laser for thick and dark hair and is used for safe laser hair removal in very dark skin patients, especially blacks [15].

8.4 Hair Removal Laser Selection

8.4.1 Hair Removal in Darker Skin

Several laser texts recommend four methods for hair removal for darker (ethnic) skin [7]. Let's review these four methods in detail.

First, a laser with a long wavelength should be chosen. Since the target tissue of hair removal is the dermis, it is better to select a wavelength above 800 nm due to the epidermal bypass effect, and longer wavelength is safer. Also, longer wavelengths are beneficial for raising temperatures deep into the dermis. For example, when comparing 800 nm (wavelength similar to diode laser) and 700 nm (wavelength similar to ruby laser), 800 nm has a sufficient melanin absorption coefficient, and since it penetrates deeper than 700 nm, the dermal–epidermal temperature ratio is higher, which is more effective at raising the dermal temperature, and the epidermal temperature is low and safe (Fig. 8.10). 700 nm leaves only ~5% of its initial energy at 3 mm depth, the location of the hair bulb, while 800 nm leaves 24%. On the other hand, 800 nm requires higher energy because the melanin absorption coefficient is lower than 700 nm, which causes more pain in treatment [2].

However, the color difference between epidermis and hair shaft is more important in determining the wavelength than the penetration depth. In case of high color differences, such as Koreans (black hair, bright skin), even shorter wavelengths such as 650–700 nm can be used without damage to the epidermis and hyperpigmentation or hypopigmentation. On the other hand, when the color difference is low (bright hair, dark skin), it is safe to use a long wavelength of 800 nm or more (Fig. 8.11).

One laser text suggested recommended skin types for hair removal lasers [17]. It should be noted that the ruby laser and IPL are only recommended for Fitzpatrick skin types III and below. In addition, the US Food and Drug Administration (FDA) only approved 810-nm diode lasers and 1064-nm long-pulsed Nd:YAG lasers for hair removal in darker skin [7]. But if the skin is not very dark as in blacks and with sufficient epider-

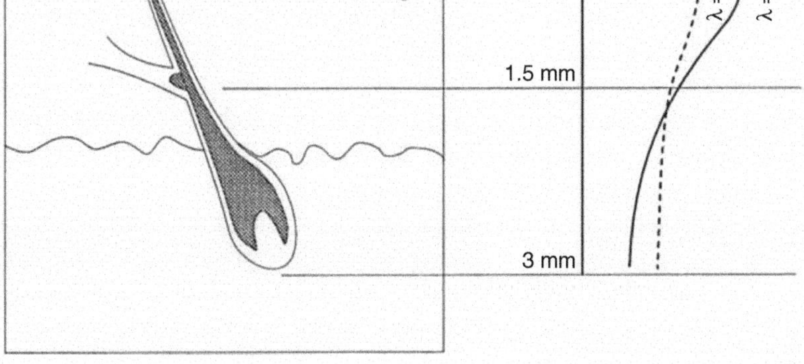

Fig. 8.10 Effect of wavelength on temperature distribution as a function of depth where other parameters are held constant. Note that the longer wavelength results in relative bulb heating and epidermal sparing. Reproduced from [2]

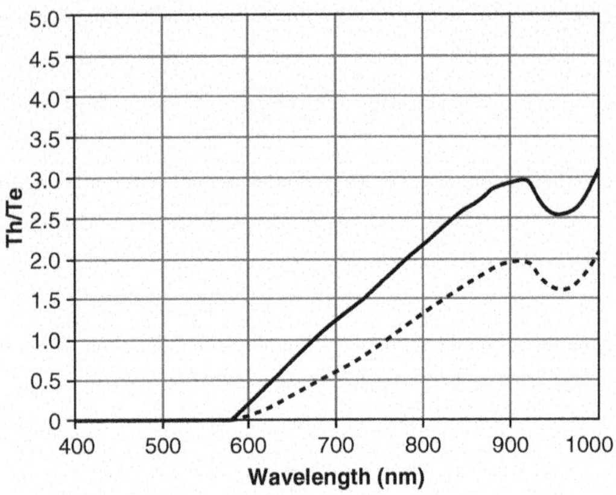

Fig. 8.11 Ration between hair bulb (Th) and epidermis (Te) temperature as a function of wavelength for hair depth of 3–4 mm. It can be seen that the temperature ratio is similar when the color difference is high at 700 nm (about 1.2) and when the color difference is low at 800 nm (about 1.3). High color difference: solid line, low color difference: dashed line. (Modified from [2])

mal cooling, alexandrite and diode lasers can be used in most skin [15].

Therefore, in Koreans, three lasers are thought to be suitable for laser hair removal. The 755-nm long-pulsed alexandrite laser, 810-nm diode laser, and the 1064-nm long-pulsed Nd:YAG laser. Of course, with the use of long-wavelength filters, IPL may also be used.

Second, a laser with a long-pulsed duration should be chosen. Due to thermal kinetic selectivity, longer pulse duration than 10 ms (epidermal TRT) is safer. (see Sect. 5.2.6 in "Chap. 5"). Longer pulse durations are also suitable for raising the temperature of hair follicle stem cells that are far from chromophores (Fig. 8.12) [2]. However, a longer pulse duration is less effective for thin hair.

Third, effective epidermal cooling should be used. Appropriate epidermal cooling must be selected depending on the laser and body region. We will review this again in Sect. 8.6.1

Fourth, the method of compacting the dermis by pressing the skin can be applied (Fig. 8.13). When the skin is pressed, blood vessels that are competing tissues disappear, epidermal pigmentations become lighter and the risk of side effects is reduced. Also, the distance between the hair follicle and epidermis becomes shorter, enabling more photons to reach the hair follicle, which

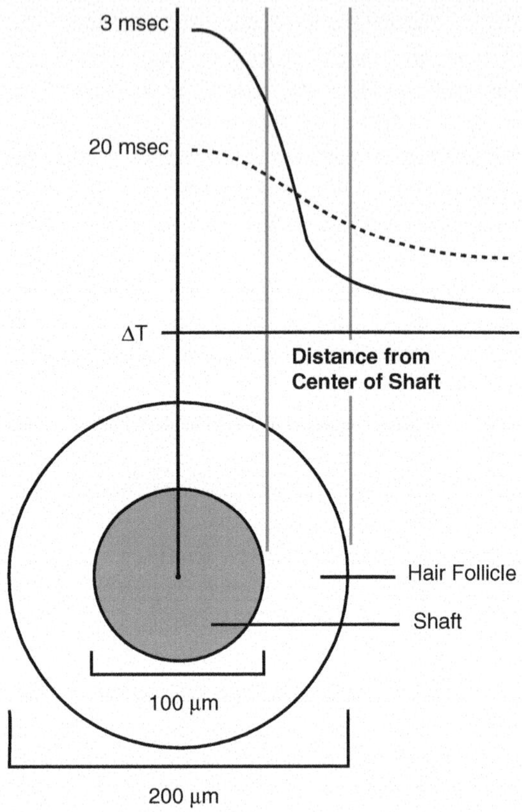

Fig. 8.12 Effect of pulse duration on the broadening of radial temperature profile. Note that longer pulse (20 ms) results in less heating of the midshaft but comparatively greater heating of the peripheral follicle. (Modified from [2])

gives hair bulb relatively high energy for the same fluence. This method may reduce the distance to the hair bulb and bulge region by 30%. However, the fluence may be variable for each procedure because the pressure may vary. Compressing dermis may also change the scattering coefficient and prevent penetration [15]. However, further studies are needed to prove this.

8.4.2 Hair Removal Laser for Koreans

Now we will compare the advantages and disadvantages of each laser, including IPL, and summarize which lasers should be selected specifically for Koreans (Table 8.4).

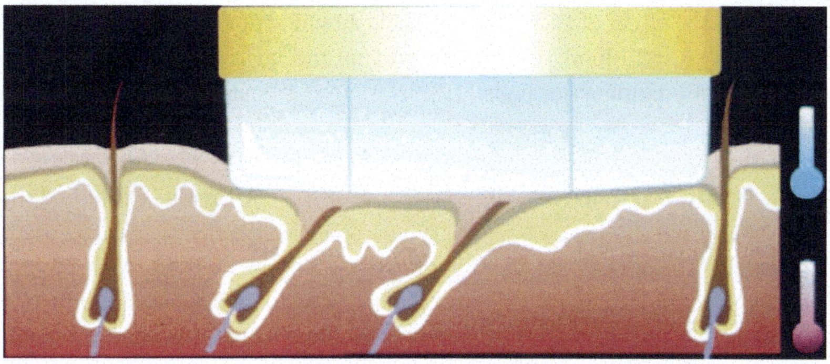

Fig. 8.13 Method of compacting the dermis. (Modified from [18])

Table 8.4 Pros and cons of hair removal laser

Category	Effect
Paradoxical hypertrichosis	IPL > others
Burn	Nd:YAG > others
Effect of fine hair removal	Others > Nd:YAG
Purchasing cost	Alexandrite > diode >IPL
Maintenance cost	Alexandrite, Nd:YAG, IPL > diode

IPL has the characteristics of divergence as opposed to collimation which is a characteristic of lasers. Thus, paradoxical hypertrichosis is most likely, due to weak energy given to the surrounding tissues. The risk of burn is present in all lasers, but long-pulsed Nd:YAG lasers have the deepest optical penetration depth (OPD), which can result in deep burns. Long-pulsed Nd:YAG lasers also have less efficacy for thin hairs. The most expensive laser is the alexandrite laser, the cost of the low-power multipass diode laser is in the middle, and IPL has the lowest cost. There is little maintenance cost for diode lasers because the laser medium and external pumping system is semiconductor and electricity, respectively. On the other hand, IPL, alexandrite lasers, and Nd:YAG lasers require lamp replacement (higher maintenance costs) because the external energy source is a flashlamp.

In summary, lower power multipass type 810-nm diode laser is effective without any side effects and with low purchase and maintenance costs. Therefore, I recommend that lower cost multipass 810-nm diode lasers for those who specialize in hair removal. However, if there is not much demand for hair removal and if you want to treat epidermal pigmentations, 755-nm long-pulsed alexandrite lasers are suitable. In addition, long-pulsed alexandrite lasers are also effective for thin hair on the face because of their short pulse duration, which also helps to whiten the face.

8.4.3 Paradoxical Hypertrichosis

The most confusing side effect of laser hair removal is paradoxical hypertrichosis. Paradoxical hypertrichosis is the phenomenon in which hair increase after laser hair removal. Paradoxical hypertrichosis is known to occur in about 5% of the Mediterranean and Middle Eastern races and is usually permanent once they occur. This occurs on or near the area where a laser removal procedure has been performed. It usually affects the jawline, cheeks, neck, shoulders, back, and upper arms, and is more likely to be closer to the torso than the treatment region. It is more common in Fitzpatrick skin types III and IV, and in people whose forehead hairline is unclear [7]. Also, it may occur if the procedure interval is more than 8 weeks, the pulse duration is short, or the wavelength or fluence is not appropriate.

The mechanism is not yet known, but LLLT (low-level laser therapy) mechanism suggests that weak light rather stimulates hair follicles and leads them to the anagen phase, resulting in thicker hair. Therefore, in order to reduce paradoxical hypertrichosis, appropriate sufficiently high fluence should be used for laser hair removal.

To prevent the effect of LLLT, a cold pack should be used to shrink blood vessels and prevent the activation of inflammatory cells [19].

8.5 Pulse Duration

The extended theory of selective photothermolysis is applied in hair removal lasers. The pulse duration (PD) should be equal to or shorter than the thermal damage time (TDT) and longer than the thermal relaxation time (TRT), i.e., TDT ≥ PD > TRT.

TRT and TDT according to the thickness of the hair shaft are shown below (Table 8.5). Laser irradiation method changes TDT value depending on rectangular temperature pulse and rectangular light pulse. In rectangular temperature pulse, the same temperature is maintained during irradiation. Most of the lasers we use are rectangular light pulses that maintain the same fluence during irradiation.

Let's look at TDT using medium coarse hair as an example. The thickness of medium coarse hair is 70 μm, which is 3 ms calculated by TRT. The TDT is 610 ms. The TRT is 27 ms based on hair follicles containing stem cells rather than hair. Therefore, the theoretical TDT ranges from 27 to 610 ms. Pulse duration should be less than or equal to TDT. Therefore, theoretically, hair removal is possible even if the pulse duration varies from 3 to 610 ms. In reality, super long-pulsed 810-nm diode laser (Super Long Pulse, Palomar, Burlington, MA) is known to have hair removal effects even though the pulse duration is very long (200–400 ms). However, the pulse duration of 50–100 ms or more can seriously damage the epidermis and upper dermis due to significant heat conduction. Heat transfer from a heated epidermis and hair follicle may cause scarring, a phenomenon called the "iron heater" effect [2]. One of the reasons for varying pulse durations in laser hair removal is due to the Arrhenius formula. I think there are various pulse durations because the denaturation of stem cells is possible with the appropriate temperature for each pulse duration. Clinically, a pulse duration of 30–40 ms is known to be appropriate. However, even 3 ms is known to be effective. However, 3 ms is known to be ineffective when the density of coarse hair is high [3].

In the Sect. 6.3 in "Chap. 6, we reviewed that "pulse durations slightly above the TRT of blood vein is suitable for vessels smaller than 0.25 mm and pulse durations same or shorter than the TRT of blood lumen is suitable for vessels smaller than 0.25 mm." Similarly, in laser hair removal, shouldn't the pulse duration be determined by adjusting thin hair to the TRT of the hair follicle and thick hair to the TRT of hair shaft? However, there is no known selection of pulse duration depending on the thickness of the hair.

The reasons why macropulse is used in vascular therapy are because (1) short pulse duration and high energy may cause purpura above 100 °C and (2) long pulse duration and low energy spare small blood vessels and cannot be treated due to thermal kinetic selectivity in the thermal phase of an optical thermal model (see Sect. 6.6.4 in "Chap. 6"). Likewise, in the case of laser hair removal, vaporization occurs over 100 °C, so that the hair removal effect due to the photothermal effect is not seen [15]. Therefore, the short pulse duration cannot be used for high energy and long pulse duration should be used for low energy. However, with long pulse durations, thin hair

Table 8.5 TRT and TDT depending on the diameter of the hair shaft (HS - hair shaft, HF - hair follicle). (Modified from [11])

Hair type	Diameter (μm)	TRT of HS (ms)	TRT of HF (ms)	TDT of stem cell (ms)	
				Rectangular temperature pulse	Rectangular light pulse
Fine	30	0.6	5.4	30	115
Medium coarse	70	3	27	170	610
Large coarse	120	9.6	87	510	1800

cannot be removed because of the thermal kinetic selectivity. This is why I think hair removal of thin hair is not effective.

Considering the above, in order to remove thin hair, pulse duration should be shortened according to the thickness so that the laser is absorbed by thin hair. Therefore, low-power multipass diode laser with long pulse duration cannot remove thin hair. And like the macropulse of blood vessels and the multipulse of IPL, I believe that hair removal laser should use multiple pulses. Ross et al. stated that when using multiple pulses for laser hair removal, 10–100 times of TRT downtime is required for sufficient cooling of the baseline temperature [2]. For example, for the epidermis, a time between 0.1 and 1 s (1–10 Hz) was required, with 10–100 times the time between repeated irradiations. Thus, I use a 755-nm long-pulsed alexandrite laser and overlap more than 70% at 1–2 Hz. Of course, precooling and postcooling must be done to prevent residual heat buildup on the epidermis.

Finally, I think that there will be thin hairs that are not treated with laser hair removal, just as blood vessels below 25.5 μm (TRT <0.296 ms) cannot be treated. Therefore, it is necessary to investigate the time and temperature of tissue degeneration for hair and stem cells like Fig. 6.17.

8.5.1 Pain and Pulse Duration

Hair follicles have pain fibers in which neurovascular bundles are arranged. Pain during laser hair removal may occur in the epidermis or the dermis. In particular, pulse duration affects pain. As pulse duration increases, heat conduction increases the temperature around the hair follicle, and pain increases [2].

8.6 Spot Size and Epidermal Cooling

In laser hair removal, using the largest spot size possible is recommended. As mentioned in "Chap. 3," the spot size effect requires the use of large spot sizes to deepen optical penetration depth and to treat dermis while protecting epidermis (Fig. 8.14). Larger spot sizes can also reduce the procedure time required for laser hair removal. However, the larger the spot size, the more overlap of the spots (Fig. 8.15).

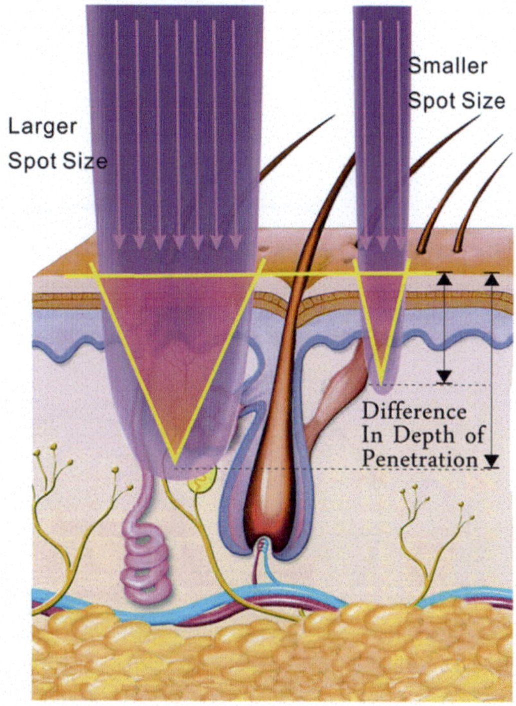

Fig. 8.14 The relationship between spot size and depth of laser beam penetration. (Reproduced from [20])

The pulse duration of hair removal laser is all in milliseconds including the IPL. That is, they are all long-pulsed lasers. In "Chap. 3," in long-pulsed lasers, pulse stacking can cause side effects due to residual heat accumulation. Therefore, to avoid pulse stacking, irradiating without overlapping is needed (an in Fig. 8.15). However, irradiating the laser without overlapping may result in missing areas. In the case of laser hair removal, the hair will grow only in this area, resulting in sparse hair growth which is not cosmetically desirable.

How can side effects be avoided while irradiating with spots overlapping (b in Fig. 8.15)? This is why epidermal cooling, especially postcooling is needed. Usually in epidermal cooling, postcooling is used to reduce pain and edema

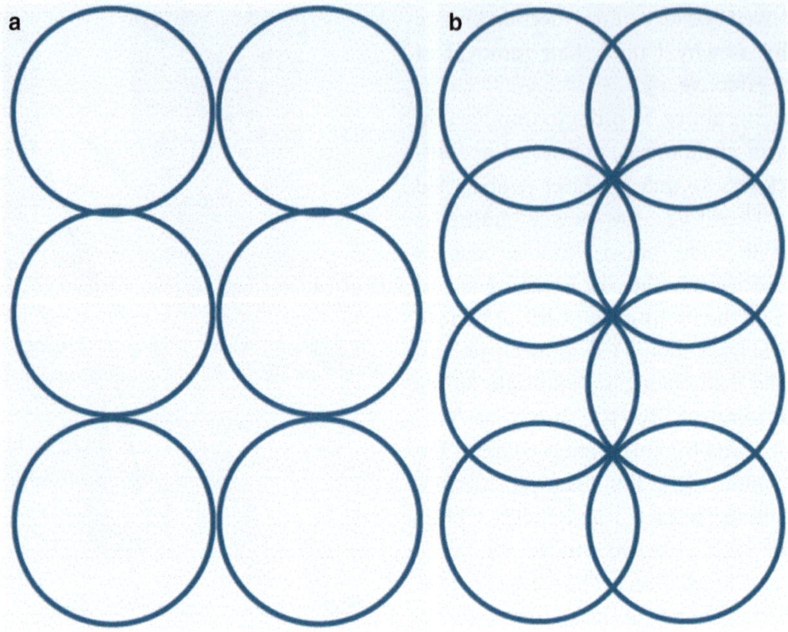

Fig. 8.15 (**a**) irradiating without spots overlapping (**b**) irradiating with spots overlapping and without missing areas

rather than affect the effect of laser. However, in laser hair removal, postcooling is important in preventing side effects of pulse stacking due to overlapping spots.

8.6.1 Epidermal Cooling

The absorption coefficient of hair shaft and hair bulb is 2–6 times higher than of epidermis [2]. So, in fact, no matter how dark the skin, the hair is darker. Thus, laser hair removal without epidermal cooling does not result in very severe epidermal damage. However, for safety reasons, epidermal cooling should be performed when laser hair removal is being done.

Epidermal cooling can be classified by various methods, but there are generally five methods [15]: (1) passive cooling by water-containing gel such as an ultrasonic gel, (2) active cooling by water flow on glass tip, (3) active conductive cooling by cooling sapphire tip with water, (4) dynamic active cooling using cryogenic spray, and (5) air cooling with a refrigerated air stream.

(1) Passive cooling. Heat exchange between the skin and the cooling mechanism is carried out through the stratum corneum which has little moisture, so heat conduction does not occur well [2]. Therefore, water or moisture-containing gel is applied to the skin to increase moisture in stratum corneum. It is very inexpensive but has a low-temperature gradient compared to other cooling methods. In other words, cooling is ineffective. In addition, since the external cooling device does not continue to draw heat, the heat drops only a little over time. Applying a lot of gel may help preserve the epidermis, as it reduces heat and reduces backscattering, but using the aforementioned method of compacting the dermis is not enough to reduce backscattering.

During (3) active conductive cooling, the sapphire tip is cooled with 2–6 °C water flow. If the 0 °C sapphire tip is in contact with the skin for 0.5 s, the temperature of the basal layer is known to drop to about 20 °C. So, you can move the handpiece relatively quickly without worrying about the basal layer being cooled enough. However, cooling in the same place for more than a few seconds cools both the bulge region and the hair shaft, reducing laser hair removal effects [2]. (2) Active cooling by water flow on glass tips, on the other hand, requires longer contact time than sapphire tips. In addition, the sapphire tip is well resistant to moisture and shock and has good thermal conductivity. A disadvantage of the cooling tip is that frost builds up on the surface in a humid environment, reducing the strength of the beam.

The ice cube method of precooling with ice can also be used for epidermal cooling. This method can achieve epidermal cooling if the contact time is sufficient. But glass, ice, and water have low thermal conductivity, resulting in longer contact time and less temperature difference between epidermis and bulge region, and less hair removal effect.

(4) Dynamic active cooling is a method in which a cryogen is sprayed immediately before laser irradiation. Cooling is efficient and the heat difference between epidermis and dermis is high. Thus, the epidermis can be sufficiently cooled while avoiding unnecessary dermal cooling. It is especially useful for cooling epidermis while treating very shallow lesions such as port-wine spots (PWS) that are 0.2–4 mm deep. However, because the bulge region and hair bulb are deeply located, this method is not mandatory for laser hair removal. When a laser is irradiated for 5–10 ms and then a cryogenic spray is sprayed for 10–50 ms, thus, the temperature of the epidermis can be kept at −10 °C for a time of 100 ms or less and the cooling is effective to a depth of 200 μm. The disadvantage is that the size of refrigerant droplets is irregular and cooling may occur unevenly. In addition, unlike conductive cooling, there is no optical coupling to prevent backscattering. In addition, condensation may occur in a high humidity environment, thereby reducing the intensity of the beam irradiated after the refrigerant is sprayed [2].

(5) Convective cooling with cold air is also useful when removing large areas of hair.

In laser hair removal, we believe that active cooling using a sapphire tip and refrigerant cooling is suitable.

8.7 Clinical End Point of Laser Hair Removal

Although several laser texts describe the clinical end point of laser hair removal as perifollicular edema (PFE) [21], PFE is not a reliable clinical end point for laser hair removal (Fig. 8.16). PFE is thought to be caused by peribulbar damage, but severe peribulbar damage does not correlate with severe edema. In addition, PFE edema does not occur during PDL procedure, so PFE is thought to only occur when the heat is applied to deep layers. In addition, PFE is more likely to occur at shorter pulse duration than at long pulse duration, so it seems that PFE occurs frequently when short and strong damage to the follicle occurs.

On the contrary, PFE does not occur with long pulse duration, but permanent hair reduction is observed. For example, super long-pulsed 810 nm diode laser (Super Long Pulse, Palomar, Burlington, MA), has a long pulse duration of 200–400 ms, so PFE does not occur, but permanent hair reduction is observed. In other words, the absence of PFE edema does not mean there is no permanent hair reduction. Therefore, there is

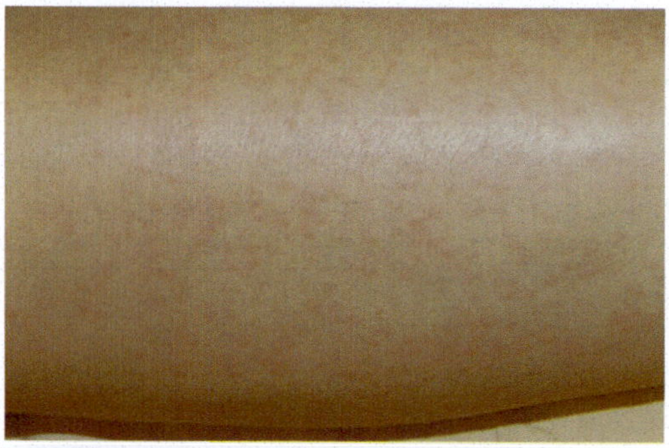

Fig. 8.16 Edema and erythema around pores after calf hair removal with 755-m long-pulsed alexandrite laser

no reliable clinical end point for laser hair removal [15], and this is why it is difficult to determine fluence in laser hair removal.

Laser hair removal is a typical procedure without a clinical end point. Then how should we determine the fluence? In procedures without clinical end points, we have no choice but to determine fluence empirically. The procedure must be repeated for several times to find the fluence that is effective without side effects.

As a result, patients may visit because of delayed side effects. For example, the fluence of the initial laser hair removal procedure is 8 J/cm^2. The problem is that after prolonged laser use, the number on the gauge does not change, but the output drops slightly. Later, when the initial fluence is ineffective, the fluence is increased up to 10 J/cm^2. After the flashlamp reaches its end of life, it is replaced by a new lamp. When 10 J/cm^2 is unintentionally used after the flashlamp change, the energy is too high, i.e., side effects occur. But it is difficult to notice in advance because there is no change immediately after a hair removal procedure. In order to avoid this, first, it should be noted that the output of laser decreases as it is used. Second, fluence should be reduced after replacing the flash lamp or calibrating the output by laser inspection. Third, patients with laser hair removal should be advised to visit the hospital immediately if erythema or papules do not disappear after 24 h. I have also been through this several times.

Sometimes immediate hair loss after laser hair removal (pop out) may be observed. Some laser physicians consider "pop out" as the clinical end point of hair removal because they can directly observe hair falling out, in front of their eyes. But "pop out" is not a clinical end point for hair removal. The reason for the "pop out" phenomenon is because due to the high fluence the temperature of hair shaft rises and vaporization occurs due to the pressure in the hair follicle. Since the energy of the laser is lost due to vaporization (phase change), heat is not transferred to stem cells. Of course, not all of the laser energy is lost by vaporization, but part of it is used for vaporization, and the rest of the energy is thermally conductive, resulting in some hair removal effect. Therefore, the "pop out" phenomenon is not a clinical end point of hair removal, and while some hair coming out is fine, if the energy is increased to the extent that all the hair comes out, the effect is not only reduced but also the likelihood of side effects, such as follicle inflammation, or scars, increases.

On the other hand, side effects such as burns do not occur even when some hairs are "popped out." I think that the reason for this is as follows. First, like fractional photothermolysis, hairs sparsely exist so that only the area around hairs are damaged and the recovery is quick. Therefore, caution should be taken in about areas where hair grows tight, such as beards and scalp hair. Second, hair follicles are epidermal appendages and may have high regenerating characteristics.

8.8 Strategy and Parameters for Laser Hair Removal

Let's summarize the strategy of laser hair removal according to Sect. 3.8 in "Chap. 3." Target tissues are the hair bulb and bulge region located in the dermis. Competitive tissue is the pigmented epidermis. First, because of the vertical relationship, epidermal cooling is more important than selective photothermolysis. Therefore, the laser physician should not neglect to check the cooling system. Second, according to the theory of selective photothermolysis and epidermal bypass effect, 800 nm or more laser should be used. 755 nm, which is close to 800 nm is safe for Koreans with light skin. 755 nm long-pulsed alexandrite laser, 810-nm diode laser, 1064-nm long-pulsed Nd:YAG lasers and IPLs with long-wavelength filters can also be used. "Dark lesions should be shot weakly and light lesions should be shot strongly." For the same reason, fluence should be lower for male beard hair removal while fluence should be higher for female philtrum hair removal. Due to thermal kinetic selectivity, the procedure will be safer if the pulse duration is longer than 10 ms, which is the TRT for the epidermis. Third, fractional photothermolysis or pinhole method has little meaning in hair removal. Finally, if there are epidermal pigmentations, it should be removed prior to the hair removal procedure.

Let's summarize the parameter of laser hair removal. First, the wavelength is described above. Second, the pulse duration of 30–40 ms is clinically used. Of course, there is also a hair removal laser that has a longer pulse duration of more than 10 ms, and in the case of long-pulsed alexandrite laser, hair removal is possible in 3 ms. Optimal pulse duration is therefore not yet known. Third, fluence should be determined empirically, not by clinical end point. Fourth, the larger the spot size, the deeper the optical penetration depth and the shorter the procedure time. That is, larger spot size is better. Fifth, because millisecond laser is mainly used, stacking may cause side effects due to residual heat accumulation and is not recommended. Therefore, the frequency should not be increased. Sixth, epidermal cooling is the most important strategy.

8.9 Effect of Laser Hair Removal

The effect of laser hair removal is summarized as follows [22]. First, laser hair removal is known to reduce 15–30% hair with each procedure, with better results after the repeated procedure [4]. With repeated procedures, the reduction in the number of hairs may be up to 40 to 80%, sometimes 100% [22]. Second, laser hair removal effect may not be permanent. Therefore, if the effect is insufficient, additional treatment is required. Third, the effect of laser hair removal differs for each body area. Effective areas are the armpits, calves, bikini lines, genital areas, foreheads, and chest. Less effective areas are the back, upper lip, and scalp [3]. Also, coarse hair like terminal hair has a better effect than vellus hair. Fourth, since laser hair removal does not remove hair but damages stem cells, hair grows again after hair removal, but the hair is thinner and brighter than before, resulting in hair removal effect is seen. Although permanent hair loss is possible, this should not be promised or guaranteed to the patient [22].

8.9.1 Effect of Laser Hair Removal Depending on Ethnicity

Factors affecting treatment outcomes in laser hair removal vary. Patients can be classified as follows, depending on skin color, hair appearance, and hormonal status (Table 8.6) [7]. First, the most ideal patient for laser hair removal is a patient with thick hair, black terminal hair, and white skin. The patient should have normal hormone levels and no hormonal abnormalities such as polycystic ovarian syndrome (PCOS). In the case of hirsutism, the effect of laser hair removal is poor [4]. Unsuccessful patients are those with thin vellus hair or whose hair is white, gray, or red (Fig. 8.17). Finally, patients with increased

Table 8.6 Hair and skin effective for laser hair removal

Patients	Hair and skin
Ideal	Thick dark terminal hairs, white skin
Not successful	Thin vellus hairs or white, grey, or red hairs
Increased risk	Dark skin types and sun exposure

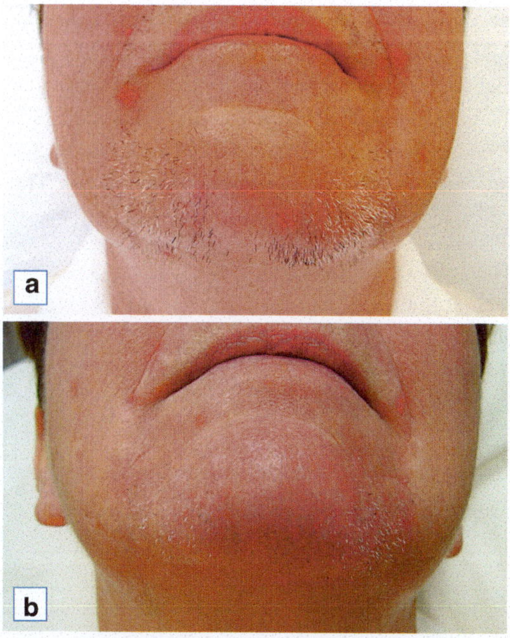

Fig. 8.17 Effective LHR (laser hair removal) can be obtained for dark, pigmented hairs but not for white hairs: (**a**) before and (**b**) after treatment. Reproduced from [10]

risks are patients with dark skin or those who received recent tanning.

In terms of ethnicity, laser hair removal is not successful in whites. Whites have no side effects because their skin is white, but their hair is red or yellow, which reduces the effectiveness of laser hair removal. In blacks the risk increases. Their hair is black, but the skin is black also, so there is a high chance of side effects. Therefore, blacks should look for methods with the least amount of side effects, in which the effect of the epidermal pigmentation is minimized. On the other hand, Koreans have light skin with black hair, making them the ideal for laser hair removal. That is why laser hair removal is especially active and popularized in Korea. However, thin hairs such as philtrum or vellus hair are less effective regardless of ethnicity.

8.10 Procedure

8.10.1 Patient Selection and Pretreatment

The most ideal patients for laser hair removal are Koreans with bright skin and thick and dark hair. Recently, many Southeast Asians live in Korea. And in people with darker skin, sufficient epidermal cooling, use of longer wavelength lasers, and increasing pulse duration to adjust parameters is needed. It is better to delay procedures for patients who have recently been tanned [7]. The effect, limitations, procedure, and side effects of laser hair removal should be explained fully before the procedure and should be performed on patients with realistic expectations. Taking oral retinoid (trade name Accutane) for the last 6 months was a contraindication but recently there are many reports that there is no significant association between oral retinoid and skin regeneration (see “Chap. 11”). I think if the patients use low-dose treatment of less than 20 mg oral retinoid and if the fluence of the laser is not high, the possibility of side effects is low. Female patients with Fitzpatrick skin type III and IV and unclear forehead hairlines may result in paradoxical hypertrichosis, but I have not observed this and think this is a rare phenomenon.

Removing the chromophore of laser (hair shaft), such as plucking or waxing before laser hair removal, may have no hair removal effect. However, unlike animals, hair cycle does not affect hair removal effects in humans, so I think that even though there is no hair there might be some hair removal effect but the effect may be reduced [4]. Nevertheless, I recommend not plucking or waxing for at least 2 weeks before the procedure and shaving only [10].

It is recommended to shave the day before the procedure. The reason for this is that blisters can occur if long hair is attached to the patient's skin. In particular, when hair is coagulated by laser irradiation and adhered to the handpiece, it is carbonized, and high heat is generated in the carbonized tissue, which may burn the skin (Fig. 8.18) [23]. Therefore, shaving should be done before

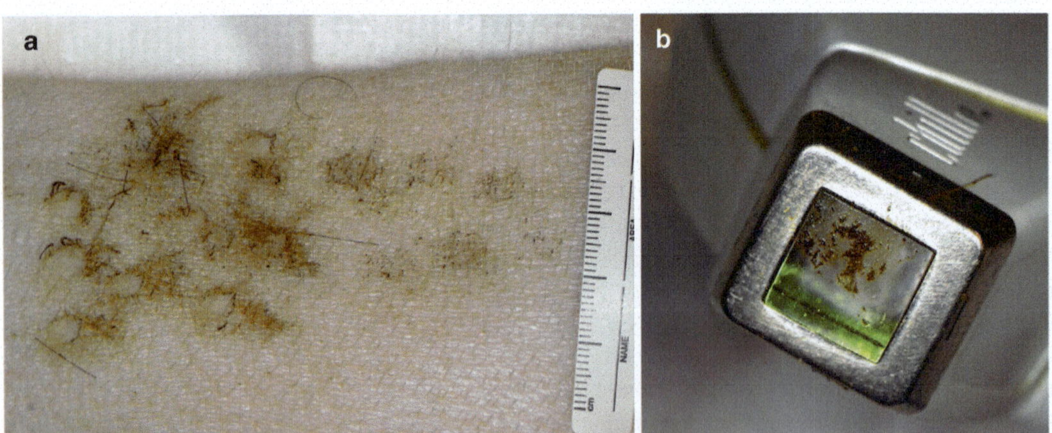

Fig. 8.18 (**a**) Stamping burn pattern after the use of an 800-nm diode laser with a dirty cold contact window. (**b**). Hair char is present on the cold window. (Reproduced from [23])

the procedure, and shaved hair should not remain in the treatment area. The handpiece should be cleaned well and should always be checked before the procedure. If the skin is damaged by shaving, the laser may further damage the skin, which is likely to cause side effects such as folliculitis. Therefore, it is important to shave without damaging the skin. Therefore, sometimes I carefully shave the patients on the day of the procedure, if they did not shave the day before.

Finally, sufficient topical anesthesia should be done before procedures that may induce pain.

8.10.2 Treatment Procedure

Immediately before the procedure, the laser should be checked for abnormalities, especially making sure that the cooling is sufficient. Everyone in the treatment room should wear safety glasses, and the patient should wear eye protection. When treating around the eyes, a metal protective device must be inserted into the eye. Laser should not be applied to the inside of the orbital rim because it can damage the eyes [7]. If pigmentations such as freckles or melanocytic nevi are present, these may be removed first or colored with a white pen before the laser procedure. Laser parameters should be appropriately adjusted according to the patient's skin type, color, area, hair thickness, and density.

8.10.3 Posttreatment Care

After the procedure, an ice pack or cool pack may be used to reduce erythema and edema. If severe erythema and edema occur immediately after the procedure, or if gray or white discoloration occurs [7], I educate the patient to return to the hospital if the side effects do not subside after applying group 1 steroid ointment three times a day for 2 days. Patients should avoid strong sunlight and tanning during the entire course of treatment and should take appropriate actions such as hats and sunscreens during outdoor activities. After the procedure, hair can come out of the skin for a week, and the patient should be told in advance that this is normal.

8.11 Recent Hair Removal Strategy

Nowadays, laser hair removal using laser or optical sources in hospitals is the mainstream of hair removal, but new hair removal methods are being developed. First, recently portable home-based devices are on the market. These devices are low-level diode lasers and IPL devices. To date, it is known that repetitive and continuous use has a transient short-term hair reduction effect for a short period [7]. Therefore, it is less effective than laser hair removal received at the clinic. However, I believe that household hair removal equipment will become mainstream in the hair removal market if the technology is developed and output increases in the future. Second is the method using photodynamic therapy (PDT). As explained in the Sect. 8.2.4 further studies are needed but it is expected that if a new photosensitizer is developed, it will be quite effective. Third, there is a method of applying eflornithine. Eflornithine (VaniqaT) is known as an enzyme that irreversibly inhibits ornithine decarboxylase, which regulates hair growth and proliferation. It can be used as an adjuvant therapy for laser hair removal. In particular, it can be used for hair that exhibits therapeutic resistance to laser hair removal on the face. The results showed that the hair removal effect was increased when used together with laser hair removal. However, there is still a lack of long-term and controlled studies of the effects and stability of eflornithine [7].

8.12 Trichostasis Spinulosa

Trichostasis spinulosa is a disease that clinically looks like black spots on hair follicles. Histologically, trichostasis spinulosa is a skin disease in which hair follicles are filled with vellus hair masses and keratin plugs. It usually occurs in the nose or forehead and is also found in the body. The exact mechanism of development is unknown but is thought to be due to abnormal hair follicle units. In other words,

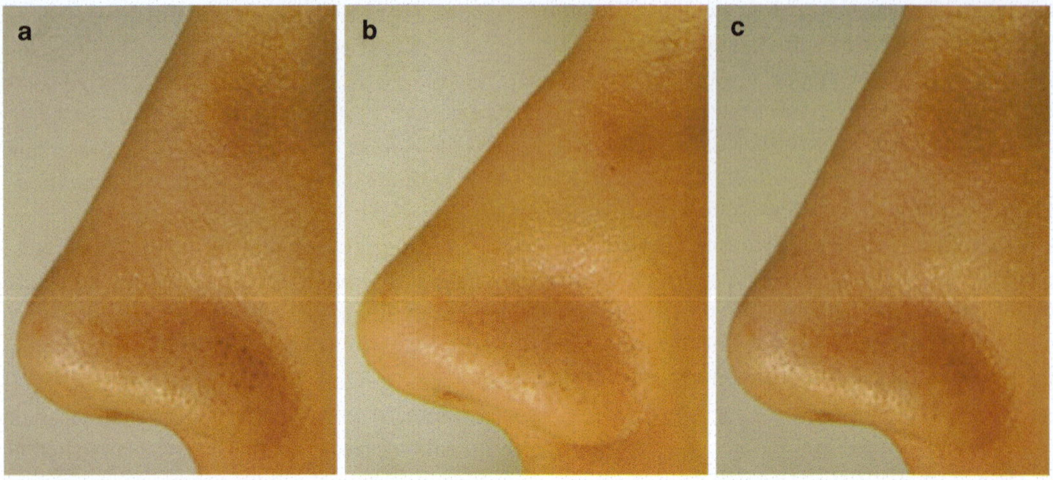

Fig. 8.19 Trichostasis spinulosa in a patient before the treatment with 755-nm Alexandrite laser (**a**). Four weeks after the first treatment showing 25–50% improvement (**b**). Twenty weeks after the second treatment showing a 50–75% improvement (**c**). Reproduced from [24]

blockage of hair follicle entrance by follicular keratosis around follicular infundibulum and the abnormal angulations of isthmus with respect to infundibulum prohibits small telogen hair coming out and the hair remains in the hair follicles. In addition, *P. acnes* is thought to be one of the causes because *P. acnes* is found in trichostasis spinulosa [24].

Thus, treatment of trichostasis spinulosa is the correction of abnormal hair follicles. Due to the presence of vellus hairs in the hair follicle, a hair removal laser treatment with a chromophore as vellus hair has been attempted. Toosi et al. used 755-nm long-pulsed alexandrite twice in 31 patients with trichostasis spinulosa [24]. The parameters were 14–18 J/cm^2 with a pulse duration of 3 ms in an 18 mm spot size. Clinical end points were considered as perifollicular erythema and edema. The results showed that 51.3% of patients showed more than 50% reduction in trichostasis spinulosa and 9.7% of patients showed more than 75% reduction (Fig. 8.19). Badawi et al. used a 755 nm long-pulsed alexandrite laser in 20 patients with trichostasis spinulosa [25]. The parameters were performed once with 1–3 passes at 5 mm spot, 0.5 ms, 15–17 J/cm^2. The clinical end point was the disappearance of "black hair dots." The results showed that trichostasis spinulosa disappeared immediately after treatment, and the follow-up of up to 3 months confirmed that it was well maintained without recurrence.

The parameters of the two papers show that the pulse duration is relatively shorter and the fluence is twice as high as that of hair removal parameter used in 755 nm long-pulsed alexandrite laser. Thus, I believe that the mechanism of treating trichostasis spinulosa with hair removal laser is due to high-energy hair follicle damage or mechanical follicle destruction through vaporization.

References

1. Textbook Compilation Committee in Korean Dermatological Association (2014) Text book of dermatology, 6th edn. (Korean). Daehanuihak, Seoul
2. Ross EV, Ladin Z, Kreindel M, Dierickx C (1999) Theoretical considerations in laser hair removal. Dermatol Clin 17(2):333–355. viii
3. Park SH, Yeo WC, Koh WS, Park JW, Noh NK, Yoon CS (2014) Laser dermatology plastic surgery, 2nd edn. (Korean). Koonja, Seoul
4. Ibrahimi OA, Avram MM, Hanke CW, Kilmer SL, Anderson RR (2011) Laser hair removal. Dermatol Ther 24(1):94–107
5. James WD, Elston D, Berger T (2011) Andrew's diseases of the skin e-book: clinical dermatology. Elsevier Health Sciences

6. Kauvar A, Hruza G (2005) Principles and practices in cutaneous laser surgery. CRC Press
7. Allemann IB, Goldberg DJ (2011) Basics in dermatological laser applications. Karger Medical and Scientific Publishers
8. Habif TP (2015) Clinical dermatology. Elsevier, St. Louis, MO
9. Goldberg DJ (2008) Laser hair removal. Informa Healthcare, London
10. Hruza GJ, Avram M (2013) Lasers and lights: procedures in cosmetic dermatology series, 3rd edn. Saunders, London
11. Altshuler GB, Anderson RR, Manstein D, Zenzie HH, Smirnov MZ (2001) Extended theory of selective photothermolysis. Lasers Surg Med 29(5): 416–432
12. Olsen EA (1999) Methods of hair removal. J Am Acad Dermatol 40(2):143–155
13. Nouri K (2018) Lasers in dermatology and medicine: dermatologic applications. Springer
14. Ahluwalia GS (2009) Cosmetics applications of laser light-based systems. Norwich, NY, William Andrew
15. Goldman MP (2006) Cutaneous and cosmetic laser surgery. Mosby Elsevier, Philadelphia, PA
16. Pai GS, Bhat PS, Mallya H, Gold M (2011) Safety and efficacy of low-fluence, high-repetition rate versus high-fluence, low-repetition rate 810-nm diode laser for permanent hair removal—a split-face comparison study. J Cosmet Laser Ther 13(4):134–137
17. Raulin C, Karsai S (2011) Laser and IPL technology in dermatology and aesthetic medicine. Heidelberg: New York
18. Alora MBT, Anderson RR (2000) Recent developments in cutaneous lasers. Lasers Surg Med 26(2):108–118
19. Lee W (2008) Principles of IPL and its uses (Korean). MDworld, Seoul
20. Lee MC, Chang CS, Huang YL, Chang SL, Chang CH, Lin YF et al (2015) Treatment of melasma with mixed parameters of 1,064-nm Q-switched Nd:YAG laser toning and an enhanced effect of ultrasonic application of vitamin C: a split-face study. Lasers Med Sci 30(1):159–163
21. Wanner M, Sakamoto FH, Avram MM, Chan HH, Alam M, Tannous Z et al (2016) Immediate skin responses to laser and light treatments: therapeutic endpoints: how to obtain efficacy. J Am Acad Dermatol 74(5):821–833. quiz 34, 33
22. Goldsmith LA, Katz SI, Gilchrest BA, Paller AS, Leffell DJ, Wolff K et al (2012) Fitzpatrick's dermatology in general medicine. McGraw-Hill Professional, New York
23. Wanner M, Sakamoto FH, Avram MM, Anderson RR (2016) Immediate skin responses to laser and light treatments: warning endpoints: how to avoid side effects. J Am Acad Dermatol 74(5):807–819
24. Toosi S, Ehsani AH, Noormohammadpoor P, Esmaili N, Mirshams-Shahshahani M, Moineddin F (2010) Treatment of trichostasis spinulosa with a 755-nm long-pulsed alexandrite laser. J Eur Acad Dermatol Venereol 24(4):470–473
25. Badawi A, Kashmar M (2011) Treatment of trichostasis spinulosa with 0.5-millisecond pulsed 755-nm alexandrite laser. Lasers Med Sci 26(6):825–829

Non-ablative Lasers

9

9.1 Skin Rejuvenation

Skin rejuvenation is a treatment that targets age-related pigmentation disorders and telangiectasia or improves wrinkles and skin texture [1]. It can be classified by treatment methods; ablative rejuvenation (AR) by CO_2 laser and erbium-doped yttrium aluminium garnet (Er:YAG) laser or nonablative rejuvenation (NAR), which induces a selective thermal reaction to the dermis and subcutaneous fat while sparing the epidermis. It can also be classified by treatment targets; type I rejuvenation targets pigmentation and vascular disorders while type II rejuvenation focuses on improving wrinkles and skin texture. For example, AR and NAR are both treatment modalities for type II rejuvenation (Table 9.1). Generally, NAR refers to rejuvenation treatment that uses nonablative methods to improve wrinkles and skin texture (type II rejuvenation).

Photorejuvenation has been also divided into four categories by targets and methods of treatment in one laser book (Table 9.2) [2].

Table 9.1 Types of skin regeneration by methods and targets of treatment

Types by treatment methods	Types by treatment targets
Ablative rejuvenation	Type I rejuvenation
Nonablative rejuvenation	Type II rejuvenation

Table 9.2 Types of photorejuvenation for the treatment of photodamaged skin

Classifications	Targets and methods of treatment
Type I Photorejuvenation	Treatment of pigmented disorders Treatment of telangiectasias Reduction of diffuse erythema
Type II Nonablative photorejuvenation	Reduction of fine wrinkles (epidermal effect) Reduction of rhytids and skin pore size (dermal effect)
Type III Ablative photorejuvenation	Ablative resurfacing using either a CO2 laser or Er:YAG laser
Type IV Photodynamic photorejuvenation	Nonablative treatment combining type I photorejuvenation with photodynamic therapy (PDT-assisted type II photorejuvenation)

9.1.1 Non-ablative Laser in Darker Skin

The clinical presentation of photoaging differs between Koreans and Caucasians in that pigmentary changes such as solar lentigines (liver spots) are major features of photoaging in Koreans, while wrinkling is a major feature of photoaging in Caucasians. Moderate-to-severe wrinkling in Koreans become apparent only at about 50 years, which is a decade or two later than age-matched

J. D. Lee et al., *Principles and Choice of Laser Treatment in Dermatology*,
https://doi.org/10.1007/978-981-15-6556-4_9

Caucasians [3]. Even though type II rejuvenation targeting wrinkles are less applicable in Koreans, improvements in skin texture, pore size, and facial erythema are still in high demand, implying the importance of type II rejuvenation in Koreans.

The use of nonablative lasers is particularly applicable to Koreans given the lesser degree of wrinkling with a demand for NAR among this population. Ablative lasers, on the other hand, are less effective and the risk of adverse effects such as pigmentation changes are high among Koreans. Therefore, nonablative lasers with a lack of downtime and lower risk of adverse effects are suitable for Koreans. Combination therapy with nonablative lasers and other procedures or lasers are also possible.

9.2 Mechanisms of Photorejuvenation

The top three mechanisms of photorejuvenation, regardless of ablation are as follows [4]. First, photorejuvenation by thermal injury with subsequent wound healing. Second, photorejuvenation by inflammatory cytokines. And third, photorejuvenation by photomodulation (Table 9.3). We will briefly discuss these three mechanisms of photorejuvenation.

First, thermal injury with subsequent wound healing is believed to be the primary mechanism for photorejuvenation. Although the exact mechanism is unknown, it is believed that thermal injury to the skin destroys collagen, resulting in recruitment and activation of fibroblasts for new collagen formation. This mechanism illustrates the paradox that in order for new collagen to form, collagen destruction must precede. This is because partial denaturation of collagen is thought to act as a trigger or scaffolding for new collagen synthesis. We will go over the details later, in Sect. 9.2.5. The target is to raise the dermal temperature to 50–70 °C.

Table 9.3 Mechanisms of photorejuvenation

1. Thermal injury with subsequent wound healing
2. Inflammatory cytokines
3. Photomodulation

This thermal injury could be confined to specific levels of the dermis so that deeper scars or wrinkles could be treated by a deeper level of heating, while with further penetration into ligaments, fascia or subcutaneous fat entire regions of skin could be tightened. Creation of this heat energy, whether by lasers, light sources such as IPL, radiofrequency, ultrasound, or microwave energy would cause collagen injury and contraction. Many have speculated that thermal injury to the dermis not only results in subsequent collagen formation by fibroblasts but also changes glycosaminoglycans (GAG) and dermal matrix resulting in dermal matrix remodeling [5].

Second, inflammatory cytokines of various origins influence the expression of extracellular matrix proteins, such as type I collagen, fibronectin, and decorin in human skin fibroblasts. These inflammatory cytokines also arise from cell injury and wound healing processes, thus taking part in the first mechanism of photorejuvenation (thermal injury with subsequent wound healing).

Some suggest that these inflammatory cytokines may be released from immune system cells, which then infiltrate after superficial capillary damage [1]. Omi et al. treated patients with pulsed dye laser (PDL, N-Lite, ICN Photonics, UK) and obtained biopsy specimens. There was no change in collagen fibers 3 h after laser exposure. Increased dermal collagen was observed 2, 4, and 5 weeks after laser exposure. This suggests that vascular laser may be helpful for photorejuvenation.

Heat shock proteins (HSP) and matrix metalloproteinases (MMP) also take part in this mechanism. Desmettre and Souil et al. observed that exposure of 60 °C for more than 1 s result in collagen denaturation, while temperatures of less than 50 °C are insufficient for thermal change but sufficient for activating HSP, thus increasing collagen production. MMP was initially thought to have a negative effect on skin rejuvenation due to its collagen degradation properties, but the opposite is found to be true. Studies by Verani et al. showed that the accumulation of partially degraded collagen observed in photodamaged skin may inhibit collagen synthesis by skin fibroblasts. Orringer et al. suggested that an increase in MMP after CO_2 laser, pulsed dye laser, and nonablative laser may remove photodamaged collagen, resulting in fibroblast activation and subsequent collagen formation.

Third, photomodulation is also known as biostimulation or low-level light therapy (LLLT). Photochemical effect can be classified by mechanism; photomodulation, photodynamic therapy (PDT), and excimer laser. Sometimes excimer laser is classified as a photoablation effect. Photomodulation may be considered as one phenomenon of the photochemical effect. Photomodulation was shown to be effective in pain control, wound healing, inflammatory acne, and skin rejuvenation. Photomodulation stimulates or suppresses normal cellular activity using the nonthermal mechanism. It occurs by controlling mitochondrial ATP production or by upregulating or downregulating the receptor. For several years, there has been much debate over the effectiveness and the mechanism of photomodulation. However, there is no longer any question over the effectiveness of photomodulation, and the underlying mechanism is unfolding as well. Still, it is considered to be less effective than other mechanisms. We will go over the details of photomodulation at the end of this chapter.

Next, we will go over the details on the first mechanism of photorejuvenation (thermal injury with subsequent wound healing) and its relation to NAR.

9.2.1 Collagen Remodeling

The target of type II rejuvenation is collagen fiber. Collagen fibers are major constituents of the dermis, it comprises about 75% of the dry weight and 18–30% of the volume of the dermis, while giving tensile strength to the skin. Collagen is synthesized in dermal fibroblasts, epidermal keratinocytes, vascular endothelial cells, and smooth muscle cells [6]. Thus, stimulating dermal fibroblasts or vascular endothelial cells will be helpful.

A collagen molecule consists of a triple helix made of three polypeptide chains hydrogen bonded to each other. Each polypeptide contains approximately 1000 amino acids. Collagen molecules form collagen fibrils, and collagen fibrils form collagen fibers.

Denaturation of collagen triple helix, loss of tensile strength, and increased collagen thickness observed by biopsy occur with skin aging. If collagen is heated, covalent bonds of collagen break leading to shrinkage of collagen. This is called heat-induced shrinkage (Fig. 9.1). This is why after NAR, such as ThermaCool TC™ system (Thermage Hayward, CA), immediate collagen molecule shrinkage leads to visible skin lifting effect.

After collagen shrinkage, macrophage and MMP remove damaged collagen, and HSP is released which triggers the wound healing process, leading to new collagen formation from fibroblasts. During the wound healing process, collagen synthesis begins approximately 3 days after injury and may continue for approximately 4 weeks. Collagen maturation and collagen remodeling begins several months after injury and may continue for approximately 1 year (Fig. 9.2). It usually lasts for 6 months.

This implies that NAR does not lead to immediate skin rejuvenation. Clinically, visible skin lifting effect is prominent after NAR due to heat-induced shrinkage (Table 9.4 process 1), but due to transient heat-induced shrinkage effect, skin lifting effect is also temporary. For up to 6 months after NAR, the skin is gradually rejuvenated, due to collagen remodeling (Table 9.4 process 2) [5]. The correlation between immediate skin lifting effect due to heat-induced shrinkage and subsequent skin lifting effect due to collagen remodeling is yet

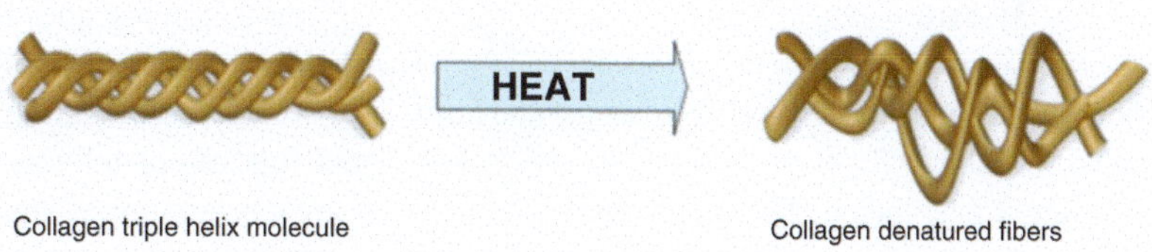

Fig. 9.1 Representation of the immediate effect of dermal heating on the collagen fibers. (Reproduced from [7])

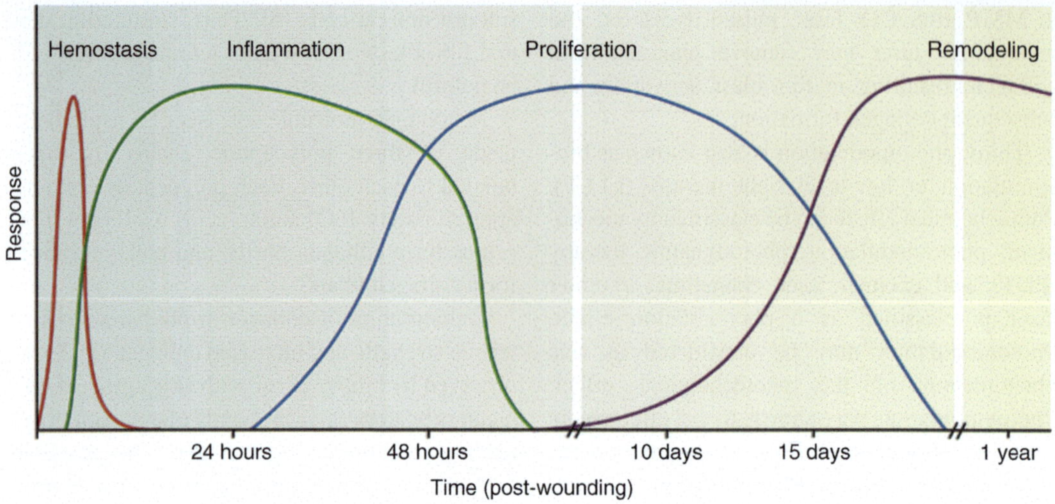

Fig. 9.2 Phases of wound healing. (Reproduced from [8])

Table 9.4 Process of collagen change by skin-tightening devices. Modified from [5]

1. Immediate collagen contraction by direct heating of collagen fibers
2. Delayed remodeling and neocollagenesis via a wound-healing response

unknown [1]. We cannot conclude that the immediate NAR lifting effect corresponds with the lifting effect after 6 months.

Further studies concerning the duration of NAR are as follows [1]. Dainich et al. observed collagen remodeling 1–2 months after 1540-nm erbium glass (Er:Glass) laser exposure, but this effect became less obvious after 1 year. Oritz et al. found that CO_2 fractional laser maintained improvement at 1–2 years compared with 3-months posttreatment. Munskiatti et al. found that CO_2 laser resurfacing also maintained considerable improvement at 2 years compared with 3-months posttreatment. This implies that AR is more effective and has a longer duration compared to NAR.

9.2.2 Thermal Reactions of Skin Tissue

Thermal reactions to elevated skin temperature are shown in Table 9.5 [2]. In nonablative laser, our main target is collagen. Thermal reactions of collagen to elevated skin temperature are as follows.

Table 9.5 Response of skin tissue to the temperature

Temperature (°C)	Thermal reactions
42–45	Beginning of hyperthermia, conformational changes, and shrinkage of collagen
50	Reduction of enzymatic activity
60	Denaturation of proteins, coagulation of the collagens, membrane permeabilisation
100	Tissue drying and formation of vacuoles
>100	Beginning of vaporization and tissue carbonization
300–1000	Thermoablation of tissue, photoablation, and disruption

- 42 °C: shrinkage of collagen
- 60 °C: coagulation of the collagen
- >100 °C: beginning of vaporization

For collagen remodeling, the temperature must exceed 60 °C for collagen coagulation. But the temperature must not exceed 100 °C, because vaporization is usually avoided in NAR. In NAR, the temperature range is between 60 and 100 °C.

The following questions arise: (1) Is the temperature of more than 60 °C the only prerequisite for collagen remodeling? Are there any other factors that might influence this? (2) Will the outcomes be similar at any temperature between 60 and 100 °C, and are there any side effects? (3) Is

100% collagen denaturation optimal? These questions will be issued.

9.2.3 Arrhenius Equation

In Table 9.5, collagen denaturation begins at 42 °C. Temperatures of less than 42 °C, regardless of exposure time, does not result in any change in skin tissue. Body temperature elevation up to 5 °C results in no prominent changes in skin tissue. On the other hand, temperatures between 42 and 50 °C triggers conformational changes in collagen. After several minutes, tissue necrosis may occur according to the Arrhenius equation.

As reviewed in "Chap. 3"; due to the Arrhenius equation, not only temperature but also exposure time must be taken into account concerning collagen denaturation. There are two ways to denature collagen for NAR: short exposure time and high temperature (method A) or long exposure time and low temperature (method B). Then, what are the differences between these two methods? We will go over the differences in the Sect. 9.2.6.

9.2.4 Tissue Damage

Thermal reactions to elevated skin temperature are diverse. Figure 9.3 illustrates thermal reactions to elevated skin temperature after CO_2 laser irradiation and might be considered as an Illustration of Table 9.5. According to the Arrhenius equation, the temperature itself is not important. The specific tissue changes itself are not clinically important. The important thing is whether the specific tissue changes are what we want, or what we do not want. That is, whether the damage is reversible or irreversible. Also, while it is not illustrated earlier, it is important to note that some irreversible damage may cause scar formation after a certain point.

Adequate energy levels of nonablative laser result in the desired effect, while higher energy levels may cause a burn, leading to scar formation. Nonablative laser rarely causes vaporization, thus most scar formation occurs during irreversible damage under 100 °C. Some irreversible damage is desired, but after a certain point, some may cause undesired scar formation.

Calderhead gave rise to the concept of damage threshold and survival threshold by taking into account tissue denaturation and cell death (Fig. 9.4) [10]. Treatments are classified as low-level light therapy (LLLT), mid-level laser therapy (MLLT), and high-level light therapy (HLLT). LLLT is also known as photomodulation. Laser resurfacing by CO_2 laser, solar lentigines treatment by Q-switched laser or IPL are examples of HLLT. Irreversible damage to the epidermis either by ablation or coagulation does not result in scar formation, but the risk of scar formation is high during ablation or coagulation of the dermis, especially the whole reticular dermis. This is why NAR by MLLT or HLLT must be treated under the survival threshold so that not all but partial layers of the dermis are damaged. This will be reviewed again in Sect. 9.4.

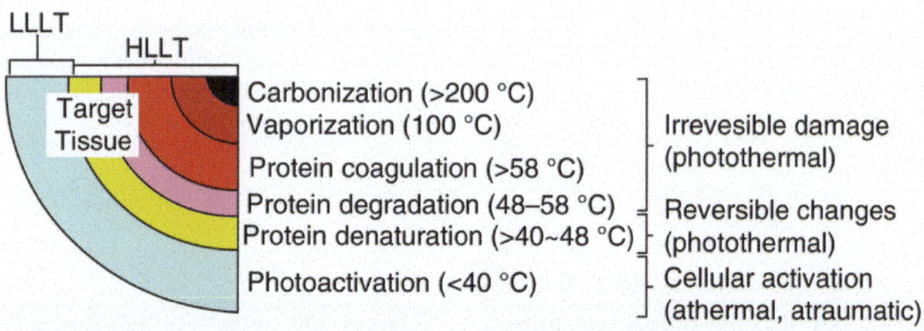

Fig. 9.3 Typical surgical laser impact on tissue. Illustration showing schematically a typical surgical laser impact on tissue with the total range of thermally-mediated reactions and the all-important athermal and atraumatic photoactivation zone at the periphery of the beam. The photoactivated cells in this zone will have a potentially beneficial effect on posttreatment pain, inflammation, and wound healing. Reproduced from [9]

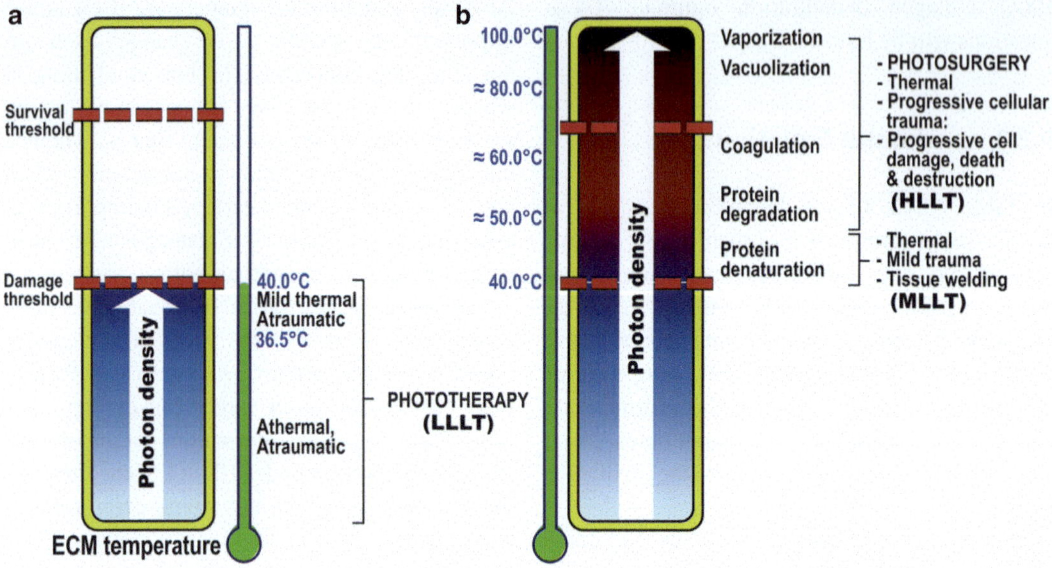

Fig. 9.4 A cell with its damage and survival thresholds indicated, together with the classification of the level of cellular reaction (Ohshiro's classification) and changes in extracellular matrix (ECM) temperature. In (**a**), as the level of the absorbed incident photon energy increases, cell activity is enhanced and is characterized as athermal and atraumatic LLLT. A slight increase in the tissue temperature would then be seen, adding mild thermal activation to the photoactivation process, although by this stage the peak in the level of cellular activity would have been reached and activity would now be dropping off. (**b**) Reactions associated with mid-level laser treatment (MLLT) (reversible damage) and high-level light therapy (irreversible damage and cell death). (Reproduced from [10])

Ross et al. treated patients with a 1550-nm erbium glass (Er:Glass) laser with a sapphire contact cooling handpiece [11]. Postauricular sites were irradiated with pulse energies varying from 400 to 1200 mJ and numbers of pulses from 4 to 40. Outcome measures included erythema, edema, and immediate epidermal whitening. In pulse energy-pulse number combinations without immediate epidermal whitening, erythema, and edema lasted less than 2 weeks, with subsequent recovery. But in combinations with immediate epidermal whitening, erosion, and ulcer led to post 1-month atrophic scar.

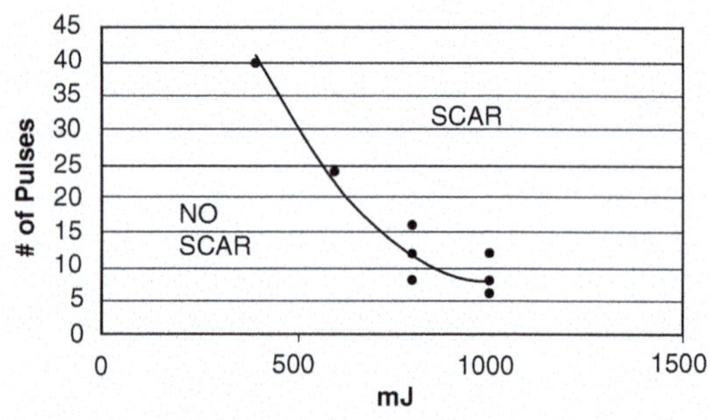

Fig. 9.5 The curved line in the graph shows where scarring was observed. Points to the right and superior of this line were associated with scarring, whereas those points to the left and inferior to the line typically did not show clinical scarring. (Reproduced from [11])

In the Fig. 9.5, a line is drawn by connecting the dots (combinations that led to scarring). The line forms a curve. The higher the pulse energy and the higher the number of pulses, the more scarring occurs. It is important to note that not only pulse energy, but also the number of pulses are important in forming scars. That is, even if the pulse energy is low, a high number of pulses may cause scarring. In other words, it can be assumed that scarring also follows the Arrhenius equation.

This paper suggests that a survival threshold for scar formation exists and that the survival threshold follows the Arrhenius equation. In one book, it has been suggested that at 80 °C, membrane permeability is compromised and the cell's chemical equilibrium is destroyed. This may imply that 80 °C may be the survival threshold [12].

This is why NAR must cause damage between the damage threshold and the survival threshold. The therapeutic window of NAR is very narrow. Damage beyond the survival threshold is irrelevant in solar lentigo treatment with IPL because it is discharged out of the skin by epidermal turnover. But in NAR the damage must be less than the survival threshold. This makes the treatment range narrower than that of IPL, which makes the treatment more challenging.

9.2.5 Partial or Total Denaturation of Collagen

Alexiades-Armenakas et al. enrolled 100 subjects with facial and neck rhytids and laxity and administered fractional bipolar radiofrequency (FRF) treatment [13]. This device (e-Prime, Korean domestic name Profound; Syneron, Yokneam Illit, Israel) can measure intradermal temperature. One single-pass FRF treatment was administered at a preselected real-time fixed temperature of 62–78 °C, energy duration for 3–5 s. The average temperature, energy duration, and collagen denaturation volume of each group were calculated by dividing the group by ≤20% and ≥20% wrinkle improvement from baseline (Table 9.6).

The higher the temperature ($p = 0.08$), the longer the energy duration ($p = 0.03$), and the larger the volume of collagen denaturation ($p = 0.05$) on biopsy, wrinkle improvement effect was statistically low (<20%, mean ± SD). Mean target temperature of 69.5 °C, energy duration of 4.9 s, and volume of denatured collagen of 3 mm^3 groups showed less than 20% wrinkle improvement, while mean target temperature of 66.7 °C, energy duration of 4.2 s, and volume of denatured collagen of 2 mm^3 groups showed more than 20% wrinkle improvement.

This paper does not verify the existence of survival thresholds, but it indicates that higher temperature and longer energy duration does not guarantee better effect, rather it is less effective. It should also be noted that larger collagen denaturation volume by biopsy, means less effect.

The author of this paper published the following paper subsequently. Alexiades et al. performed FRF as previously described [14]. Fifteen patients were divided into three arms and the degree of improvement in rhytids and skin laxity was evaluated (Table 9.7). The results showed that the improvement of rhytids was best in arm 3 with 25%, 29%, and 40% in arm 1, 2, and 3, respectively. Skin laxity improvement relatively effective in arms 2 and 3, with 25%, 36%, and 34% in arm 1, 2, and 3, respectively. In subjective satisfaction, patients in arms 2 and 3 were satisfied.

After 6 months, the Pearson coefficients, which correlate with the improvement of rhytids and skin laxity in relation to the temperature change, were 0.56 and 0.47, respectively, implying mild correlation. The optimal target dermal temperature for facial and neck rhytids and laxity treatment is 67 °C and a duration of 3–4 s.

By combining the results of these two papers, the treatment group can be classified into four groups. They are 52–57 °C group, 62 °C group, 67 °C group, and 69 °C group. The results showed that the higher the temperature (the more severe the collagen damage), the better the effect on rhytids and skin laxity, with the exception of

Table 9.6 Statistical analysis: console setting and corresponding volumes

Improvement from baseline	Target temperature (°C)	Duration (s)	Volume (mm^3)
≤20%, mean ± SD	69.5 ± 4.5	4.9 ± 0.3	3.02 ± 1.36
>20%, mean ± SD	66.7 ± 4.5	4.2 ± 1.0	2.00 ± 1.49
p Value	0.08	0.03	0.05

SD standard deviation. (Reproduced from [13])

Table 9.7 Target temperature and energy duration of three arms. (Reproduced from [14])

	Target temperature (°C)	Duration (s)
Arm 1	52–57	3
Arm 2	62	3
Arm 3	67	3

the 69 °C group. The 69 °C group had a high collagen denaturation volume, but the effect was low.

Although there was no scar formation, the larger the extent of collagen damage, the less effective. The authors speculated that the underlying reasons for this were first, the smaller extent of damage led to a better oxygen supply, resulting in better wound healing, resulting in higher collagen remodeling. Second, it was speculated that at lower temperatures, more partially denatured collagen is produced leading to more collagen formation. Partially denatured collagen may trigger new collagen formation. Ross et al. describe this hypothesis as scaffolding instead of triggering [11]. It is speculated that the heat contracted collagen becomes the framework for new collagen and is the basis for collagen remodeling. Conversely, in in vivo and in vitro porcine experiments, the complete denaturation of the collagen and visible shrinkage led to scarring. This implies that all denatured collagen must be avoided.

9.2.6 Two Methods in Nonablative Rejuvenation

Based on the earlier results, Alexiades-Armenakas et al. presented Fig. 9.6 in the paper. The zone was divided into three according to treatment temperature and exposure time. Zone of no denatured collagen, zone of partially denatured collagen, and zone of all denatured collagen. The zone of partially denatured collagen showed the best effect.

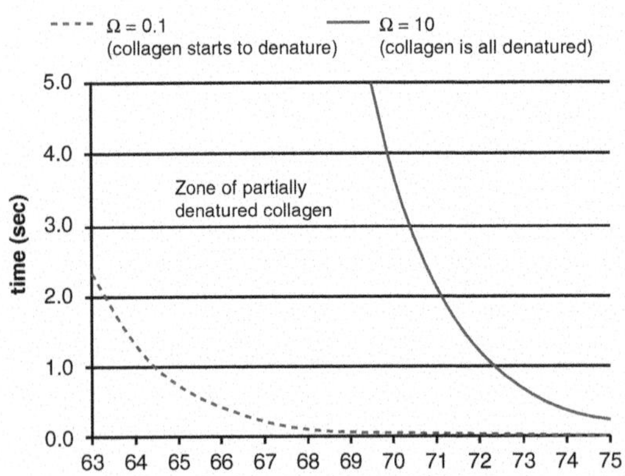

Fig. 9.6 Thermal dose threshold showing the conditions where collagen starts and completes its denaturation process (dotted and solid curves, respectively). Settings of 67 °C for 3–4 s are optimal conditions to create partially denatured collagen. (Reproduced from [14])

The curve between partially denatured collagen and all denatured collagen may follow the Arrhenius equation, so I redrew Fig. 9.7 by applying Fig. 3.12 from the Arrhenius equation.

As reviewed earlier, there are two methods for NAR applying the Arrhenius equation: short exposure time and high temperature (method A) or long exposure time and low temperature (method B). Figure 9.7 shows the characteristics of each method. These are summarized in Table 9.8.

Partial denaturation of collagen will be the same in either method: Short exposure time and high temperature (A) or long exposure time and low temperature (B). However, method A has a narrow therapeutic window. Therefore, it may not be effective and side effects such as scarring are likely. Also, severe pain is a clinical problem. In contrast, method B can be implemented without worrying about side effects because of its wide therapeutic window. However, the procedure takes a very long time. For example, if the temperature is maintained at 45 °C, it takes at least 1 h for it to be effective.

We will now review important papers on A and B methods for NAR.

Taylor et al. performed a split-face study [16]. Patients with sagging skin were treated once with laser (long-pulsed 1064-nm neodymium:yttrium–aluminium–garnet (Nd:YAG) laser, three pass, 10 mm spot, 50 ms, 50 J/cm^2, left side) and once with radiofrequency (RF, Thermage®, right side). Improvement was greater for wrinkles and laxity on the laser-treated side and essentially the same with both modalities for texture, pores, and pigmentation. Improvement was maintained for at least 2–6 months on both facial sides (Figs. 9.8 and 9.9).

This paper implies that the effect of the "5050 technique" of long-pulsed Nd:YAG laser is similar or better than Thermage®, a representative device of NAR. Thermage® and the 5050 techniques are both A method that uses high energy in

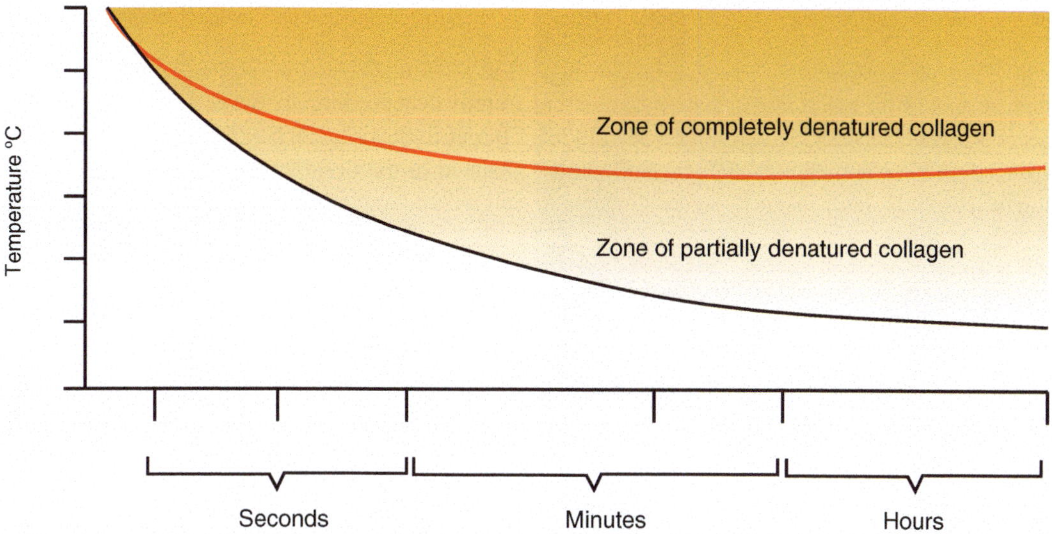

Fig. 9.7 Relationship between time and temperature in tissue damage. Zones can be divided into two: zone of completely denatured collagen and zone of partially denatured collagen. (Modified from [15])

Table 9.8 Two ways of nonablative rejuvenation

Method	Time and temperature	Therapeutic window	Drawback
A	Short time and high temperature	Narrow	Pain, side effect
B	Long time and low temperature	Wide	Long procedure time

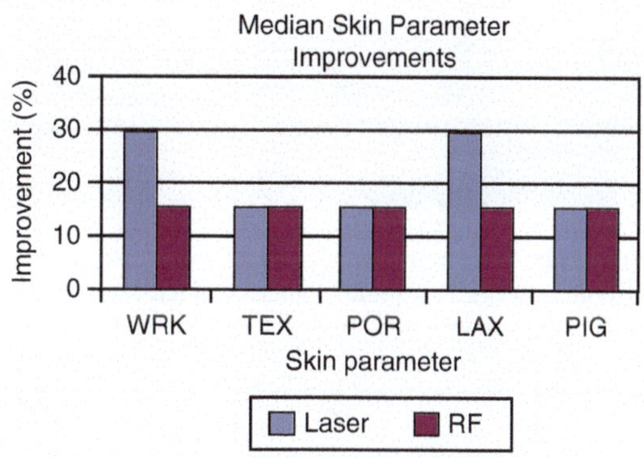

Fig. 9.8 Median improvement (%) in skin parameters of seven patients treated once with laser energy (left side of the face) and once with radiofrequency (RF) energy (right side). Overall improvements in wrinkles and laxity were higher on the laser-treated side than on the radiofrequency-treated side. (Reproduced from [16])

a short time. Since I did not have Thermage®, I tried the 5050 techniques with long-pulsed Nd:YAG laser based on this paper. However, these days I rarely perform the procedure because the pain is so severe that the patient is reluctant. At one time, blisters formed due to inadequate epidermal cooling.

Schmults et al. performed long-pulsed 1064-nm Nd:YAG laser on nine patients, 3 times at 2 week intervals [17]. The parameters were 5 mm spot, 300 μs, and 13 J/cm^2, but because of 2–4 cm distance from the skin, the actual parameters on the skin were 6–7 mm spot, 7–9 J/cm^2, 12,000–14,700 shots and the total procedure time was about 30 min. Photographic evaluation showed that those patients with preexisting erythema showed improvement in erythema along with an associated improvement in skin quality. Electron microscopy showed improved solar elastosis.

This paper is also known as the "Genesis technique," method B that uses low energy for a long time. This is the method I currently use.

9.3 Genesis Technique

There is still much debate about the effects and mechanisms of the Genesis technique. In this section, the effects and mechanism of the Genesis technique will be summarized.

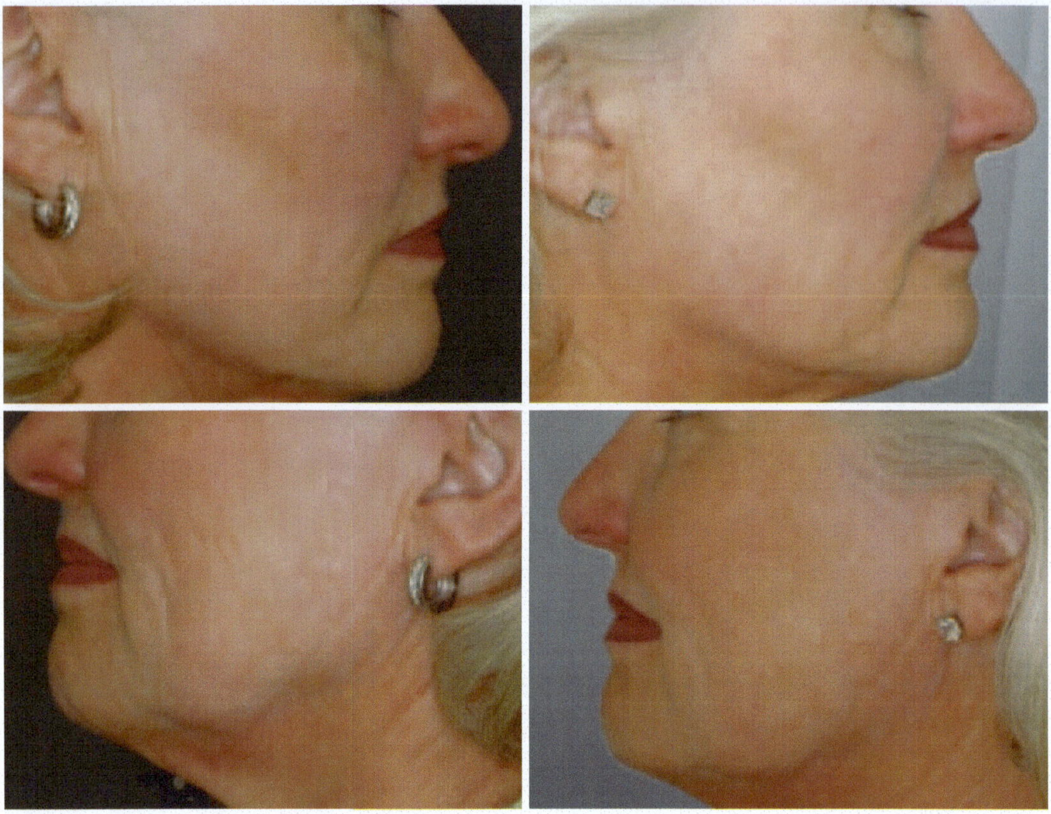

Fig. 9.9 The top two photographs show the radiofrequency-treated side of the face of patient 3 before (left) and 6 months after (right) a single treatment. The bottom two photographs show the laser-treated side of the same face before (left) and 6 months after (right) a single treatment. In this patient, blinded observers considered improvements in wrinkles, texture, pores, laxity, and pigmentation to be slightly greater on the laser-treated side of the face. (Reproduced from [16])

Chiba et al. treated a total of 19 female Japanese patients with Fitzpatrick skin types III or IV with long-pulsed 1064-nm Nd:YAG laser [18]. The parameters were spot size 8 mm, pulse duration 0.3 ms, and 13 J/cm^2 at 7 Hz with no cooling. The handpiece was placed at a distance of 2 cm from the skin with a repetitive painting motion technique. For the face, 4200 shots for 10 min, two to seven times every 3–4 weeks, and for the right arm, 1680 shots for 4 min and five times every 3 weeks.

The results showed that more than 50% improvements in wrinkles, skin laxity, skin texture, and fine lines were observed in 10 of 19 patients (53%). In addition, histological examination showed an increase in the density of collagen fibers in the papillary dermis.

This study measured skin surface temperature while performing the Genesis technique. Facial skin temperature was elevated from 33.5 to 42 °C by the Genesis technique, while the right arm skin temperature was elevated from 32 to 42.7 °C by the Genesis technique. The paper cites that the dermal temperature of 55–65 °C at which collagen is denatured correlates to 40–48 °C skin surface temperature [19]. Therefore, this paper suggests that the clinical end point for the Genesis technique is the skin surface temperature of 40–48 °C. When one has a high fever during a common cold, the body temperature is usually about 40 °C. By touching the patient's skin with the operator's hand after the Genesis technique, and feeling the similar warmth, it can be assumed that it is the clinical end point of the Genesis technique. However, there is no evidence that the skin surface temperature ranges from 40 to 48 °C when the dermal temperature is 55–65 °C. Also, there is still no consensus on the clinical end point of the Genesis technique.

Badawi et al. performed long-pulsed 1064-nm Nd:YAG laser on 22 patients with Fitzpatrick skin types III-VI [20]. The parameters were fluence of 14–16 J/cm^2, pulse duration of 300–500 μs, and repetition rate of 5–7 Hz. The handpiece was above 1–2 cm from the skin surface. Shots ranged from 8000 to 13,900 with an average of 11,700 shots. An average of six treatments was performed on each patient approximately 3 weeks apart and the mean follow-up time after the final treatment was 9 months (range of 3–10 months). Clinically and statistically significant median improvement of 2 in scarring, 2.3 in texture, and 2 in pigment were observed. The paper implies that the effects of the Genesis technique improved not only scars and skin texture but also pigmentation.

In Table 9.9, I summarized the effects and related cytokines of the Genesis technique from various papers.

So far, we have discussed that the Genesis technique is an effective NAR method. The mechanism of the Genesis technique is not fully known, but the mechanism of the laser can be used to make the assumption. Let's first consider what the chromophores of the Genesis technique are. In order to know the chromophore, the wavelength and pulse duration of the laser parameters must be considered. The wavelength of the Genesis technique is 1064 nm. The absorption coefficients of the three major chromophores are all low, but out of these three, the absorption coefficient for melanin is the highest, followed by blood and finally water. I think the primary chromophore for the Genesis technique is the basal layer. The basal layer has the most pigmentations and this is where the laser reaches before contacting blood. Also, the basal layer's thermal relaxation time (TRT) is about 0.1–0.3 ms, which is consistent with the Genesis technique's pulse duration of 0.3 ms. However, the fluence is around 10 J/cm^2, implying that rather than treating the basal layer directly, it may be intended to transfer heat to the papillary dermis, which is near the basal layer, through heat diffusion by repeatedly irradiating with low energy.

Table 9.9 Effects and related substances of the Genesis technique [16, 17, 21, 22].

Effects of Genesis technique	Related cytokines
1. Increased collagen synthesis—Improvements in scar, pore, texture, wrinkle, laxity 2. Reduced flushing 3. Reduced inflammation 4. Reduced pigmentation	1. Elevation of wound healing related substances: Heat shock protein(HSP), tumor necrosis factor-β(TGF-β) 2. Decrease of inflammatory cytokine: Interleukin-8 (IL-8)

The second chromophore of the Genesis technique is thought to be small, invisible blood vessels. If the blood vessel's TRT is less than 4.5 ms (vessel thickness 0.1 mm), these are very thin blood vessels that cause flushing. Among these, there could be a blood vessel corresponding to 0.3 ms, and like the basal layer, if repeatedly irradiated with low energy, it may transfer heat to the blood vessels, especially the papillary dermis. However, for long-pulsed 1064-nm Nd:YAG laser, a fluence of 20–40 J/cm^2 is usually required for laser hair removal while a fluence of 140–160 J/cm^2 is usually required for vascular therapy. That is, the fluence used in the Genesis technique is insufficient for generating heat through the blood vessels. However, it may help stimulate the blood vessels of the papillary dermis and releasing inflammatory cytokines, which is the second mechanism of NAR.

The 1064-nm wavelength can generate heat throughout the dermis, including the epidermis, because of the absorption coefficient of water, but since the absorption coefficient is lower than that of melanin and blood, I believe that the main chromophore of the Genesis technique is the basal layer and vessels of the papillary dermis. The target tissue is thought to be the basal layer, basement membrane, and papillary dermis.

Heat loss consists of three mechanisms: heat conduction, convection, and radiation. First, heat conduction (heat diffusion) transfers heat to surrounding tissues while chromophores are the main way in which heat dissipation occurs. Second, heat convection is a method of depriving the heat of chromophores as blood passes through blood vessels in tissues. Third, there is radiation [4]. In the Genesis technique, the main mechanism of heat loss is thought to be heat diffusion and convection. While heat loss takes place sufficiently and energy continues to be supplied by repeatedly irradiating several passes of low energy, Genesis Technique balances its heat to a relatively low temperature. However, high energy or stacking on the same spot may result in a burn. That is why (1) when the patient complains of feeling hot the energy must be reduced and (2) to avoid repeated exposures the handpiece should be moved faster or the exposure range must be extended to a larger area.

Genesis techniques have long been known at private practice, but there are debates regarding its efficacy. Why are there controversies over its effectiveness when theoretically it should be effective? First, the problem is that the procedure is not done for a long enough time. According to the papers, the procedure should be performed for 30 min. But in private practice, it is difficult to perform a laser procedure for 30 min. What should be done? I suggest that instead of performing on the entire face, reducing the area and performing only on important parts such as melasma, malar area, and cheeks may reduce time. Second, NAR is significantly less effective than AR [1]. In some patients, it may be effective, but to some, it may have no effect at all. Third, there is no clinical end point in NAR [23]. For example, there are clinical end points such as darkening, vessel disappearance, and purpura in vascular therapy, but there are no clinical end points in NAR. Clinical changes such as blanching may occur, but this is not a clinical end point, but rather a warning end point meaning tissue necrosis. In NAR there is no special clinical end point other than erythema. But even this is unclear because we do not know how red the erythema should be or how long it should be maintained.

Earlier we reviewed that the clinical end point for the Genesis technique is the skin surface temperature, and by touching the patient's skin with the operator's hand after the Genesis technique and feeling the warmth similar to a high fever during common cold is the clinical end point. But this is not yet a consensus, and it is very inaccurate. However, when the patient feels hot we should take that as a warning end point since this might indicate the possibility of a burn. In this case, we should stop the Genesis technique or move the handpiece quickly so that the temperature rises slowly.

9.4 Fibroblasts in Papillary and Reticular Dermis

We already know that during mechanical dermabrasion or CO_2 laser AR (skin resurfacing) permanent scarring may occur if the skin is removed beyond the papillary dermis to the reticular dermis. We know that during CO_2 laser AR we should stop when we see a layer that seems yellow. The reason it looks yellow is because of the sebaceous gland. This is the boundary between the papillary and reticular dermis. Going deeper than this boundary and damaging the reticular dermis, similar to a full-thickness burn wound, results in the skin becoming hard and forms permanent scars without epidermal appendages such as hair follicles, sebaceous glands, and eccrine glands [24]. Why is there a high risk of scarring when the reticular dermis is damaged?

Fibroblasts synthesize all the components of the dermis. It regulates and replaces collagen synthesis and dermal extracellular matrix(ECM) components [24]. Fibroblasts are known to play a particularly important role in wound healing. When tissue damage occurs, fibroblasts are known to migrate to the damaged area, create new collagen, and promote the wound healing process. Fibroblasts differ in the papillary and reticular dermis, in that there are more fibroblasts in the papillary dermis and are known to be more active. Let's take a closer look at the difference between fibroblasts in the papillary and reticular dermis.

Through research, Ryan R. Driskell et al. revealed that fibroblasts in the papillary dermis and fibroblasts in the reticulated dermis have different lineages. In other words, the fibroblasts of the papillary dermis play an important role in hair growth by forming the papillary dermis and controlling the hair follicle and the arrector pili muscle, whereas the fibroblasts of the reticular dermis forming the reticular dermis and the underlying adipose layer (hypodermis) [24].

Let's review the experiment by Ryan R. Driskell et al. Nineteen antibodies known as "fibroblast markers" were injected into the rats before delivery and examined on the second day after birth to confirm that the fibroblasts of the papillary and reticular dermis had different fibroblast markers (Table 9.10).

Table 9.10 Selected fibroblast marks staining the papillary dermis and reticular dermis in late gestation/postnatal skin

Cell marker	Papillary dermis	Reticular dermis
PDGFR alpha	Positive	Positive
CD34	Positive	Positive
BLIMP 1	Positive	Negative
CD26	Positive	Negative
Lrig1	Positive	Negative
Sca1	Negative	Positive
DLK1	Negative	Positive

BLIMP B-lymphocyte-induced maturation protein, *CD* cluster differentiation, *DLK1* Delta-like homolog 1, *Lrig1* leucine-rich repeats, and immunoglobulin-like domains protein 1, *PDGFR alpha* platelet-derived growth factor receptor alpha, *Sca1* stem cells antigen 1. (Reproduced from [24])

The results showed that fibroblast markers PDGFR-α and CD34 were both found in fibroblasts of the papillary and reticular dermis, but BLIMP-1, CD26, and Lrig1 were found only in fibroblasts of the papillary dermis while Sca1 and DLK1 were found only in fibroblasts of the reticular dermis.

The two fibroblasts with fibroblast markers were then extracted from the skin and mixed together. This time, a silicone chamber was inserted into the back of the experimental rat and the mixed fibroblasts were injected (Fig. 9.10). Surprisingly, they found that fibroblasts in the chamber produced skin-like tissue. Similar to epidermis and dermis, it was composed of two layers divided by the basement membrane, composed of type VII collagen and anchoring fibril.

When CD26+, BLIMP+, and Sca 1-cells (fibroblasts derived from the papillary dermis) were injected into the silicone chamber, papillary dermis was produced. When cells with other

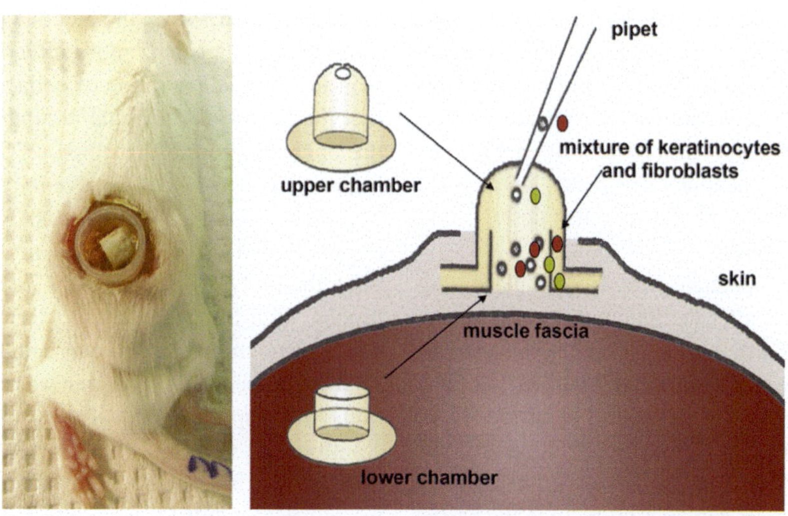

Fig. 9.10 Cell-sorted skin equivalent to SCID mice. Mouse model of human skin cell suspensions sorting themselves into a human skinlike tissue with an epidermal layer, basement membrane, and dermis. A silicon chamber is sewn over the *panniculus carnosus* of the mouse. The chamber is filled with a culture medium and then suspensions of human keratinocytes and human fibroblasts are injected into the chamber. Within a week, the injected keratinocytes have formed an epidermal layer and the injected fibroblasts have formed a neodermis. (Reproduced from [24])

markers (fibroblasts derived from the reticulated dermis) were injected, reticular dermis and the subcutaneous fat layer were produced. CD26+, BLIMP+, and Sca 1-cells (fibroblasts derived from the papillary dermis) play an important role in hair follicle formation, while CD26-, BLIMP-, and DLK1+ cells (fibroblasts derived from the reticular dermis) play an important role in the reticular dermis and subcutaneous fat formation.

Based on these findings we could conclude that the origins of the fibroblasts of the two dermal layers are different and play different roles in the wound healing process.

Wound healing can be divided into two types. Reparative wound healing and regenerative wound healing. Reparative wound healing refers to wound healing in which wounds, such as burn scars, as they heal, leave scars and change into tissues without epidermal appendages such as hair follicles, eccrine glands, and sebaceous glands [24]. Examples of regenerative wound healing are salamanders and human fetuses. Salamanders can regenerate a fully functioning new leg after their original leg is cut off. In the first trimester of pregnancy, even if the fetus gets wounded in the uterus they do not leave a scar.

In summary, if the damage is limited to the epidermis and the papillary dermis, regenerative healing takes place, which is the role of fibroblasts of the papillary dermis, and a completely new epidermis and papillary dermis are formed. On the other hand, if the reticular dermis is damaged, reparative healing takes place, which is the role of fibroblasts of the reticular dermis, thus scarring takes place.

Why does reparative healing take place, thus creating a scar, after the reticular dermis is damaged? I think the reason for this is because the most important function of the skin is barrier function; to protect our body from the outside world. When the damage is limited to the epidermis and the papillary dermis, the reticular dermis acts as a barrier, so there is no major problem in the barrier function even if regenerative healing takes place. But if the reticular dermis is damaged, reparative healing would be needed to rapidly recover barrier function despite the scarring (Table 9.11).

We should choose a laser considering the differences in fibroblasts between the papillary and reticular dermis and the differences in wound healing. Which laser would be most effective? The most effective laser for rejuvenation of papillary dermis is CO_2 laser resurfacing. Then what is the most effective laser for the reticular dermis?

Table 9.11 Comparison of fibroblasts of papillary and reticular dermis

	Fibroblast from papillary dermis	Fibroblast from reticular dermis
Wound healing	Regenerative	Reparative
Scarring	Without scarring	With scarring
Examples	Newts, salamanders Human fetus(first trimester)	Burn scar
Meaning	Esthetics	Survival
Ablative lasers	CO_2 laser resurfacing	CO_2 fractional laser
Nonablative lasers	Genesis technique Vascular laser	Needle RF Er:Glass fractional laser

The damage to the reticular dermis should be limited as much as possible because reparative healing may cause scarring. However, collagen remodeling in the reticular dermis may be effective for elasticity, deep wrinkles, and scars. In other words, the reticular dermis may also be a treatment target. Given the fact that partial denaturation of collagen is more effective and safe than the total denaturation of collagen, I believe that the theory of fractional photothermolysis is the most appropriate method. CO_2 fractional lasers are known to be effective in treating scars. The most effective method for NAR of reticular dermis should also follow the theory of fractional photothermolysis. Therefore, using invasive bipolar high-frequency needle RF or 1550-nm Er:Glass fractional laser seems suitable.

It would be ideal if collagen was remodeled in both the papillary and the reticular dermis. Combination therapy is needed for this to happen. If so, what combination should we use? If we review Table 9.11, we could see that several combination therapies are possible. The most effective method would be a CO_2 laser resurfacing with a CO_2 fractional laser treatment. However, if these procedures are performed on the same day there would be a high risk of serious side effects. It would be better to perform them on different days. The most effective NAR method would be the combination of the Genesis technique and needle RF. AR and NAR may also be used in combination. For example, a CO_2 laser resurfacing may be followed by needle RF.

Earlier, we had raised three questions in the Sect. 9.2.2. Now we shall address these three questions. First, in skin rejuvenation, time should be considered. According to the Arrhenius equation, the temperature is important but time is also important. Second, the damage must be taken into account. In addition to the damage threshold, there is also a survival threshold at which scarring can occur. High energy does not guarantee efficacy. Therefore, there are two methods for NAR, and I recommend method B. Third, the treatment layer should be considered. The reticular dermis should not be treated too strongly. Fractional treatment is recommended because it is effective and safe.

9.5 Nonablative Lasers

9.5.1 Absorption Curve of Collagen and Water

Collagen absorption curves exist only in far-infrared (FIR, > 3 μm) and peaks between 6000 and 7000 nm (Fig. 9.11). There is a "free-electron laser" that uses this wavelength to directly heat collagen, but it has not been commercialized yet [4]. Therefore, skin rejuvenation involves heat conduction indirectly from water using lasers with absorption coefficients for most water, such as CO_2 lasers, Er:YAG lasers, and mid-infrared (MIR) lasers.

Absorption curves of water show very low absorption in the ultraviolet and visible light ranges, and forms small peaks at 980 nm, larger peaks at 1060 and 1480 nm, and absorption curves gradually increase from midinfrared (MIR) (Fig. 9.12) [4].

9.5.2 Nonablative Laser Classification by Mechanism

The final target tissue of NAR is collagen, but indirect methods are used because we cannot directly target collagen by laser. There are two indirect target tissues of NAR: First, water. By raising the temperature of water in the dermis by using mid-infrared, the temperature of collagen could also be raised. Second, blood vessels. By raising the temperature of the blood vessels by using a vascular laser, the temperature of collagen could also be raised. (Fig. 9.13) [27].

The target tissue and mechanism of NAR can be summarized as shown in Table 9.12. First,

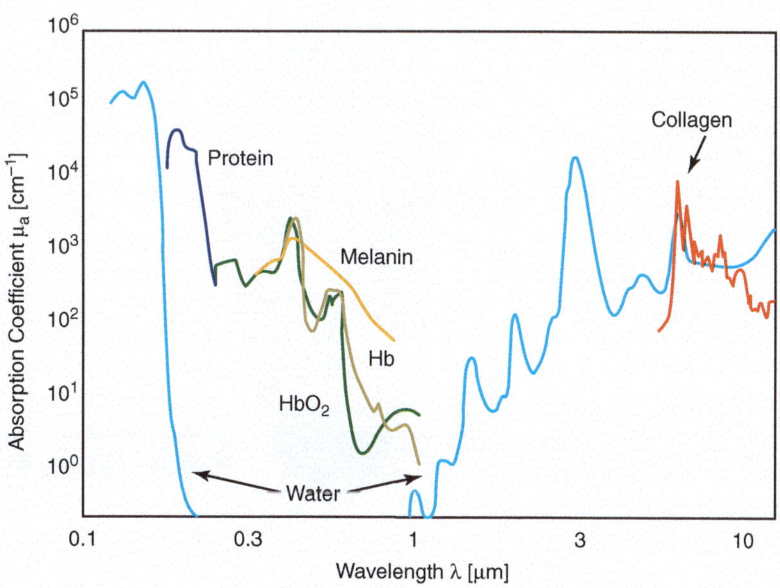

Fig. 9.11 Optical absorption coefficient of principle tissue chromophores in the 0.1–12 μm spectral region. Adapted with permission from Chemical reviews. 2003;103(2):577–644. Copyright 2020. American Chemical Society [25].

indirect collagen remodeling is achieved by direct dermal heating, i.e., applying heat to the water of the dermis using a wavelength with a high absorption coefficient for water. Second, indirect collagen remodeling is achieved by indirect dermal heating, i.e., applying heat to the blood vessels by vascular laser with a high absorption coefficient for hemoglobin, and then indirectly applying heat to the water of the dermis. Third, heat is applied to the cutaneous vessel and surrounding tissues by vascular laser, which in turn releases cellular mediators and growth factors, thereby creating collagen through a wound healing process. Finally, there is a photomodulation.

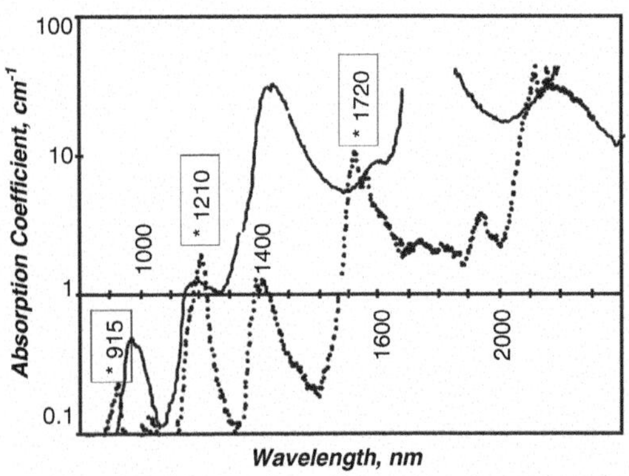

Fig. 9.12 Infrared absorption spectra of water (solid line) and human fat (dotted line). (Reproduced from [26])

9.5.3 Nonablative Lasers for Koreans

Based on the earlier findings, nonablative laser can be classified as a mid-infrared laser and vascular laser. Also, although not a laser, nonablative methods could be added to this list (Table 9.13).

Then what is the best device for NAR in Koreans? Except for vascular lasers with 500–600 nm wavelengths, neither mid-infrared lasers nor nonablative devices are related to skin color. Therefore, both may be used safely regardless of skin color. But what works best? Theoretically, the vascular laser seems less effective, because it has to first heat the blood vessels and then the water second before it finally reaches collagen. But there are no papers on this yet. Mid-infrared lasers were mostly withdrawn from private practice due to severe pain and side effects.

Table 9.12 Mechanisms of NAR by targets

Target	Mechanisms
Water	Direct dermal heating → new collagen
Hb and/or melanin	1. Indirect heating of the dermis → new collagen 2. Cutaneous vessels and/or adnexal structures → cellular mediators and growth factor → wound-healing response → new collagen
Photomodulation	LLLT – LED, PDT

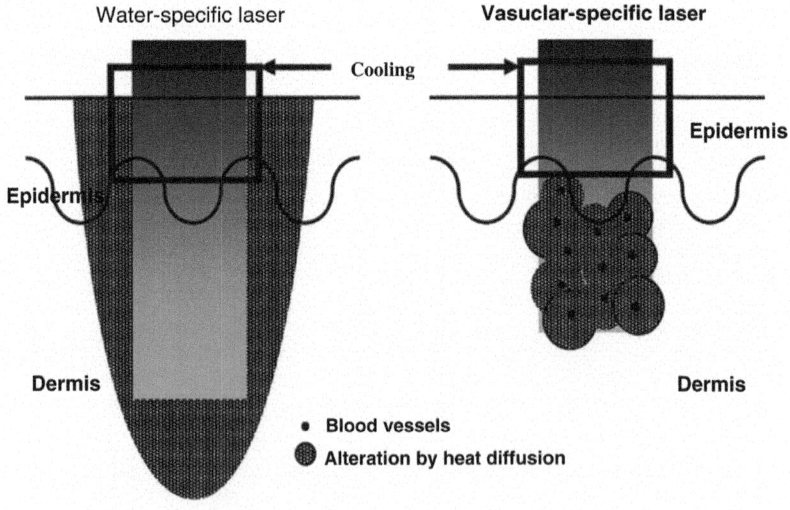

Fig. 9.13 Nonablative lasers used for skin rejuvenation. Water-specific laser induces thermal changes in water-containing tissues, while vascular-specific laser induces thermal changes in the surrounding tissues around blood vessels. Cooling devices must be associated to prevent thermal injury of the skin surface. (Reproduced from [27])

Table 9.13 Types of lasers and devices in NAR

Lasers and devices of NAR	Wavelength	Proprietary name
Mid-infrared lasers	1540-nm Er:Glass	Aramis
	1450-nm diode	Smoothbeam
	1320-nm Nd:YAG	CoolTouch
Vascular lasers	IPL, PDL, 532-nm long-pulsed KTP, and 1064-nm Long-pulsed Nd:YAG laser	
Nonablative devices	RF, needle RF, focused ultrasound	Thermage, LDM, and Ulthera

And as we saw in the previous Table 9.11 (Comparison of fibroblasts of the papillary and reticular dermis), the treatment should be divided into the treatment of the papillary dermis and the reticular dermis. I believe that the Genesis technique is most appropriate for the treatment of the papillary dermis. In the treatment of reticular dermis, needle RF fits the theory of fractional photothermolysis and is considered most suitable in terms of price and accuracy.

9.6 Drawbacks of Nonablative Lasers

NAR has no downtime and few side effects. Despite these advantages, NAR has several disadvantages. Let's review the disadvantages of NAR.

First, NAR is significantly less effective than ablative rejuvenation [1]. Second, the results are not consistent. Some patients find it effective, while others do not. Third, despite topical anesthesia, there is considerable discomfort. Pain may be severe in method A. Fourth, the procedure time is the very long (15–20 min) for method B, so the operator is reluctant to perform the procedure. But if we shorten the procedure time, then it is less effective [4]. Fifth, there is no clinical end point [23]. The only visible symptom is erythema, but we do not know how long the erythema should last and how red it should be. The next symptom observed on the skin is immediate epidermal whitening, a warning end point that indicates scar formation. This is not a clinical end point, but a warning end point. Therefore, in NAR the maximum energy, the maximum number of shots and procedures should be set in advance.

So why is NAR significantly less effective than AR?

First, NAR has a very narrow therapeutic range compared to AR. NAR has to adjust the temperature between the damage threshold and the survival threshold, which is very narrow. On the other hand, in AR, if the temperature is above 100 °C, skin tissue that is above the survival threshold at any temperature is generally vaporized or falls out of the skin during the wound healing process, leaving only the tissue between the damage threshold and the survival threshold.

Second, biopsy after AR by a CO_2 laser or Er:YAG laser shows a thin band of heat distribution. NAR, on the other hand, has a wide thermal distribution in the dermis. Solar elastosis, found in aged skin, is observed in a shallow layer (depth of 100–400 μm). Mechanical peeling, chemical peeling, or CO_2 laser resurfacing removes this layer and initiates collagen remodeling. In other words, the range of AR is narrow, but it definitely removes the shallow layer that we want to target and creates definite tissue regeneration. But the range of NAR is wide and deep, and sometimes it may not affect or insufficiently affect the layer we want to target. In addition, it is almost impossible to generate heat only in the subepidermal zone by NAR. Epidermis cooling is required in NAR, making it difficult to cool the epidermis while generating heat just below the epidermis. Rather, there is a high risk of developing a pitted scar while trying to generate sufficient heat under the epidermis [4].

Third, is my personal assumption. AR, such as a CO_2 laser, will result in both ablation and thermal damage (Thermal damage can be divided into irreversible thermal damage and reversible thermal damage. Irreversible thermal damage is sometimes considered the same as residual thermal damage. See "Chap. 10"). Chemical peeling or mechanical peeling only results in ablation. NAR only results in thermal damage (Table 9.14).

Table 9.14 Skin rejuvenation and damaged tissue

Method	Damaged tissue
Ablative rejuvenation	Ablation, irreversible, and reversible thermal damage
Chemical peeling, dermablation	Ablation
Nonablative rejuvenation	Irreversible and reversible thermal damage

The most effective skin rejuvenation procedure is in the order of AR, chemical peeling, mechanical peeling, and NAR.

In conclusion, we can assume that ablation is the tissue damage that has the greatest effect on collagen synthesis. Ablation may be most effective because the wound healing process is most activated. This may be the reason why NAR might be the least effective since there is no ablation.

9.7 Conclusion for Nonablative Laser

In Korea, there is not much demand for wrinkles, and NAR is less effective than AR. These are the factors that sometimes make us disregard NAR. But NAR is a necessary procedure. The reason is as follows: First, there is still a demand for skin texture, pore size, and facial erythema. Second, NAR does not have downtime, and the demand for this is gradually increasing. Third, and the most important reason is because of melasma. In the treatment of melasma, the only way to improve the dermal layer without stimulating the epidermal layer (where the melanocytes are) is NAR. Therefore, NAR is very useful in Koreans, because the prevalence of melasma and the activity of melanocytes are both high in Koreans.

9.8 Photomodulation

9.8.1 Arndt–Schultz Curve

Now we will discuss the mechanism and effects of photomodulation.

We will first discuss the Arndt–Schultz law, which is considered as the basic principle of photomodulation. The Arndt–Schultz law is the theory that all drugs and toxic substances stimulate vital activity at low doses but inhibit and destroy vital activity at moderate doses. Substances that cause irritation below harmful levels include antibiotics, snake venom, heat, radiation, and magnetic fields. Fig. 9.14 makes it easier to understand. There is no change in cells from A–B, but when more than a certain amount of stimulation is applied, cellular activity increases (B–C). Then cell activity plateaus (C–D) and falls (D–E), and finally cell activity falls below normal level and causes cell damage (E–F), and cell death (F–G) [10].

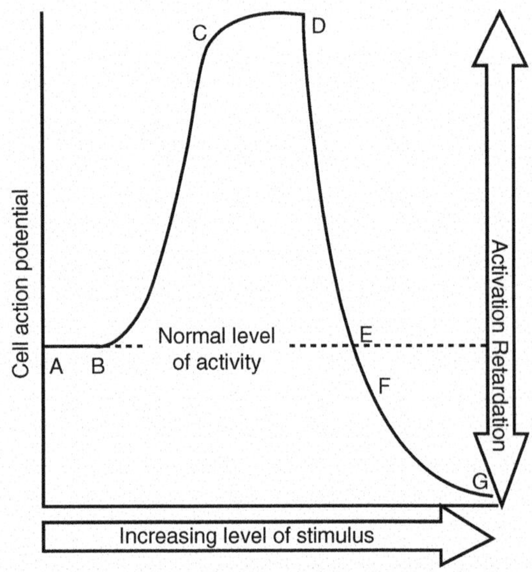

Fig. 9.14 Ohshiro and Calderhead's LLLT-adapted version of the Arndt–Schultz curve. From point A to B there is very little change in the cell action spectrum, but there is a rapid increase from point B to C concomitant with the increasing stimulus level. The activity plateaus out at C to D and after D drops sharply back down to normal levels at point E. As the strength of the stimulus increases beyond point E to point F, activity drops below the normal level with mild retardation and cell damage, which further drops until cell death at point G. The highest increase in cell activity, and most effective LLLT treatment, would, therefore, be induced by the parameters that could achieve section C to D on the curve. *HLLT* high-level light therapy. (Reproduced from [10])

In terms of low-level light therapy (LLLT), mid-level laser therapy (MLLT), and high-level light therapy (HLLT), the E–F and F–G sections may be seen as MLLT or HLLT, respectively. The corresponding section for photomodulation is section B–E, to which LLLT is applied. In other words, photomodulation is a therapeutic method that stimulates cells using photons to increases cell activity rather than causing cell damage or cell death.

Considering Calderhead's concept of damage threshold and survival threshold, photomodulation occurs below the damage threshold. Photomodulation is known to generate no heat, and although it is defined on the premise that no heat is generated, actually it may generate some heat.

Photomodulation is thought to have three effects at the cellular level. First, if the photoactivated cells are damaged and inhibited, photomodulation treats these cells. Second, photomodulation makes cell activity better and faster. For example, it promotes collagen synthesis of fibroblasts. Third, if there are not enough cells, photomodulation recruits the cells elsewhere and promotes existing cells to proliferate [10].

9.8.2 Light-Emitting Diode

In 1988, a new LED (aka NASA LED) was developed by Professor Harry Whelan from the National Aeronautics and Space Administration (NASA). Since then LED has been used for photomodulation due to its wound-healing effect and LLLT effect.

LEDs have a small semiconductor chip in the center that generates light when current flows. Thus, LEDs are light, not lasers. Four characteristics of light, that define them from lasers are polychromaticity, incoherence, divergence, and low intensity. NASA LEDs were able to overcome two of the four light characteristics. First, the higher the quality of the LED, the narrower the bandwidth, so that it can create a wavelength range that is only slightly out of a specific wavelength. This is called quasimonochromaticity. Second, a parabolic reflector can be used to slightly suppress dispersion from 60° to 110°. However, unlike the CO_2 lasers, focusing is not possible because it does not create perfect collimation. However, NASA LEDs could not overcome incoherence and low intensity, but this is not a problem in photomodulation [10].

Rather, there are several advantages to LEDs. First, very little current is needed to produce light. Second, since LEDs are solid semiconductors, there is no need for flash lamps such as filaments or fluorescent lamps. That is, there is no need for consumables. This is why signs and indoor lamps are changed to LEDs these days. Third, due to quasimonochromaticity (light with a wavelength range of several nanometers) LEDs have target specificity, like a laser. Fourth, a hands-free operation is possible because the LEDs can be closely arranged in a large area so that the entire face can be irradiated at once. Fifth, the biggest advantage is the low price. Another advantage is that there are no pains and side effects and it can be used at any age from infants to the elderly, which is not necessarily an advantage of LEDs, but the advantage of photomodulation [10].

9.8.3 Karu's Photo-Biomodulation Band

Photomodulation must also determine the three parameters of the laser (wavelength, pulse duration, and fluence). Wavelength is the most important parameter in photomodulation because without absorption no reaction is possible [28]. Then what wavelength is the most effective wavelength for photomodulation for skin rejuvenation?

Tiina Karu, a well-known Russian photobiologist, stated that photo-biomodulation band suitable for photomodulation is from visible red (around 620 nm) to near infrared (around 1000 nm) [10].

The better the wavelength is absorbed, the shallower the depth of penetration. Conversely,

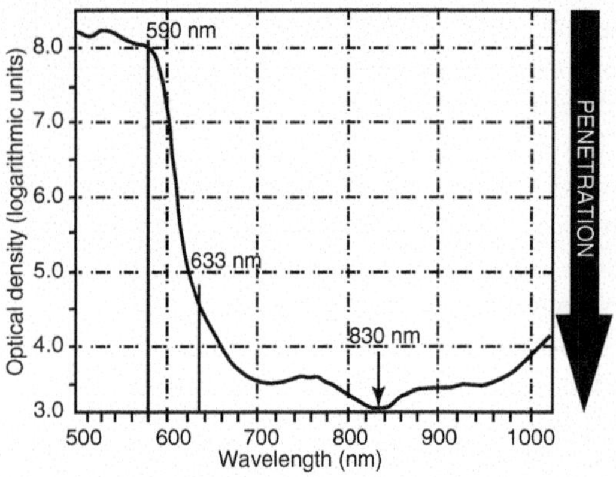

Fig. 9.15 Penetration of broad waveband light through a human hand in vivo. Note that the optical density units are logarithmic. (Reproduced from [10])

the poorer the absorption, the deeper the penetration depth. In the Fig. 9.15, the *y*-axis is the optical density (OD), indicating the absorption of the entire skin according to the wavelength regardless of the chromophore. The lower the absorption rate, the deeper the depth of penetration, so as it goes down on the *z*-axis, the penetration depth deepens. The green and yellow wavelengths (500–600 nm wavelengths) are absorbed blood and melanin, making them difficult to penetrate in the living tissue. Therefore, green and yellow wavelengths are not suitable for deep penetration. Photomodulation for skin rejuvenation requires a wavelength that can penetrate the dermis for wound healing and rejuvenation. In Fig. 9.15, we can see that wavelength from 620 to 1000 nm is a suitable photo-biomodulation band.

While 633 nm is a slightly longer wavelength than 590 nm by 43 nm, the optical density decreases by 3 OD, from 8 OD to 5 OD. Although only 3 OD has decreased, the y-axis is reduced by 1000 times because it is expressed in logarithmic units. Also, 830 nm is 5 OD difference than 590 nm and can penetrate the deepest. LEDs used for the skin rejuvenation mainly use 630 and 830 nm wavelengths, which is under the Karu's photo-biomodulation band [10]. LEDs are used not only for the purpose of skin rejuvenation but also for acne treatment (400 nm) and rejuvenation of the epidermis and papillary dermis (590 nm) [29].

9.8.4 Mechanism of Low-Level Light Therapy by LED

The mechanism of photomodulation can be divided into (1) visible light including 630 nm, under Karu's photo-biomodulation band, and (2) near-infrared including 830 nm (Fig. 9.16). Visible light targets the cytochrome C oxidase (CCO) of the mitochondria, and near-infrared light targets the cell membrane. Cytochrome C oxidase or complex IV (CCO) is an end-terminal enzyme of the mitochondria and is involved in the synthesis of adenosine triphosphate (ATP). ATP is used as a fuel for cells and whole organisms [28].

First, visible light is absorbed by the CCO to produce ATP by photochemical cascade and promote cell wall transport mechanisms such as a sodium-potassium pump (Na1/K1-ATPase). Then intracellular/extracellular exchanges between cells and extracellular matrixes increase calcium ions (Ca^{++}) and hydrogen ions (H^+), both potent cell–cell signaling compounds. Eventually, the DNA and RNA of the nucleus are made leading to cell proliferation.

Second, near-infrared rays are absorbed by the cell walls and change the electronic state of the cell wall molecules through photo-physical responses such as a rotational and vibrational exchange. It then promotes cell transport mechanisms, allowing calcium ions (Ca^{++}) to increase hydrogen ions (H^+) and produce more ATP in the mitochondria. Near-infrared light, unlike visible light, causes an indirect photo-physical response rather than a photochemical cascade. Eventually, it induces photomodulation such as cell proliferation.

9.8.5 Nonablative Rejuvenation by Photomodulation

Photomodulation also plays a role in skin rejuvenation. However, the effect is not immediately visible and gradually increases over 12 weeks [10].

Lee et al. studied the patient's subjective satisfaction by dividing the group into three: 633, 830, and 633 and 830 nm combination. The

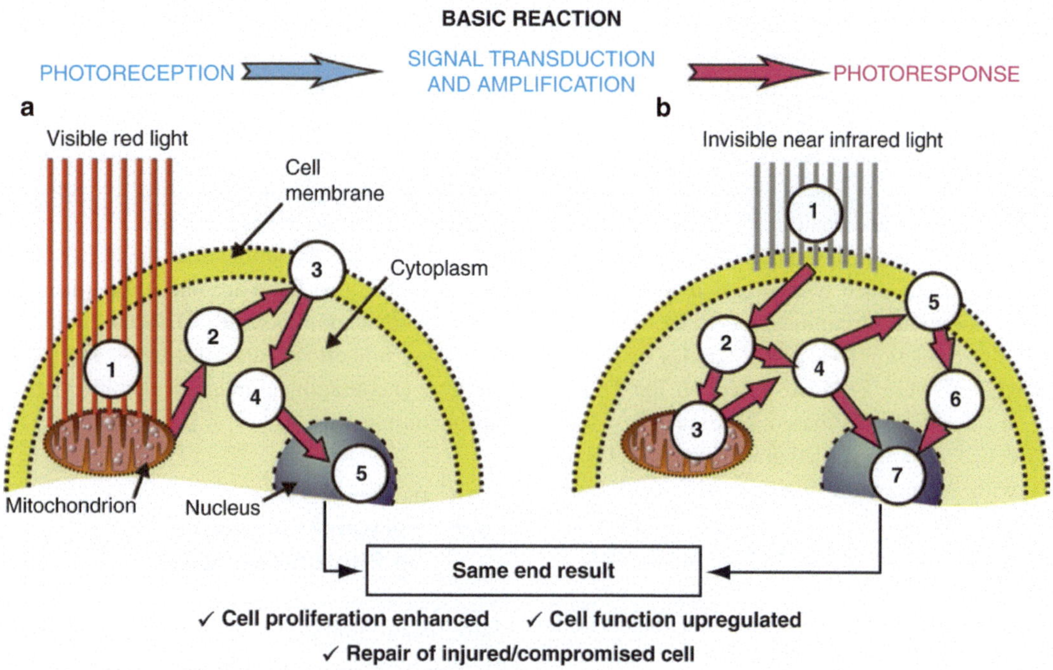

Fig. 9.16 Mechanism of photomodulation. (Reproduced from [30])

results show that all three groups were not "very satisfied" during the first 4 weeks. But 12 weeks later, the "very satisfied" response increased. In particular, the "very satisfied" total number and increase speed was highest in the 830-nm group. The reason for the gradual increase in satisfactory response seems to be because photomodulation by LED also rejuvenates the skin through collagen remodeling. The results of histology showed increased collagenesis and elastinogenesis. Cutometer results show that the 830-nm group showed higher skin elasticity than the other groups. In addition, photomodulation by 830-nm LED was effective not only when used alone but also when used as an adjunctive modality.

Trelles et al. studied 60 patients who underwent full-face ablative resurfacing, 30 of whom received LED-LLLT as adjuvant therapy, and 30 did not [4]. The results showed that LED–LLLT had statistically less pain, erythema, bruising, and edema, and faster wound recovery, and fewer complications than the non-LED group.

LED adjuvant therapy recover wound more than 50% faster, reducing side effects and downtime. The LED adjuvant therapy protocol is as follows. Perform LED as soon as possible immediately after the procedure. The energy is about 60 J/cm^2. For severe trauma or extensive surgical procedures, at least six procedures are recommended over 3 weeks (twice a week). The procedure interval should be at least 2 days.

The 830-nm LED-LLLT can be used as adjuvant therapy after any procedure, from mild microdermabrasion to rhytidectomy. It also benefits the patient with its parasympathetic rest and relax response.

9.8.6 Consensus on LED

Despite these studies, we rarely find clinically noticeable effects of LED. Does LED really work?

In the past, many doubted photomodulation (LLLT) including LED. There were many doubts regarding its clinical efficacy because most studies on photomodulation used cell culture models, and only a few were clinical studies [4]. But recently, there are many clinical studies regarding photomodulation of LED. However, there is no consensus by objective research.

Jagdeo et al. analyzed the effects of LEDs in 31 randomized controlled trials (RCTs): acne vulgaris (eight trials), herpes simplex and zoster (HSV, HZV) (three trials), skin rejuvenation (six trials), acute wound healing (five trials), psoriasis (three trials), atopic dermatitis (one trial), chronic wound healing (two trials), oral mucositis (one trial), radiation dermatitis (one trial), and thigh cellulite reduction (one trial). Grades of recommendation were assigned based on the Oxford Centre for Evidence-based Medicine-Levels of Evidence. Recommended grades are A, B, C, and D, with A being the highest [31]. The results showed that acne vulgaris, herpes simplex and zoster, and acute wound healing were grade B, and the rest were C or D.

This paper analyzed only the RCTs, which is an objective research method, but the number of papers is too small to make a clear conclusion about the effect of all LEDs. However, we can say LEDs are relatively effective against acne vulgaris, herpes simplex and zoster, and acute wound healing compared to other diseases. But our main interest—skin rejuvenation and thigh cellulite reduction—are grade C and D, respectively, i.e., we cannot yet say that LED is effective for these indications.

Jagdeo et al. proposed a protocol for each disease based on the analysis results. (1) For acne, blue and red light LEDs are recommended for 20 min with the energy of 6–40 and 8–100 mW/cm^2, respectively. The treatment interval should be 4–8 weeks twice a week. (2) For herpes simplex and herpes zoster, near-infrared LEDs are recommended. Recovery time can be reduced by at least 2 days when the LED is used. In addition to oral antiviral drugs, 3 days a day at-home LED is recommended. The parameter should be 33 J/cm^2 for 10 min at 55 mW/cm^2 at 830 nm (3). For acute wounds, treatment with yellow light (590 nm) or near-infrared LEDs every day until the wound is healed can reduce the duration and erythema of the acute wound, regardless of the cause. Yellow light LEDs are recommended 50 mW/cm^2 for 1–2 min and near-infrared LEDs 5–40 J/cm^2 for 20 min at 50 mW/cm^2 [31].

For skin rejuvenation, daily use of near-infrared LED and red-light LED for 8–10 weeks was most effective in improving wrinkles. The parameters vary from paper to paper, making it difficult to present a protocol. Several papers state that yellow-light LEDs are effective for skin rejuvenation, but no RCTs are found.

Jagdeo et al. recommended the LED use, despite the fact that there are only three diseases with Recommendation Grade B, because LEDs have fewer side effects, are affordable, and more and more encouraging clinical results are continuously coming out.

9.8.7 Personal Comments on Photomodulation

Many recent studies on photomodulation have revealed many facts regarding photomodulation effects and its mechanism. However, the exact mechanism is still unknown, and there are many debates about parameters such as energy, distance, and treatment intervals. The main problem is its efficacy. In my personal experience, I have not seen any photomodulation effect through monotherapy with LEDs, and thus use it as adjuvant therapy. As with the paper mentioned earlier [31], I believe that the LED is effective for acne, herpes simplex and herpes zoster, and acute wound healing. Therefore, I use LED for acute wound healing after an ablative procedure such as the CO_2 fractional laser or severe erythema after laser treatment, and PDT treatment for acne.

References

1. Park SH, Yeo WC, Koh WS, Park JW, Noh NK, Yoon CS (2014) Laser dermatology plastic surgery, 2nd edn. (Korean). Koonja, Seoul
2. Raulin C, Karsai S (2011) Laser and IPL technology in dermatology and aesthetic medicine. Heidelberg: New York
3. Allemann IB, Goldberg DJ (2011) Basics in dermatological laser applications. Karger Medical and Scientific Publishers
4. Goldman MP (2006) Cutaneous and cosmetic laser surgery. Mosby Elsevier, Philadelphia, PA

5. Hruza GJ, Tanzi EL (2018) Lasers and lights. Elsevier, Edinburgh
6. Textbook Compilation Committee in Korean Dermatological Association (2014) Text book of dermatology 6th edition (Korean). Daehanuihak, Seoul
7. Issa MCA, Tamura B (2018) Lasers, lights and other technologies. Springer
8. Ogawa R (2020) Total scar management. Springer, Singapore
9. Nouri K (2014) Handbook of lasers in dermatology. Springer
10. Calderhead RG, Vasily DB (2016) Low level light therapy with light-emitting diodes for the aging face. Clin Plast Surg 43(3):541–550
11. Ross EV, Sajben FP, Hsia J, Barnette D, Miller CH, McKinlay JR (2000) Nonablative skin remodeling: selective dermal heating with a mid-infrared laser and contact cooling combination. Lasers Surg Med 26(2):186–195
12. Niemz MH (2007) Laser-tissue interactions. Springer, New York
13. Alexiades-Armenakas M, Newman J, Willey A, Kilmer S, Goldberg D, Garden J et al (2013) Prospective multicenter clinical trial of a minimally invasive temperature-controlled bipolar fractional radiofrequency system for rhytid and laxity treatment. Dermatol Surg 39(2):263–273
14. Alexiades M, Berube D (2015) Randomized, blinded, 3-arm clinical trial assessing optimal temperature and duration for treatment with minimally invasive fractional radiofrequency. Dermatol Surg 41(5): 623–632
15. Berlien H-P (2003) Applied laser medicine. Springer Science & Business Media
16. Taylor MB, Prokopenko I (2006) Split-face comparison of radiofrequency versus long-pulse Nd-YAG treatment of facial laxity. J Cosmet Laser Ther 8(1):17–22
17. Schmults CD, Phelps R, Goldberg DJ (2004) Nonablative facial remodeling: erythema reduction and histologic evidence of new collagen formation using a 300-microsecond 1064-nm Nd:YAG laser. Arch Dermatol 140(11):1373–1376
18. Chiba C, Usui A, Hara H, Ishi Y (2009) Clinical experience in skin rejuvenation treatment in Asians using a long-pulse Nd:YAG laser. J Cosmet Laser Ther 11(3):134–138
19. Alam M, Dover JS (2003) Nonablative laser and light therapy: an approach to patient and device selection. Skin Therapy Lett 8(4):4–7
20. Badawi A, Tome MA, Atteya A, Sami N, Morsy IA (2011) Retrospective analysis of non-ablative scar treatment in dark skin types using the sub-millisecond Nd:YAG 1,064 nm laser. Lasers Surg Med 43(2):130–136
21. Lipper GM, Perez M (2006) Nonablative acne scar reduction after a series of treatments with a short-pulsed 1,064-nm neodymium:YAG laser. Dermatol Surg 32(8):998–1006
22. Tanaka Y, Matsuo K, Yuzuriha S (2011) Objective assessment of skin rejuvenation using near-infrared 1064-nm neodymium: YAG laser in Asians. Clin Cosmet Investig Dermatol 4:123–130
23. Wanner M, Sakamoto FH, Avram MM, Chan HH, Alam M, Tannous Z et al (2016) Immediate skin responses to laser and light treatments: therapeutic endpoints: how to obtain efficacy. J Am Acad Dermatol 74(5):821–833. quiz 34, 33
24. Woodley DT (2017) Distinct fibroblasts in the papillary and reticular dermis: implications for wound healing. Dermatol Clin 35(1):95–100
25. Vogel A, Venugopalan V (2003) Mechanisms of pulsed laser ablation of biological tissues. Chem Rev 103(2):577–644
26. Anderson RR, Farinelli W, Laubach H, Manstein D, Yaroslavsky AN, Gubeli J III et al (2006) Selective photothermolysis of lipid-rich tissues: a free electron laser study. Lasers Surg Med 38(10):913–919
27. Watanabe S (2008) Basics of laser application to dermatology. Arch Dermatol Res 300(Suppl 1):S21–S30
28. Calderhead RG (2007) The photobiological basics behind light-emitting diode (LED) phototherapy. Laser Ther 16(2):97–108
29. Opel DR, Hagstrom E, Pace AK, Sisto K, Hirano-Ali SA, Desai S et al (2015) Light-emitting diodes: a brief review and clinical experience. J Clin Aesthet Dermatol 8(6):36–44
30. Nouri K (2018) Lasers in dermatology and medicine: dermatologic applications. Springer International Publishing
31. Jagdeo J, Austin E, Mamalis A, Wong C, Ho D, Siegel DM (2018) Light-emitting diodes in dermatology: a systematic review of randomized controlled trials. Lasers Surg Med 50:613

Ablative Lasers and Fractional Lasers

10

10.1 Wavelength and Types of Ablative Laser

Absorption curves for water are very low in the ultraviolet and visible range and the absorption curve rises in the near-infrared range and is the highest in the far-infrared. The absorption curve of water in far-infrared peaks at 2940 nm and then decreases, then gradually increases (Fig. 10.1) [2].

There are three far-infrared lasers. There is the erbium-doped yttrium aluminum garnet (Er:YAG) laser with the highest absorption coefficient of water at 2940 nm and there is the 10,600 nm CO_2 laser which has an absorption coefficient that is 1/10 lower than the absorption coefficient of Er:YAG laser. Finally, there is the 2790 nm erbium:yttrium–scandium–gallium–garnet (Er:YSGG) laser with an absorption coefficient between Er:YAG and CO_2 laser. Er:YSGG lasers have three times the absorption coefficient of CO_2 lasers and one-third times the absorption coefficient of Er:YAG lasers [3].

A commercialized 2790-nm Er:YSGG laser is the "Pearl" laser, which is not widely used in private clinics [4]. I think this is because the laser is "in between." Both the effect and the side effects are "in-between," making it ambiguous.

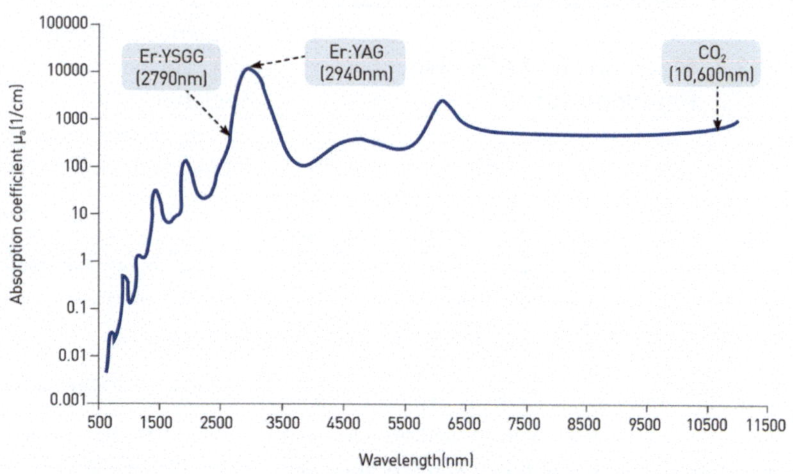

Fig. 10.1 Absorption coefficient of pure water. (Modified from [1])

J. D. Lee et al., *Principles and Choice of Laser Treatment in Dermatology*,
https://doi.org/10.1007/978-981-15-6556-4_10

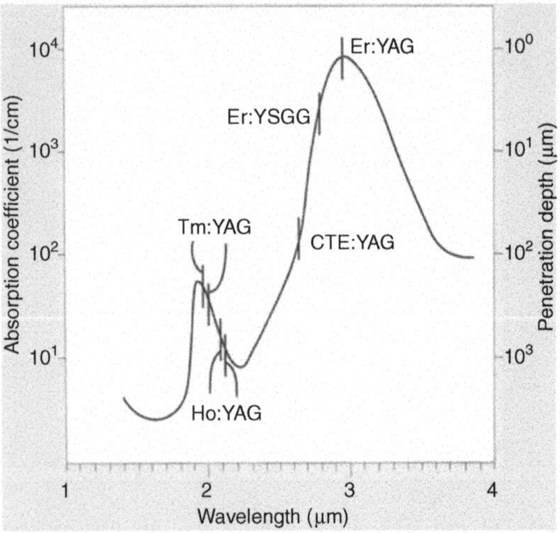

Fig. 10.2 Absorption coefficient and penetration depth of water. Tm:YAG; thulium laser. (Reproduced from [1])

The same applies to the 1927-nm thulium laser which is in between mid-infrared and far-infrared. The absorption coefficient for water for 1927 nm is in between ablative rejuvenation (AR) and nonablative rejuvenation (NAR) (Fig. 10.2). It is not very effective because it does not completely ablate and if the energy is a little high, it frequently causes postinflammatory hyperpigmentation (PIH).

10.2 Mechanism of Ablative Laser

10.2.1 Mechanism of Ablative Rejuvenation

Although the mechanism of AR can be thought of as vaporizing skin tissue, it is not. When energy accumulates in the skin in a very short time and the water temperature rises, vaporization occurs, increasing the volume of the water and increasing the pressure. At 300 °C, the water rises to 1000 atm. As the water pressure increases in the tissue, the water in the tissue is exploded due to the pressure difference with the atmosphere, and the skin tissue is removed by explosive removal. The mechanism of AR is not to vaporize all skin tissue, but to use water to forcibly eject skin tissue from the surface [2]. Therefore, AR should be described as "cutting" or "digging" rather than "burning" (Fig. 10.3).

Therefore, ablation due to vaporization removes not only the target area but also surrounding tissues, causing damage to the surrounding tissues causing side effects. CO_2 lasers are known to have the highest side effects in treating epidermal pigments than long-pulsed lasers or Q-switched lasers [6].

10.2.2 Water Vaporization Threshold

Water vaporization and explosion is needed for explosive removal of tissue. The energy for this should be greater than the energy for water vaporization. The energy needed for water vaporization at the epidermis is 2500 J/cm^3. Therefore, more than 2500 J/cm^3 of energy is required.

The energy needed for water vaporization at the dermis is 4300 J/cm^3, which is about twice the energy needed than the epidermis [2]. The reason for this is because of the high tensile strength of the collagen fibers. If the dermis is treated with the energy needed for water vaporization at the epidermis, ablation will be inadequate. It will only cause dry skin, which will make the area of residual thermal damage (RTD) become larger, which is likely to cause side effects. Therefore, when treating the dermis, twice the energy needed than the epidermis.

The energy needed to vaporize water (E_v) is known as the following equation:

$$E_v = \text{fluence} \times \mu_a$$

The absorption coefficient of water of a CO_2 laser is 500 cm^{-1}, so if we substitute this into the formula:

$$\text{Fluence} = 2500/500 = 5\left(\text{J/cm}^2 \text{in } CO_2 \text{ laser}\right)$$

At least 5 J/cm^2 of energy is required when using the CO_2 laser for AR. Vaporization does not happen below 5 J/cm^2. This is called the water vaporization threshold of the CO_2 laser [2].

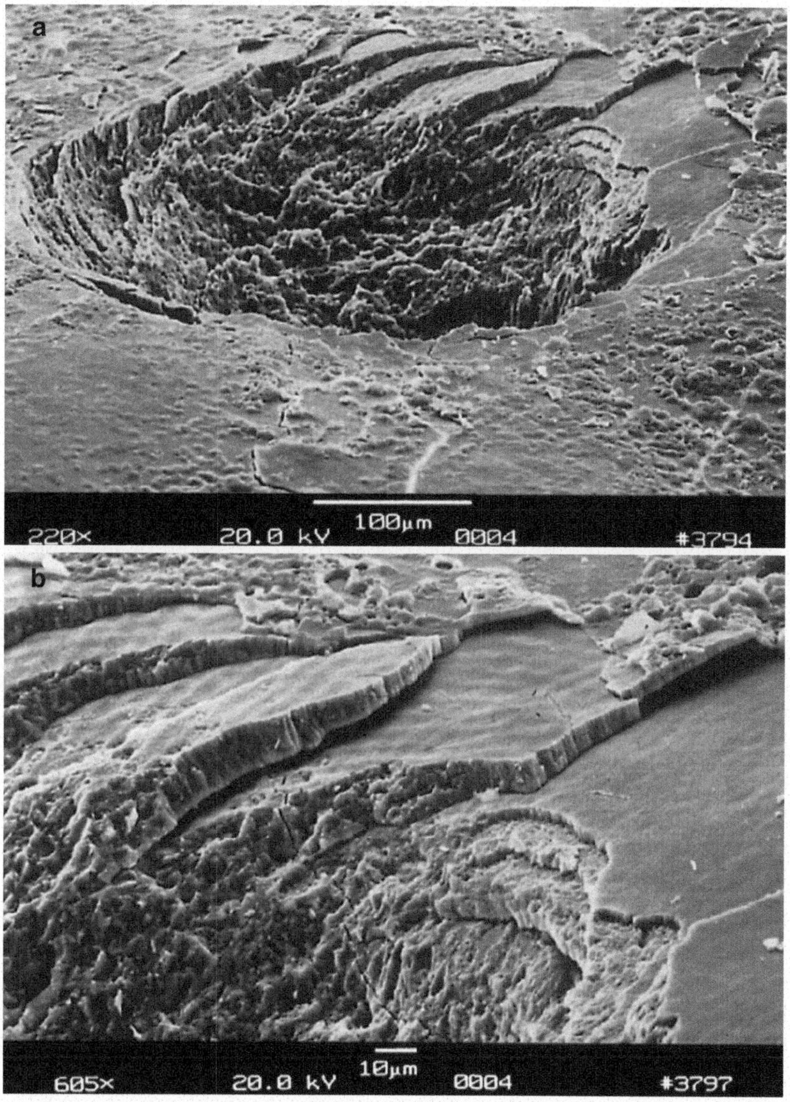

Fig. 10.3 (**a**) Human tooth vaporized by 20 pulses from an Er:YAG laser (pulse duration: 90 µs. Pulse energy: 100 mJ, repetition rate: 1 Hz). (**b**) Enlargement showing the edge of ablation. (Reproduced from [5])

10.2.3 Residual Thermal Damage

Ohshiro presented the laser apple concept in 1995 [8]. The laser apple concept is that not all photons irradiated with ablative laser are used for ablation, but some are absorbed in the remaining tissue, elevating the temperature, and influencing tissue response. The remaining tissue shows a series of temperature-dependent bioreactions in tissue [9]. As shown in Fig. 10.4, when CO_2 laser is irradiated on the skin most photons are irradiated on the skin surface making the temperature highest. As we go deeper into the skin, there are fewer photons resulting in lower temperatures.

The thermal reactions of skin tissue are as follows:

- >100 °C: vaporization
- >60 °C: coagulation
- >55 °C: protein degradation
- >40 °C: protein denaturation.

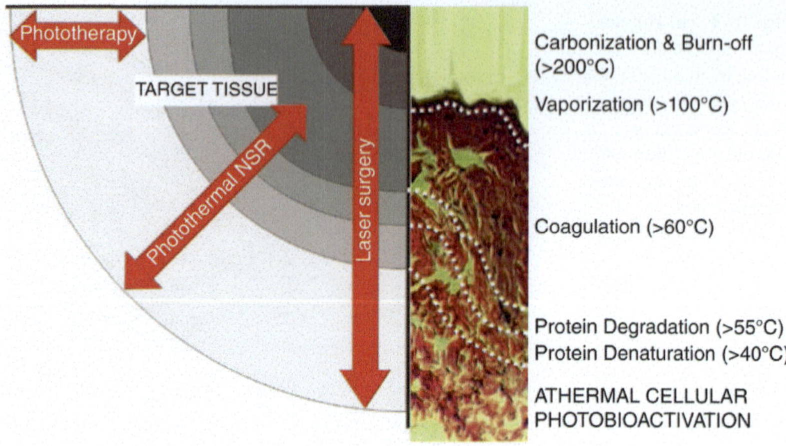

Fig. 10.4 Range of photothermal and athermal photobioreactions in tissue following a typical surgical laser impact, e.g., a CO_2 laser. (Reproduced from [7])

Ohshiro assumed that irreversible damage occurs above 40 °C. Residual thermal damage (RTD) refers to the tissue that has not been vaporized and has been irreversibly damaged. RTDs are not normal tissue and are eventually discharged out of the skin. This means that even RTDs are eventually removed later. For example, when removing melanocytic nevus by CO_2 laser, even if the operator takes care to remove the nevus only and does not remove surrounding tissue, the surrounding tissue is damaged anyway, because of RTDs. These tissues are eventually removed, resulting in undesirable side effects. That is why, when removing nevi, the operator should not try to remove them all at once but should rather leave a little bit of nevus tissue behind. If there is remnant nevus tissue, it can be removed later. This is why I perform nevus removal at two different times.

10.3 Determining Pulse Duration

10.3.1 Absorption Coefficient and Optical Penetration Depth

In "Chap. 3," we reviewed that the optical penetration depth (OPD) is described by the following equation [7].

$$\delta = \frac{1}{\sqrt{3\mu_a\left(\mu_a + \mu_s\left(1-g\right)\right)}}$$

δ: the wavelength dependent optical penetration depth of light, or the depth at which there is attenuation to 37% of the surface value (37% = 1/e, where e = 2.7, the base of the natural logarithm),

g: anisotropy coefficient (a measure of the "mean" direction of the scattered photons). $g = 0.9$ for the skin,

μ_a: absorption coefficient,

μ_s: scattering coefficient.

If we look into this equation closely, we can see that the optical penetration depth is inversely proportional to the absorption coefficient and the scattering coefficient. That is, the optical penetration depth becomes shallower as the absorption (μ_a) and scattering (μ_s) become larger. Since scattering does not occur in ablative lasers, the equation above can be simplified as follows [2]:

$$\delta \fallingdotseq \frac{1}{\mu_a}$$

In ablative lasers, the absorption coefficient and the optical penetration depth are inversely proportional. In other words, ablative lasers with wavelengths that are absorbed well have shallower optical penetration depths. For example, the Er:YAG laser has a higher water absorption coefficient than CO_2 lasers. Many photons are absorbed on the surface, so the depth of penetration becomes shallower, making the ablation thinner. Therefore, the Er:YAG laser with high absorption coefficient enables a more precise procedure.

If we know the absorption coefficient, we can substitute this in the equation above, and calculate the optical penetration depth. For example, the absorption coefficient of water in a CO_2 laser is 500 cm^{-1}. The optical penetration depth is calculated to be 20 μm. This is consistent with the actual ablation depth of 20–60 μm [2].

10.3.2 Thermal Relaxation Time in CO_2 Laser

$$\text{TRT} \fallingdotseq d^2 / g\kappa$$

g: geometric factor, κ; thermal diffusivity.

In CO_2 laser, the diameter *d* in the TRT formula is the depth of penetration (Sect. 3.4.2 in "Chap. 3") which is 20 μm g is a geometric factor, and since the skin is on a plane it is 4. The thermal diffusivity constant κ is about 1.3×10^{-3} cm^2/s. If we substitute these in the equation above, the TRT is approximately 800 μs. Therefore, the pulse duration of the CO_2 laser should be 800 μs or less, approximately 1 ms or less [2].

In summary, the pulse duration for a CO_2 laser should be less than 1 ms when the fluence is at least 5 J/cm^2. In this case, the optical penetration depth is 20 μm, and the actual ablation depth is 20–60 μm. The residual thermal damage is known to be 3–4 times the optical penetration [10], and the actual residual thermal damage depth is about 60–100 μm.

10.3.3 Comparison of Ablative Lasers

Here we will compare CO_2 and Er:YAG laser, wherein both are ablative lasers (Table 10.1). CO_2 lasers have a photothermal effect with a TRT of less than 1 ms. The Er:YAG laser originally had a subpulse of 1 μs but extended the pulse duration to 250 μs by using macropulse. Er:YAG lasers have a photomechanical effect due to their high absorption coefficient and short pulse duration [2].

Table 10.1 Comparison of CO_2 laser and Er:YAG laser [2].

	CO_2 laser	Er:YAG laser
Wavelength	10,600 nm	2940 nm
Pulse duration	<1 ms (~800 μs)	<1 ms (250 μs, macropulse) 1 μs (subpulse)
Mechanism	Photothermal	Photomechanical
Absorption coefficient(μ_a)	790 cm^{-1}	8000–9000 cm^{-1}
Skin containing 70–80% water	500 cm^{-1}	12,800 cm^{-1}
Depth of penetration($1/\mu_a$)	20–60 μm	2–5 μm
Residual thermal damage	60–100 μm	20–50 μm
Water vaporization threshold	5 J/cm^2	0.5–1.5 J/cm^2

CO_2 and Er:YAG lasers have wavelengths of 10,600 nm and 2940 nm, respectively. The absorption coefficients differ in ten times, 790 and 8000–9000 cm^{-1}, respectively. Er:YAG laser is known to have ten times higher absorption coefficient than the CO_2 laser, but since the skin contains 70–80% of water, the absorption coefficient considering this differs more than ten times by 500 and 12,800 cm^{-1}. Since the absorption coefficient of Er:YAG laser is more than ten times higher than the CO_2 laser, the penetration depth is ten times less than that of a CO_2 laser. The depth of penetration for CO_2 and Er:YAG is 20–60 μm and 2–5 μm, respectively. RTD is generally known to be three to four times the OPD. Since the Er:YAG laser has a shallower OPD and less RTD than the CO_2 laser, fewer side effects occur. The water vaporization threshold is E_v = fluence × μ_a. Since the Er:YAG laser has a high absorption coefficient, the water vaporization threshold is rather low (0.5–1.5 J/cm^2) [2].

10.4 Spot Size

10.4.1 Spot Size in Ablative Laser

Which spot size should be used in ablative lasers? The use of small spot sizes results in remnant tissues because the results are irregular and uneven

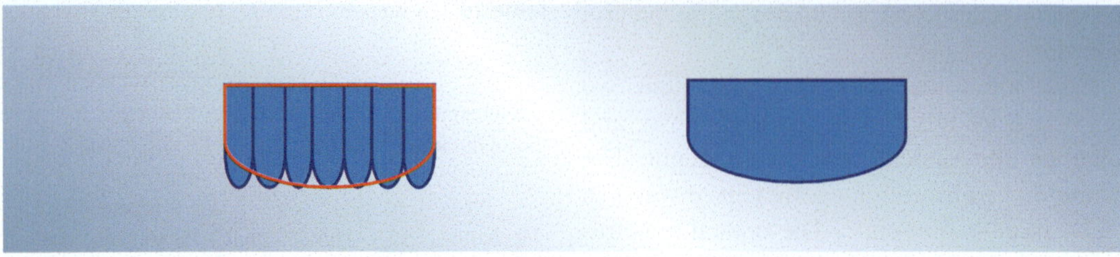

Fig. 10.5 Differences in spot size in ablative lasers. When small spot sizes are used to remove the same volume of tissue (e.g., nevi, depicted as red boxes) some tissues remain while some are excessively removed

(Fig. 10.5). Poor hemostasis is a problem because bleeding from blood vessels larger than the spot size cannot be stopped. The use of large spot sizes results in a smoother, more even ablation of tissues. Therefore, small spot sizes should be used to make incisions, and large spot sizes should be used to remove nevi or for skin rejuvenation [2]. But if the spot size is larger the power density decreases, and longer pulse duration is needed to achieve the same effect. This may result in the risk of heat buildup and charring, and eventually scarring. To avoid this, an ablative laser with a high output must be used or the spot size should be adjusted according to the output.

In "Chap. 1." we reviewed that as the spot size becomes larger, the optical penetration depth (OPD) becomes deeper. But the ablation depth is the same even though the spot size increases. What is the reason for this phenomenon? The reason that the OPD becomes deeper as the spot size becomes larger is due to scattering. Since scattering is almost nonexistent in far-infrared lasers, the OPD is determined by the absorption coefficient regardless of the spot size change. Therefore, if the laser is a far-infrared laser of the same wavelength, the ablation depth is the same regardless of spot size.

10.5 Fluence

10.5.1 Parameters on the Panel

In CO_2 lasers, the water vaporization threshold is 5 J/cm^2, so CO_2 laser treatment should be performed with fluence higher than 5 J/cm^2. However, the instrument panel of our CO_2 laser

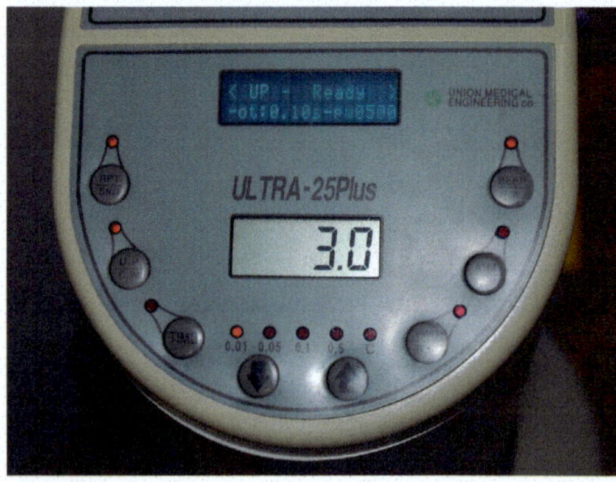

Fig. 10.6 The panel of a CO_2 laser. The parameters are shown on the panel: pulse duration 500 μs, on-time 0.01 s, off-time 0.1 s, and 3 W. Fluence is not shown on the panel

does not show the unit of fluence (J/cm^2) but shows Watt, which is the unit of power (Fig. 10.6). Therefore, we must convert power to fluence, so we know how much fluence we use. For example, when the spot size is 0.1 mm and the pulse duration is 500 μs, how many Watts is 5 J/cm^2?

$$W = \text{fluence} / \text{s} = \left(\text{J}/\text{cm}^2\right) \times \pi R^2 / \text{s}$$

$$5\,\text{J}/\text{cm}^2 \times 3.14 \times \left(0.05\,\text{cm}\right)^2 / 0.0005\,\text{s} = 0.785\,\text{W}$$

In other words, at least 0.8 W of power must be used for ablation. When less than 0.8 W power is used, ablation does not occur. Only coagulation occurs.

10.5.2 Defocusing Methods (Low Fluence Methods)

After the laser is made in the optical cavity, it reaches the handpiece through the delivery

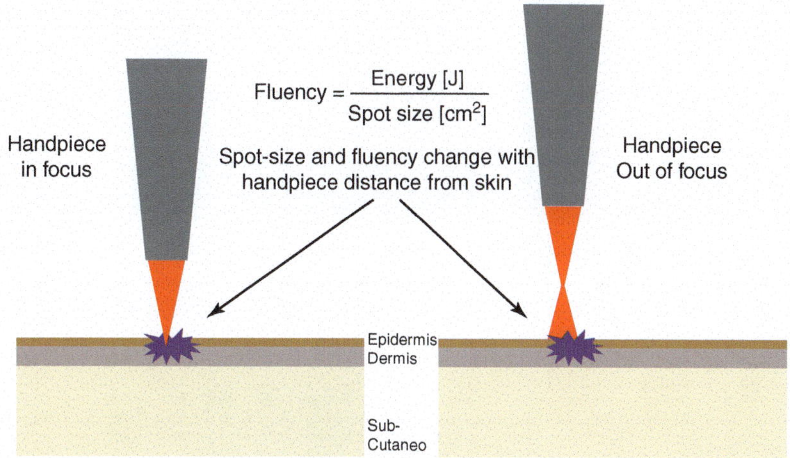

Fig. 10.7 Focused headpiece. Laser in focus: power density is at its maximum (vaporizing, cutting). Out of focus: power density is reduced (coagulation, milder treatment). (Modified from [11])

system. After that, the convex lens refracts the photons to a focal point of the skin, creating a high-power density. This is called focusing. The distance at this time is called a focal length. On the other hand, defocusing is a method of lowering the power density by lifting the handpiece from the skin and making the actual distance longer than the focal length (Fig. 10.7).

Now we will review the fluence and the power density during focusing and defocusing.

For example, during CO_2 laser focusing with 3 W and 0.1 mm spot size, the fluence is 13.461 J/cm^2. During CO_2 laser defocusing with 3 W and 0.8 mm spot size, the fluence is 0.2086 J/cm^2 (Table 10.2). In other words, focusing leads to ablation because it exceeds the water vaporization threshold of 5 J/cm^2 while defocusing results in coagulation only because it is less than 5 J/cm^2.

$$\text{Power density} = W / \pi R^2$$

Since power density is inversely proportional to the square of the diameter, defocusing increases the diameter by 8 times but the power density decreased by 64 times.

Therefore, by moving the handpiece up and down in perpendicular to the skin, focusing and defocusing may easily be selected to either ablate or coagulate. The coagulation effect of defocusing can be used to treat shallower epidermal pigments, such as solar lentigines. This method is called the defocusing method or low fluence method. However, this method has a very narrow therapeutic window between 3.7 and 4.4 J/cm^2. If the fluence is higher than the therapeutic window, ablation occurs but if it is less than the therapeutic window it is ineffective. The procedure requires extreme accuracy and careful attention. Also due to heat conduction, there is a possible risk of side effects [12]. Therefore, I use the defocusing method mainly for hemostasis and for small epidermal pigmentations for a very short time, but not for most epidermal pigmentations. One thing to note is that the defocusing method is intended to only coagulate, not ablate. That is why tissue should not be ablated with this procedure.

Table 10.2 The comparison of energy density and power density of CO_2 laser when spot size is 100 and 800 μm at 3 W

	3 W, Ø = 100 μm (focusing)	3 W, Ø = 800 μm (defocusing)
Energy density	13.461 J/cm^2	0.2086 J/cm^2
Power density	38,460 W/cm^2	596 W/cm^2

10.6 Power Density

10.6.1 High- Versus Low-Power Density Laser

$$\text{Energy} = \text{Power} \times \text{Pulse duration}$$

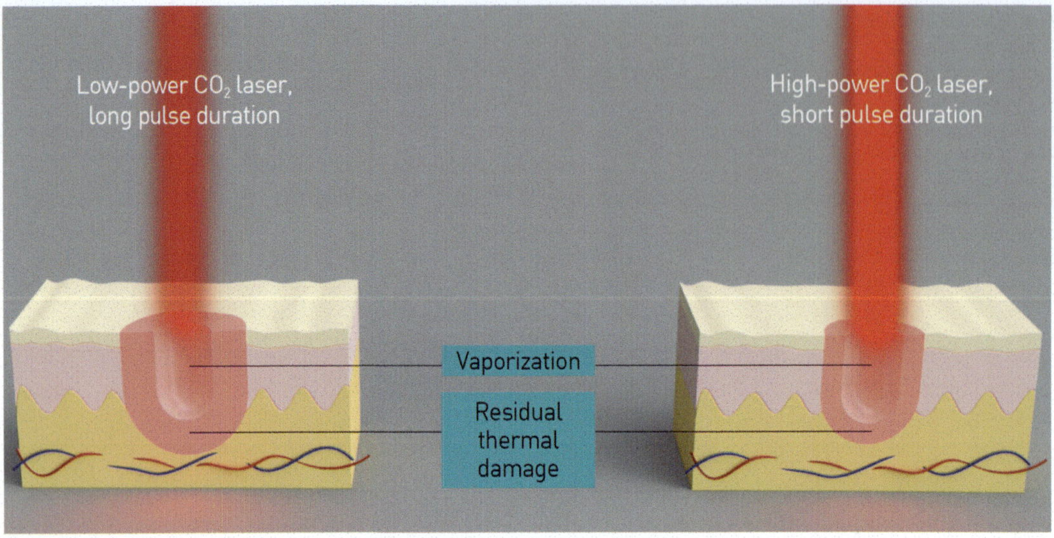

Fig. 10.8 Comparison of tissue response between low-power and high-power CO_2 laser. Although the area of vaporization may be the same in both lasers, the area of residual thermal damage is different. Published with kind permission of © Jin Kwon Cho 2019

The volume of ablation by the ablative laser is proportional to the total energy [2]. Since energy is the multiplication of the power and pulse duration (the equation above), the total energy is the same even if the power is increased and pulse duration is shortened or the power is decreased and the pulse duration lengthened. In other words, the volume of ablation is the same either in using expensive high-power CO_2 lasers and using high watts and shortening the pulse duration or by using cheaper low-power CO_2 lasers and using low watts and lengthening the pulse duration.

However, longer pulse duration at lower watts results in wider RTD (Fig. 10.8). Also, in longer pulse duration at low watts, the water in the tissue does not explode with high pressures, but slowly evaporates with low pressure. This causes the tissue to dry up and vaporize the tissue itself rather than the water. The vaporization temperature of the tissue is higher than the vaporization temperature of the water and should be raised to 600 °C or higher. Because vaporization occurs at a much higher temperature, the RTD is even deeper [2]. That is why a high-power ablation laser should be bought if possible and shorter pulse duration at high watts will reduce damage to the surrounding tissue.

In AR, power density is the most important parameter in determining RTD and ablation depth, not fluence. For example, the minimum fluence of CO_2 laser in evaporating water is 5 J/cm^2 in 1 ms, but even if the pulse duration is longer than 1 ms, increasing fluence to 15 J/cm^2 and thus increasing the power density results in ablation. Even if the fluence is low as 1–4 J/cm^2, the pulse duration could be reduced to microseconds, then the power density will increase, also resulting in ablation [10].

The high-power CO_2 lasers on the market are now known to have a power density of 10,000–50,000 W/cm^2, and when the power density drops to 2000 W/cm^2, vaporization occurs slowly increasing RTD and side effects. Therefore, the power density should be at least 2000 W/cm^2 and should be about 10,000–50,000 W/cm^2.

10.6.2 Charring

Another disadvantage of low-power CO_2 laser is charring. Long exposure time with low-power CO_2 laser causes the tissue to dry up and eventually cause charring. The ultimate end product of all heated living tissue is carbon. The carbon becomes a new heat sink, which, when irradiated with a laser, rapidly increases the temperature to 300–600 °C, resulting in deeper RTD. As a result, the damage to the surrounding tissue becomes more severe [2]. In AR, high-power lasers should be used to reduce the exposure time so that only vaporization and no charring occur. If charring occurs, the treatment should be discontinued until the carbonized tissue is removed with wet cotton.

10.7 Fluence Adjustment and Multiple Passes

10.7.1 Depth of Ablation and Residual Thermal Damage

What is the relationship between fluence, ablation depth, and the depth of RTD? Ross et al. biopsied pigskin after CO_2 laser exposure of 10 J/cm^2 [10]. Since CO_2 is a Gaussian beam, it has the highest fluence (20 J/cm^2) in the middle. The middle portion is the deepest, indicating that ablation depth is the deepest in the middle. Therefore, we can see that the higher the fluence, the deeper the ablation depth.

From the end of the laser beam to the center, the RTD area initially becomes a little thicker, but after it reaches 3 J/cm^2 (this fluence probably corresponds to the vaporization energy of water in pigskin) the thickness is relatively constant. That is, when the energy is lower than the water vaporization threshold, higher fluence increases the depth of RTD, but when it is higher than the water vaporization threshold, the depth of RTD is relatively constant. The reason why the depth of RTD is relatively constant above the water vaporization threshold is because of Beer's law [10]. In other words, as the depth increases, the subsurface photons decrease exponentially, and the optical penetration depth does not increase in relation to an increase in fluence. However, this phenomenon only occurs when the pulse duration is shorter than 1–5 ms. Otherwise, if the pulse duration is longer, the depth of RTD increases as fluence increases.

10.7.2 Multiple Passes

What happens to the ablation depth or the RTD depth after multiple passes of a CO_2 laser or Er:YAG laser?

In Fig. 10.9, when multiple passes are administered in the same place with a CO_2 laser, the ablation

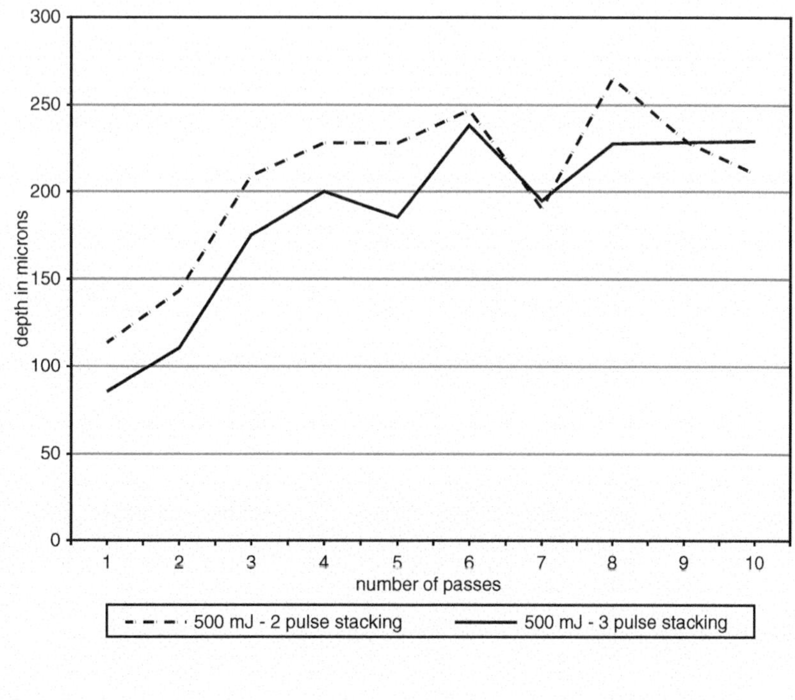

Fig. 10.9 Depth of vaporization with pulse stacking. (Modified from [13])

depth increases gradually, but after the fourth pass, the ablation depth does not increase significantly but plateaus [2]. "Pulses stacking" means stacking in the same place. For example, two passes with three pulse stacking mean, three laser exposures in the same place without moving the handpiece, and then moving the handpiece somewhere else, and then coming back again for two laser exposures.

On the other hand, the depth of RTD gets deeper without a plateau as the number of passes increases. Also, as the number of pulses (stacking) increases, the depth of RTD increases.

Generally, RTDs deeper than 100–150 μm are known to be associated with side effects [2]. In other words, they are associated with prolonged erythema, postoperative pain, delayed wound recovery, infection, and scarring. In Fig. 10.10, one pass without stacking is not a problem because the depth of RTD is less than 100 μm, but three passes with three pulses stackings may be a problem.

In summary, when using a CO_2 laser to remove melanocytic nevi, after four passes the depth of ablation does not get deeper. Only the depth of RTD gets deeper increasing the likelihood of side effects. Therefore, if there is a remnant nevus after four passes, the procedure should be stopped. The procedure for the remnant nevus should be continued at the next session. Also, stacking in the same place will deepen the RTD, so the handpiece should not stay in one place but should move to a different place.

Unlike CO_2 lasers, however, Er:YAG lasers do not have ablation depth plateaus after four passes. The depth of ablation for Er:YAG lasers increase as passes increase. Therefore, Er:YAG laser can remove deep nevi all at once by repeat-

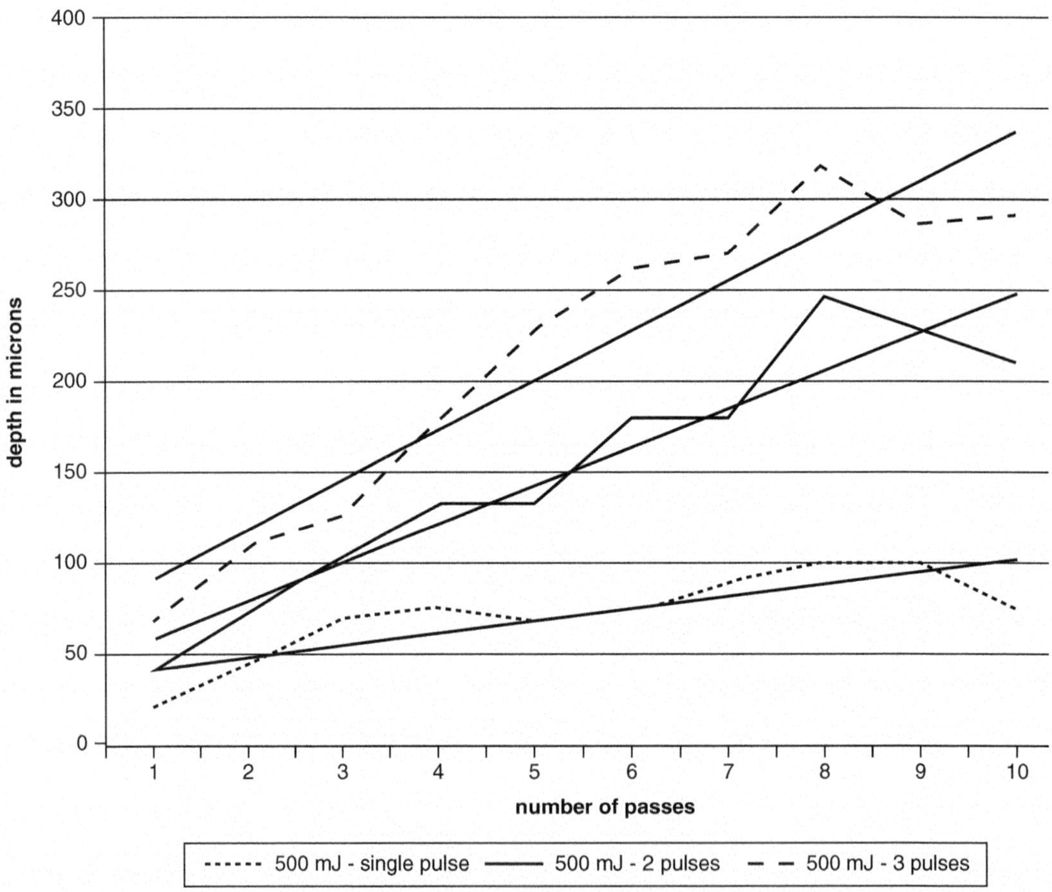

Fig. 10.10 Residual thermal necrosis: 500 mJ pulses. (Reproduced from [13])

ing several passes. For example, Er:YAG laser can remove most pigmentations in the dermo-epidermal junction or upper dermis and junctional nevi through 4–10 passes of fluence 5.2–14.4 J/cm^2 [14].

10.8 Er:YAG Laser

10.8.1 Er:YAG Laser

Er:YAG lasers have a ten times higher absorption coefficient than CO_2 lasers, with a penetration depth of 1/10 of CO_2 lasers, 2–5 μm, and lower water vaporization threshold of 0.5–1.5 J/cm^2 (Table 10.1). Pulse duration is short, 250 μs, thus showing a photomechanical effect. Tissue particles are removed at supersonic velocities because of the more explosive pressure than CO_2 lasers. Due to this phenomenon, the skin is pushed down when using Er:YAG lasers and the RTD is 20–50 μm, which is less than that of CO_2 lasers [2]. On the other hand, due to the explosive pressure, there is more hemorrhage with Er:YAG lasers (Fig. 10.11).

In summary, Er:YAG lasers compared to CO_2 lasers have shallower ablation depths, less RTD, and therefore less chance of charring. In the past, in order to reduce RTD and minimize damage to surrounding tissues, expensive high-power CO_2 lasers drew attention. However, with the introduction of Er:YAG lasers with much less RTD, the market for an ablative laser is now divided into Er:YAG laser and low-power CO_2 laser.

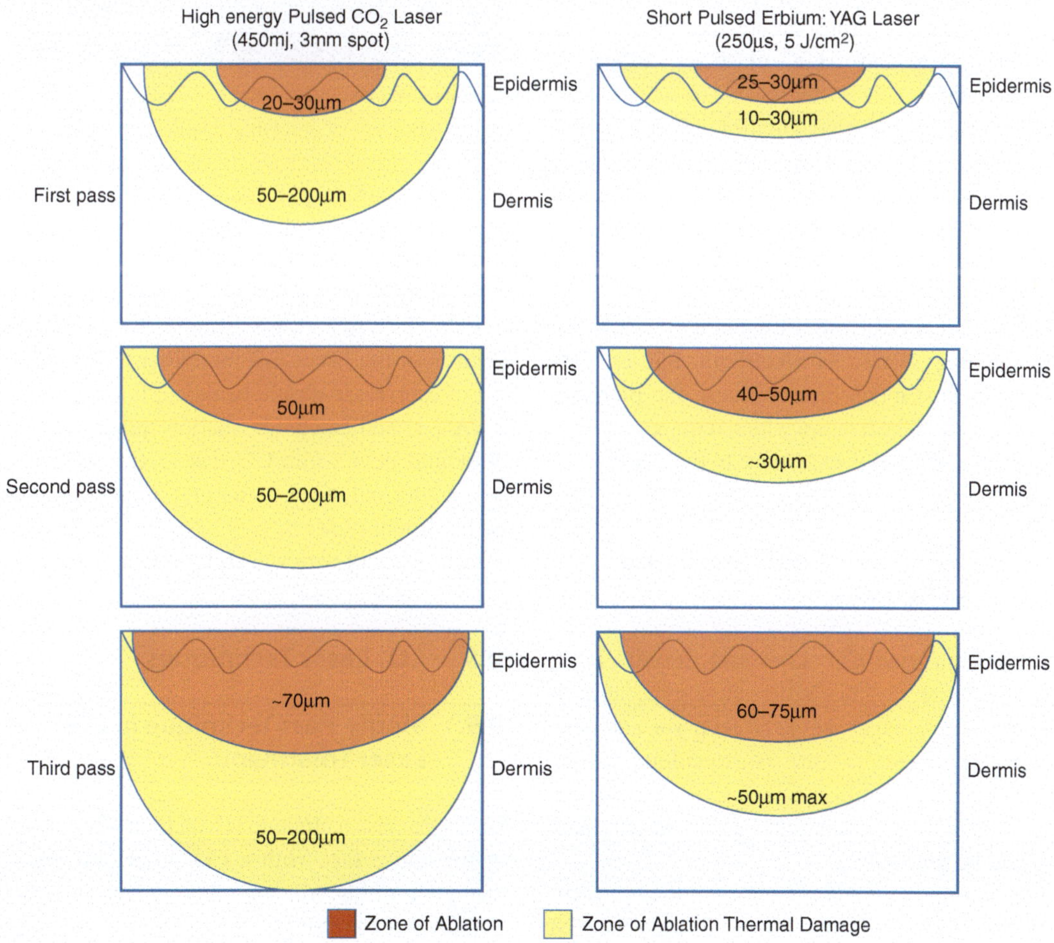

Fig. 10.11 Depth of ablation and thermal injury produced by the high energy pulsed CO_2 laser and the short-pulsed Er:YAG laser. (Reproduced from [15])

10.8.2 Pros and Cons of Er:YAG Laser

The followings are the pros and cons of Er:YAG laser.

1. The depth of RTD in Er:YAG laser is much less than that of CO_2 laser, which means fewer side effects and faster wound healing.
2. Er:YAG laser has a shallow penetration depth, allowing precise depth adjustment (Fig. 10.12).
3. Due to less RTD and explosive pressure, bleeding occurs very well in Er:YAG lasers. The disadvantage is that this makes deep ablation difficult, but the advantage is that it may be safe because ablation beyond the papillary dermis (where the blood vessels are) is difficult. However, with pulse stacking, it is possible to go deeper than the papillary dermis.
4. The depth of ablation and RTD is shallow in Er:YAG lasers, thus unlike CO_2 lasers, skin shrinkage, and skin elasticity effect is minimal.
5. Due to the nerve coagulation effect of RTD, there is less pain during CO_2 lasers, unlike Er:YAG lasers, which do not have this effect and are more painful during the procedure.
6. Er:YAG lasers are loud due to photomechanical effects.
7. CO_2 lasers cost little to maintain because the pumping system is electricity, but Er:YAG lasers cost much more because the pumping system is a flash lamp, which requires replacement costs and is expensive to purchase.

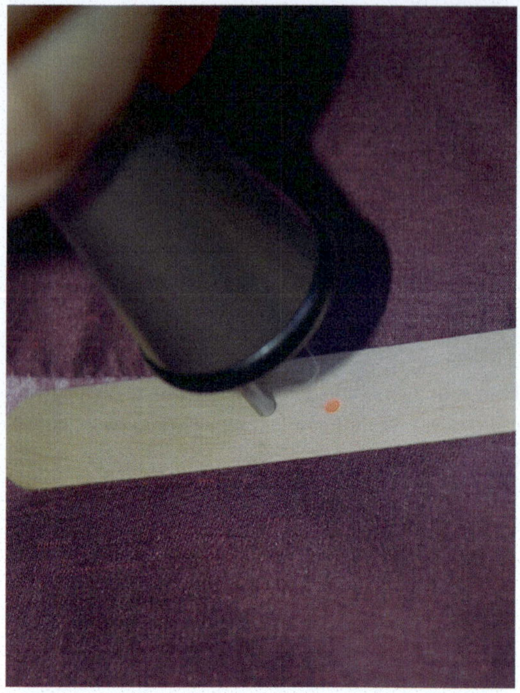

Fig. 10.12 Er:YAG lasers with suctioning properties have the advantage of observing ablation in real time

10.8.3 Selection of Ablative Lasers in Koreans

When comparing CO_2 laser and Er:YAG laser, Er:YAG laser is the better choice because it focuses the damages on the target tissue and minimizes damage to the surrounding tissue. However, CO_2 lasers are better for AR effects, such as wrinkle treatment. Then which laser should be selected?

Selecting Er:YAG lasers would be ideal because there are fewer side effects, but the cost of Er:YAG lasers are high, whereas CO_2 lasers are very cheap to purchase. That is why CO_2 lasers are recommended first. Then ways to minimize the side effects of CO_2 lasers should be sought. Later when CO_2 lasers are not enough, Er:YAG lasers should be selected. When both the lasers are there then full advantage of each laser should be taken. For example, Er:YAG is indicated for shallow junctional or compound nevi while CO_2 lasers are indicated for intradermal nevi or dermal pigmentations and treatment of scars.

Next, we will review CO_2 laser techniques.

10.9 CO_2 Laser Techniques

10.9.1 Single-Pass Technique in CO_2 Laser Treatment

The single-pass technique is a method of irradiating the entire face with a CO_2 laser only once when performing AR, and then leaving it alone without dressing. Single-pass is known to accelerate reepithelialization and has fewer side effects because the ablation depth and RTD are shallow. The remnant tissue acts as a biologic wound dressing, eliminating the need for dressing. An additional pass should be done in only the part with severe photoaging. Several papers have shown that the single-pass technique is considerably better in terms of side effects than the existing multiple-pass method [7].

Then which parameter should we use? The ablation depth in which wound healing occurs without side effects is the epidermis and the papillary dermis layer. How much fluence should be used to single-pass to this depth?

My parameter for the CO_2 laser is 3 W, pulse duration 500 μs, and 0.1 mm spot size. 3 W was sufficient to remove epidermal pigment lesions such as solar lentigo and freckles with only a single pass. This also had fewer side effects. Let's check if this is theoretically correct.

$$\text{Fluence} = \text{W} \times (\text{pulse duration}) / \pi R^2$$

$$3\,\text{W} \times 0.0005\,\text{s} / 3.14 \times (0.05\,\text{cm})^2 = 19.1\,\text{J} / \text{cm}^2$$

In the formula above, 3 W is about 20 J/cm² in fluence,

In Table 10.3, 20 J/cm² is four times the water vaporization threshold for the CO_2 laser. Increasing fluence does not increase the depth of penetration in direct proportion, but assuming a fourfold increase in penetration depth, approximately 80 μm will be ablated, and because the RTD is 60 μm, this will add up to 140–180 μm. The thickness of the epidermis is 100 μm, so 140–180 μm is expected to damage the entire epidermis and part of the papillary dermis. This is why in pigmented lesions limited to the epidermis, I only use a single-pass technique of 3 W, and if the lesion is not larger than 2–3 mm, I do not apply the dressing.

The power density is 19.1 J/cm²/0.0005 (s) = 38,200 W/cm², which corresponds to the power density of 10,000–50,000 W/cm² previously mentioned. This also corresponds to the power density without side effects which is more than 2000 W/cm². Since the watts vary depending on the spot size or pulse density, you should not use the 3 W used by myself but should try to calculate or use the single-pass technique on an epidermal pigment lesion to find the watt which is effective with fewer side effects.

For reference, my parameter for the Er:YAG laser is 6 J/cm² and less than eight passes. In Table 10.3, the water vaporization threshold for the Er:YAG laser is about 1 J/cm². The fluence of 6 J/cm² is six times this, so the penetration depth should be about 12 μm, which is six times the depth of penetration. Eight passes will add up to 96 μm and adding up 20 μm of RTD will result in 120–150 μm. Therefore, I use 6 J/cm² with Er:YAG laser and perform a maximum of eight passes unless the nevus is very deep.

Table 10.3 Brief comparison of CO_2 laser and Er:YAG laser

	CO_2 laser	Er:YAG laser
Depth of penetration ($1/\mu_a$)	20–60 μm	2–5 μm
Residual thermal damage	60–100 μm	20–50 μm
Water vaporization threshold	5 J/cm²	0.5–1.5 J/cm²

10.9.2 Dermo-Epidermal Sliding Effect

In Ohshiro's laser apple concept (Fig. 10.4), the ablation zone and RTD zone are drawn as semicircles schematically. The actual model is different, as we will review in this chapter.

Fulton et al. histologically examined the zone of vaporization and the zone of thermal damage after CO_2 laser exposure [16]. In Fig. 10.13, the figure above is drawn based on the laser apple concept and the figure below is redrawn based on the biopsy results. The difference between the two figures is that there is a zone of cavitation, in addition to the zone of vaporization and the zone of thermal damage. The zone of cavitation is between the epidermis and the dermis and also between epidermal appendages such as hair follicles and the dermis. The cavities develop 2–3 times the diameter of the target tissue, between the epidermis and the dermis, and along the hair follicle up to a depth of 300–400 μm [3].

This cavitation phenomenon may be useful for AR. After CO_2 laser exposure to the skin,

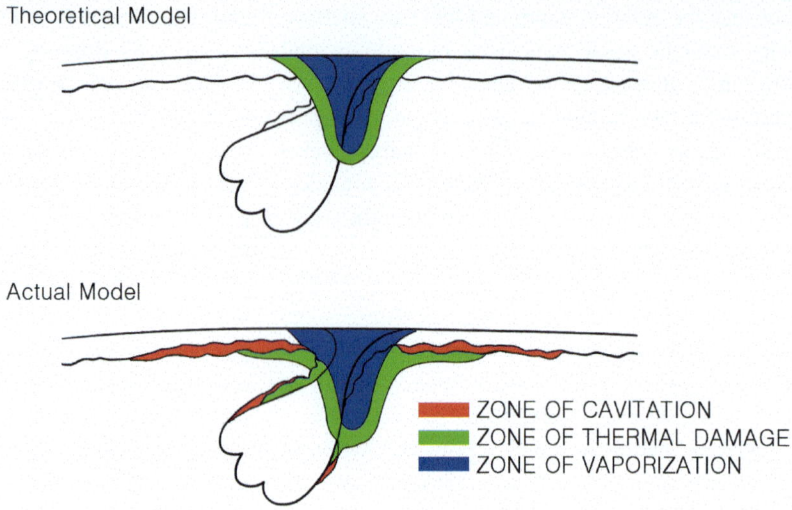

Fig. 10.13 Reaction of skin and tissue with CO_2 Laser exposure. Theoretical Model (above) and Actual Model (below). Modified from [16]

only the epidermis can be peeled off by gently pushing it with cotton or gauze soaked with boric or normal saline. I call this phenomenon "dermo-epidermal sliding effect." This also removes some of the zones of thermal damage and can be used to check whether epidermal pigments are removed and may be useful for removing nevus of unknown depths or lentigines. For example, after a single-pass technique with a CO_2 laser to treat junctional nevus, the skin may be pushed gently so that a portion of the nevus and only the epidermis of the surrounding tissue may be removed, resulting in fewer side effects. If there is any remnant nevus, CO_2 laser may be used again and the skin may be gently pushed again. Repeating this process removes only the nevus while sparing the surrounding tissues.

10.9.3 Q-Switched Nd:YAG Laser Treatment for Removing Melanocytic Nevus

Most think that only ablative lasers are used to remove melanocytic nevus. But long-pulsed lasers are also used by adjusting the pulse duration to the thermal relaxation time (TRT) of the nevus, which is in milliseconds. Then how about Q-switched lasers? Could we use them to break the nevus itself?

Yoon et al. attempted melanocytic nevi removal (flat, <10 mm in diameter) by 1064-nm Q-switched Nd:YAG laser [17]. The lesions were delivered over a spot 2 mm in diameter with a frequency of 10 Hz and fluence of 10–12 J/cm^2. It took about 2–4 s per nevus. After the procedure, sterile tissue paper was attached for hemostasis and hydrocolloids dressing (Tegasorb®) was applied. Dressing change was undertaken every other day. After 6 weeks, about 70% of the nevi were completely removed after one session. The remaining 30% were completely treated within three sessions. But in the figures in the paper, PIH can be seen.

Based on this paper, when removing melanocytic nevi, I initially use CO_2 laser or Er:YAG laser and then for the remnant nevi, use 1064-nm Q-switched Nd:YAG laser. However, fluences 10–12 J/cm^2 is high and may break cells and burst blood vessels, leading to PIH. That is why I use fluences 5–6 J/cm^2, which break cells but does not damage blood vessels.

Is it possible to remove nevi completely with Q-switched lasers? There are two problems in removing nevi by Q-switched lasers alone. First, some nevus cells do not have melanin. For example, some cells on the dermal side of compound nevus and most of the cells of the intradermal nevus do not have melanin. Thus Q-switched lasers targeting melanin cannot remove these nevi. Second, in nevus, the nevus cells are gathered in one place to form a nest. Because the photons of the laser move from outside of the skin to the inside of the skin, even if all the cells have melanin, only the cell on the surfaces can be affected by the Q-switched laser. The cells situated deep are not affected, because no photons are able to reach it (mass effect). Therefore, like the results of the paper earlier, there are some that can be removed at once by the Q-switched laser, but there are some that need to be removed several times, and there are some that are not affected at all.

10.9.4 My Protocol of CO_2 Laser in the Removal of Melanocytic Nevus

Based on the above, my protocol of CO_2 laser in removing melanocytic nevus is as follows:

1. Use fluence that is high enough only to damage the epidermis and parts of the papillary dermis. It also uses short pulse duration with high power. Specifically, 3 W is used at 0.1 mm spot size with a pulse duration of 500 μs.
2. For shallow lesions, use the single-pass technique, and dressing is not needed unless the size is greater than 2–3 mm.
3. For thick lesions, use the dermo-epidermal sliding effect and gently push the skin with gauze.
4. After pushing the skin with gauze, use the CO_2 laser or Q-switched Nd:YAG laser (see Sect. 7.7.2 in "Chap. 7").
5. Use CO_2 laser defocusing for hemostasis.
6. If the size of the lesion is larger than 3 mm, use the pinhole method.
7. Use Duoderm® for occlusive dressing.
8. If there is a remnant nevus, repeat the procedure after 3 months.

Which is the most important of the eight methods above? I think number 8 is the most important. Attempting to remove all nevus at once may deepen the RTD and damage the surrounding tissues. Therefore, it's alright to leave some nevus tissue behind. The remnant nevus can be removed next time. And the next time, the size of the nevus will be smaller and shallower than the last time, resulting in fewer side effects.

10.10 Ablative Rejuvenation

10.10.1 Skin Resurfacing or Rejuvenation

Sometimes, patients complain that their faces are dirty and they want to "grind" their entire face. Will grinding the face really result in better skin? Yes. After CO_2 laser resurfacing the skin will look 10 years younger (Fig. 10.14). This method is called skin resurfacing or ablative rejuvenation (AR), and there are chemical and physical meth-

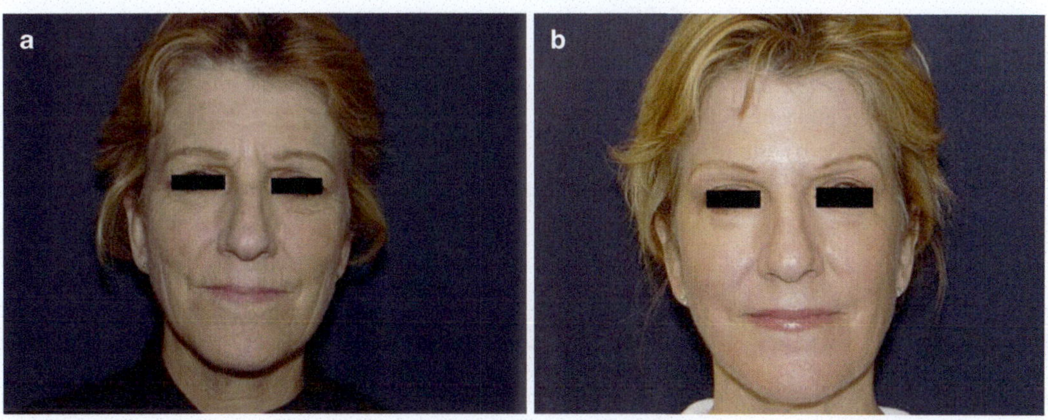

Fig. 10.14 (**a**) Female patients with deep static rhytides and skin laxity at baseline. (**b**) Dramatic improvement in rhytides and laxity 6 months after traditional CO_2 ablation. (Reproduced from [18])

ods and methods that use lasers. Chemical methods include phenol peeling and physical methods include dermabrasion using sandpaper or grinder. Lasers include laser resurfacing using CO_2 lasers or Er:YAG lasers. Here, we will review AR by CO_2 laser.

10.10.2 Traditional Skin Resurfacing of CO_2 Laser

The mechanism of traditional skin resurfacing with CO_2 lasers is the synthesis of collagen through wound healing processes by ablation and thermal damage. Here we will only review the wound healing processes by thermal damage [18].

Irradiation of the CO_2 laser onto the skin results in a series of temperature-dependent bioreactions in tissue, as in Ohshiro's laser apple model (Fig. 10.4).

When heat is applied to collagen, cross-link bonds in the collagen triple helix are broken without damaging the collagen molecules, resulting in immediate contraction and visible skin tightening. The shrinkage without collagen fibril damage occurs between 57 and 65 °C. The temperature range is very narrow and areas that this phenomenon occurs in tissues are also very narrow. The ideal temperature is known to be 63 °C. The higher the temperature, the more covalent hydrogen bonds are broken. I think the site corresponding to this temperature is the same as the site where the AR took effect.

When the temperature rises to 65–70 °C, the structure of the triple helix is broken into an amorphous form. When the temperature rises above 70 °C, denaturation of collagen molecules occurs. The denatured collagen molecule is released from the skin within a few days after the CO_2 laser procedure.

Full reepithelialization of the skin takes 1 week and new collagen and fibroblast proliferation occur through the wound healing process over 3–6 months. Fibroplasia through fibroblast proliferation and the transformation of fibroblasts into myofibroblast induces skin contraction. Thirty to forty percent of contractions occur, which is clinically dramatic in terms of skin laxity. The RTD depth that does not cause scarring is known to be less than 300 μm.

Traditional skin rejuvenation using CO_2 lasers has a dramatic effect, but also may cause serious side effects. Persistent erythema, the most common side effect, is known to last about 4.5 months. The most serious side effects are scar formation and delayed-onset hypopigmentation. Scars occur in areas with thin skin and lack of epidermal appendages, such as the eyelids, neck, and chest. The neck is known to cause scarring in 10% with only one pass. Delayed-onset hypopigmentation is known to occur in about 15% of cases.

Sriprachya-anunt et al. performed AR on 22 Asians with Fitzpatrick skin type IV [19]. The subjects were divided into three groups depending on what laser they received: CO_2 laser alone, Er:YAG laser alone, or both lasers. The average patient achieved greater than 50% improvement. PIH occurred in 68% of patients, starting 1-month postoperative and lasting 3.8 months. There was no correlation to pretreatment or type of laser used as far as the incidence of PIH was concerned.

As in the paper aforementioned, AR using CO_2 laser shows high PIH incidence in Asians (Fig. 10.15). The entire face darkens because the procedure was done on the entire face. Also, the face looks uneven due to mixed areas of severe PIH areas and hypopigmentation areas. If the duration of the PIH is short, this should not be a problem, but it lasts for an average of 3.8 months, making the patient uncomfortable for a long time.

Fig. 10.15 (**a**) 40-year-old Asian patient with persistent melasma in spite of more than 1 year of treatment with tretinoin 0.05%, topical 15% vitamin C, 4% hydroquinone, and full-spectrum sunscreen with Parsol 1789, SPF 30. (**b**) Marked PIH 2 weeks after full-face laser resurfacing with the ultra-pulse CO_2 laser, using two passes. (**c**) Three months after resurfacing, the PIH has improved with treatment but still persisted. (**d**) One year after treatment, the PIH has resolved after 9 months and there has been no recurrence of the melasma. Reproduced from [19]

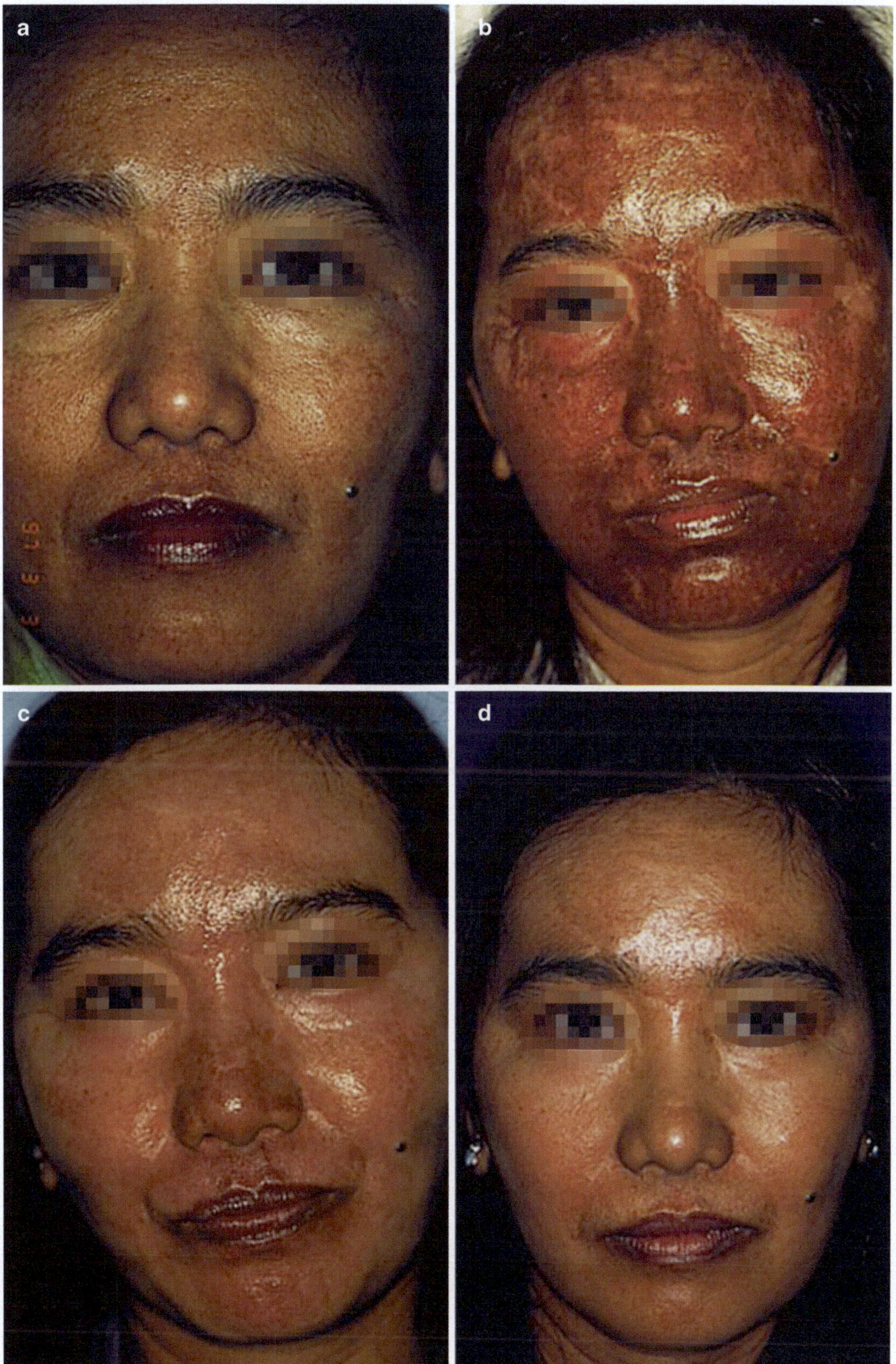
a
b
c
d

10.10.3 Comparison of Rejuvenation Methods

In the past decades, AR using CO_2 lasers has been recognized as the gold standard for skin resurfacing [20]. However, due to serious side effects such as long downtime and scarring, and long PIH duration (especially in Koreans), the procedure is not as popular as it used to be.

This is why NAR, which has no side effects, have been developed. But NAR is much less effective. This brings us to the recently developed fractional laser. Fractional lasers have fewer side effects than AR but are more effective than NAR. The first fractional laser to be developed was 1550 nm Er:Glass laser, which did not induce ablation but only coagulation (which is why it is called nonablative fractional rejuvenation). This fractional laser was thought to lack efficacy, and hence the use of CO_2 laser, for ablative fractional rejuvenation (Fig. 10.16). As we go through the history of lasers and consider the reasons why lasers were developed, the effects and the side effects of each laser can be understood.

You et al. compared the results of treatments for facial atrophic acne scars using CO_2 laser and Er:YAG laser (both ablative lasers) and Er:Glass laser (nonablative fractional laser, NAFL) and CO_2 fractional laser (ablative fractional laser, AFL) [22]. Clinical improvement was assessed with a scale graded from 0 to 10. Adverse events were also noted. Mean improvement scores of the CO_2, Er:YAG, NAFL, and AFL groups were 6.0, 5.8, 2.2, and 5.2, respectively (Fig. 10.17). The NAFL group showed a significantly lower score than the other groups. It should be noted that the effect of AFL is not significantly different from the AR using a CO_2 laser or Er:YAG laser.

The pain was more severe in NAFL than in AFL, and PIH incidence was 10% in NAFL and 20% in AFL (Table 10.4). PIH incidence was higher in AFL than in NAFL, but significantly lower than CO_2 laser (80%) or Er:YAG laser (60%). Therefore, we can say that CO_2 fractional laser, which is AFL, is effective with relatively few side effects.

Ablative rejuvenation > ablative fractional rejuvenation > nonablative fractional rejuvenation > nonablative rejuvenation.

The order of effectiveness is as given earlier. The reverse order will be the ones with the least adverse effects. At present, ablative fractional rejuvenation (AFL) is considered the gold standard for skin resurfacing. We will see why in the next article.

10.10.4 Laser Selection in Rejuvenation

As seen in the paper above, a laser that is effective with relatively fewer side effects, which is adequate for rejuvenation in Koreans is AFL. But do

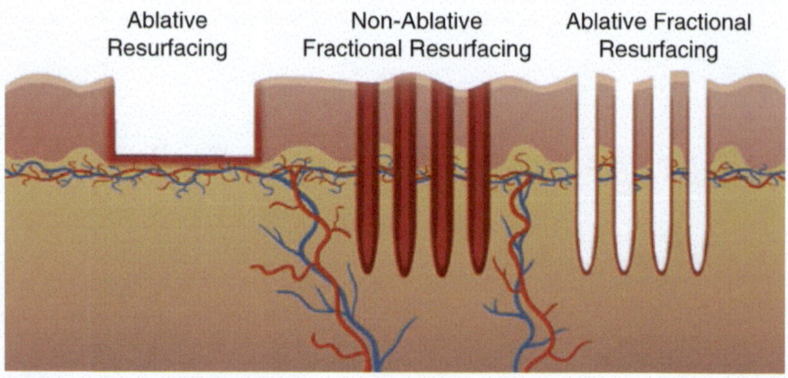

Fig. 10.16 Schematic figure of the zone of damage in ablative and fractional lasers. (Reproduced from [21])

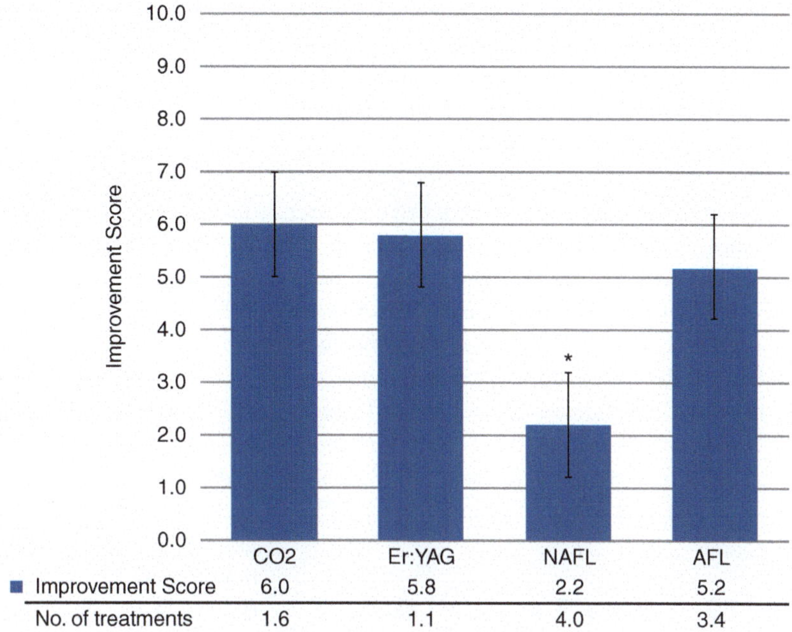

Fig. 10.17 Mean clinical improvement scores (*$p < 0.05$). (Reproduced from [22])

Table 10.4 Comparison among lasers

	Resurfacing		Fractional	
Laser	CO_2 ultrapulse	Er:YAG	NAFL	AFL
Pain	+++	+++	++	+
Oozing	++	++	–	+
Epithelialization (days)	5–10	4–7	1	2–3
Erythema	1–3 months	2–4 weeks	2–3 days	1–2 weeks
Social downtime	1 month	1–2 weeks	1–2 days	3–4 days
PIH				
%	80%	60%	10%	20%
Degree	++++	+++	±	+
Immediate collagen shrinkage, %	25	1–2	–	11.5
Late collagen contraction, %	–43	–14	–4.3	–9

AFL ablative fractional laser, *CO_2*, carbon dioxide, *Er:YAG*, erbium-doped yttrium aluminum garnet, *NAFL* nonablative fractional laser, *PIH* postinflammatory hyperpigmentation. (Reproduced from [22])

we need to buy NAFL later, to have a laser that does not have side effects? Personally, I think it's better to buy a nonablative laser rather than NAFL. In NAFL, 10% PIH occurs, resulting in less PIH than AFL (20%), but nonablative lasers have almost no side effects, including PIH. It is better not to buy lasers that are "in between." Therefore, if you want to buy a fractional laser, then a CO_2 fractional laser is recommended. But if you are concerned about side effects, you should buy a nonablative laser instead of a fractional laser.

10.11 Fractional Laser

10.11.1 Fractional Laser in Ethnic Skin

Fractional lasers do not irradiate the entire skin but irradiate parts of the skin leaving normal tissue between the beams. It is a method of reducing side effects by speeding up the rejuvenation of the irradiated necrotic tissue from normal surrounding tissues [23].

Fractional rejuvenation is known as a relatively safe laser in ethnic skin because it uses a mid-infrared or far-infrared laser that is not selective to melanin. Er:Glass fractional lasers are known to have few side effects except for slight erythema even in, Fitzpatrick skin types IV and V [24].

Alster et al. performed 1550 nm Er:Glass laser (Fraxel) on atrophic facial acne scars in 53 patients with Fitzpatrick skin types I to V. Ninety-one percent of patients improved by 25–50% on a single procedure and 87% of patients who underwent three procedures showed an improvement of 51–75%. Since there were no differences in results regarding skin type, it can be concluded that Fraxel is a safe laser for patients of all skin types and an effective laser for acne scars [24].

10.11.2 Types of Fractional Lasers

Fractional lasers can be classified into two types: ablative and nonablative. The ablative fractional laser (AFL) is available in three laser types: 10,600-nm CO_2 fractional laser, 2940-nm Er:YAG fractional laser, and 2790-nm Er:YSGG fractional laser. Nonablative fractional lasers (NAFL) include lasers of various wavelengths including 1410, 1440, 1540, 1550, and 1927 nm (Table 10.5) [23].

10.11.3 Parameters in Fractional Laser

There are four major factors that influence the outcome of fractional laser treatment (Table 10.6) [25]. First, it is the ratio of the fraction where the fractional laser is irradiated and the fraction that is not irradiated. The higher the proportion of the irradiated area, the greater the efficacy and the greater the likelihood of side effects. The parameter of the fractional laser that determines this ratio is "density." Sometimes "%" is used or "spot/cm^2" is used as well. "spot/cm^2" indicates how many beams are irradiated in 1 cm^2. Of the two units, "%" is a more accurate unit because "spot/cm^2" varies depending on the damage range and the spot size of the beam.

Table 10.5 Types of ablative and nonablative fractional lasers

Ablative fractional laser	Nonablative fractional laser
1. 10,600nm CO_2 (Fraxel re:pair, Reliant)	1. 1,410nm Erbium fiber (Fraxel re:fine, Reliant)
2. 2,940nm Er:YAG (Lux2940, Palomar)	2. 1,440nm Nd:YAG (Affirm, Cynosure)
3. 2,790nm Er:YSGG (Pearl, Cutera)	3. 1,540nm IPL powered laser (Lux)
	4. 1,550nm Er:Glass laser (Fraxel re:store, Reliant)
	5. 1,550nm Er:Glass/1,927nm thulium laser (Fraxel re:store DUAL, Reliant)

Table 10.6 Factors affecting results in fractional laser procedures and corresponding parameters

Points to consider in parameters	Parameters in fractional laser
Percentage (cross-section area) of skin ablated	Density
Diameter of the individual microwounds	Spot size and energy per MTZ
Depths of the individual injuries	Energy per MTZ
Ration of ablation of coagulation	Kinds of fractional laser (laser medium)

Second, the ratio of the fraction may be changed according to the damage diameter of the irradiated area. The parameter corresponding to this is also the spot size of the beam, but the damage diameter also varies depending on the energy. If the energy per MTZ is higher, the diameter of the damage is larger.

Third, the depth of damage also influences the outcome. Depending on the depth of damage, different effects can be seen. If the depth of damage is deeper, it is more effective but the likelihood of side effects is also high. Therefore, the depth should be determined according to the effect desired by the operator. The corresponding parameter is energy per MTZ.

Finally, it is the ratio of ablation and coagulation. The parameter corresponding to this is the laser wavelength (medium), i.e., the type of laser. It is known that CO_2 fractional lasers have an ablation:coagulation ratio of 70:30, which is most effective. Both Er:YAG fractional laser (90:100) or nonablative fractional laser (0:100) are known to be less effective than the CO_2 fractional laser.

10.11.4 Fractional Laser Parameter Selection in Koreans

CO_2 fractional lasers are the most appropriate lasers in Koreans, but side effects still occur. What parameters can be used to increase the effectiveness of fractional lasers and reduce side effects? Patient satisfaction and procedure results in fractional lasers are associated with high energy, but the risk of side effects is associated with high treatment density, i.e., irradiating the beam densely [20].

Several papers also indicate that treatment density, rather than energy, is an important factor in PIH. In one paper, the total treatment density was lowered (the number of passes—1 pass means one full-face treatment—was reduced to four passes rather than the eight) and the treatment session was increased from three to six times and the incidence of PIH in Asians has decreased from 18.2% to 6% [26]. In other words, lowering the treatment density reduces side effects, while increasing energy and increasing the treatment session result in better effects.

Jung et al. enrolled ten male patients with moderate to severe acne scars and pores and used CO_2 fractional laser to treat half the face with high-fluence, low-density (70 mJ, 150 spots/cm^2), and the other half of the face with low-fluence and high-density (30 mJ, 250 spots/cm^2) [27]. Three months of follow-up showed that in the low-fluence and high-density parameter, four out of ten patients improved by 51–75%, while in the high-fluence and low-density parameter, five out of ten patients improved by over 76% (Fig. 10.18). It can be seen that the high-fluence and low-density parameters have a better effect. Also, the subjective satisfaction of patients was higher in the high-fluence and low-density parameter as well (Fig. 10.19).

In ablative fractional laser (AFL) one pass is generally recommended and one pass is known to be effective in scar treatment and skin rejuvenation of Asians.

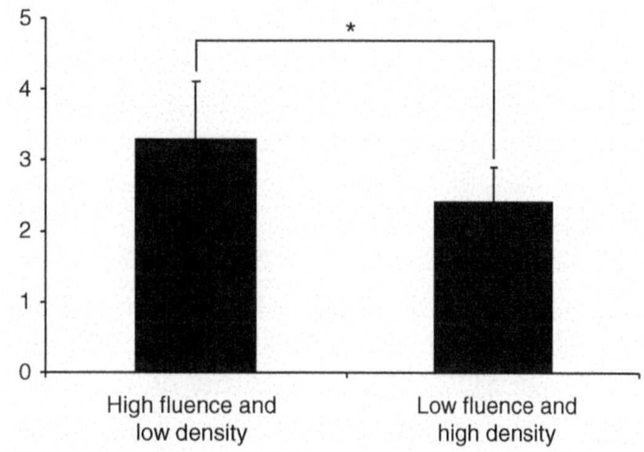

Fig. 10.18 Mean grade of clinical improvement according to laser settings; low-fluence, high-density (70 mJ and 150 spots/cm^2) versus high-fluence, low-density (30 mJ and 250 spots/cm^2). $p = 0.02$. (Reproduced from [27])

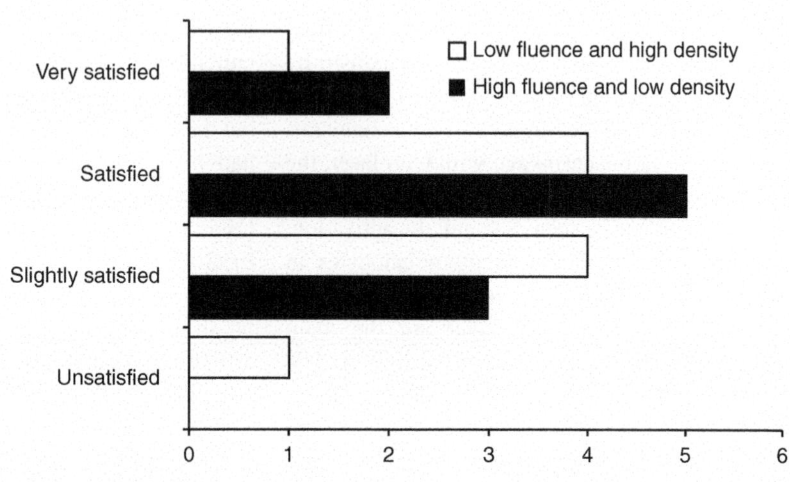

Fig. 10.19 Patient satisfaction levels according to treatment settings. (Reproduced from [27])

10.11.5 Fractional Laser Techniques

Finally, here are some tips when using a fractional laser in indications other than skin rejuvenation, such as skin diseases.

Fractional lasers do not treat the entire skin, unlike AR by CO_2 lasers. This is why combination therapy with nonablative lasers for vascular/pigmentation treatment or superficial peeling is possible. Generally, nonablative lasers are administered first followed by an ablative fractional laser later. However, superficial macroablation, such as nevus removal should be done after fractional laser that goes deeper, such as the 1550 nm Er:Glass laser, to avoid side effects [4].

During fractional laser treatment, the skin needs to be pulled so that it is. Flat skin allows uniform treatment and easy access to deep lesions. For this reason, botulinum toxin may also be helpful prior to fractional laser treatment [4].

Hélou et al. conducted a CO_2 fractional laser on ten patients with refractor non-segmental vitiligo (NSV) [28]. The parameters were 100 mJ energy per MTZ, 125 Hz, a density of 3, and an initial spot size of 6 mm (later adjusted according to lesion size). The procedure was performed three times, 1 month apart. Five days after the procedure, the patient basked in the sun for 2 h between 3 pm and 6 pm. Vitiligo in the joints, such as elbow and armpit, was less effective, but vitiligo on the face, neck, and legs improved.

Gold standard treatment for vitiligo is known as the 308-nm excimer laser, but this paper suggests that vitiligo treatment is possible with fractional lasers. Although the exact mechanism by which CO_2 fractional laser improved vitiligo is unknown, the authors suggest two mechanisms. First, due to tissue shrinkage with CO_2 laser, the size of vitiligo lesions is reduced, thus visual improvement can be seen. Second, the activation, proliferation, and migration of melanocytes in the outer root sheath of the hair follicles and the surrounding normal basal layer are the main mechanisms for the treatment of vitiligo via UV treatment or excimer laser. MMP-2 (matrix metalloproteinase-2) is known to promote the migration of melanocytes from the surrounding normal tissues. Experimentally, it was observed that MMP-2 activity was increased in melanocytes after narrowband UVB. Also, after laser ablation, narrowband UVB, and steroid use, vitiligo was improved. Thus, the authors believe that exposure to sunlight after CO_2 fractional laser treatment improves MMP-2 activity and improves vitiligo.

Yang et al. enrolled 24 ethnic South Korean patients with varying degrees of atrophic striae alba in the abdomen [29]. On a randomly selected half side of the abdomen skin lesion, the patients were treated with 1550-nm fractional Er:Glass laser at a pulse energy of 50 mJ and a spot density of 100 spots/cm^2, using a scan area of 5 × 10 mm in a static mode with one pass administered per treatment site without overlapping. The other half side was treated with ablative fractional CO_2 laser resurfacing at a pulse energy of 40–50 mJ and a spot density of 75–100 spots/cm^2, using a scan area of 8 × 8 mm in a static mode. The procedure interval was performed three times at 4-week intervals. Each half of the abdominal lesion was randomly selected and treated three times at intervals of 4 weeks using the same parameters.

The results show that both Er:Glass and CO_2 fractional lasers significantly increase the elasticity of the stretch marks (19.1 ± 16.4%, 23.0 ± 19.5%, respectively) and decreased the width of the stretch marks (32.4 ± 19.9%, 29.7 ± 27.4%). In addition, the degree of visual improvement, patient satisfaction, and histology showed significant improvement. When comparing the two groups, both the evaluator and the patient evaluated the CO_2 fractional laser to be more effective than the Er:Glass fractional laser, but there was no statistical difference. Both lasers had high PIH rates, eight patients (36.4%) in Er:Glass laser and 18 patients (81.8%) in CO_2 laser. PIH rate was higher in CO_2 laser than Er:Glass laser.

This paper studied the effect of fractional laser on striae distensae, which is known to be very difficult to treat. All of the fractional lasers were effective, but the PIH incidence was very high. Therefore, patients with stretch marks who are planning to undergo fractional lasers should be informed in advance that they are very likely to develop PIH.

References

1. Berlien H-P (2003) Applied laser medicine. Springer Science & Business Media
2. Goldman MP (2006) Cutaneous and cosmetic laser surgery. Mosby Elsevier, Philadelphia, PA
3. Allemann IB, Goldberg DJ (2011) Basics in dermatological laser applications. Karger Medical and Scientific Publishers
4. Raulin C, Karsai S (2011). Laser and IPL technology in dermatology and aesthetic medicine. Heidelberg: New York
5. Niemz M (2019) Laser-tissue interactions. Springer International Publishing
6. Kauvar A, Hruza G (2005) Principles and practices in cutaneous laser surgery. CRC Press
7. Nouri K (2018) Lasers in dermatology and medicine: dermatologic applications. Springer International Publishing
8. Ohshiro T (1996) The laser apple: a new graphic representation of medical laser applications. Laser Ther 8(3):185–190
9. Omi T, Numano K (2014) The role of the CO2 laser and fractional CO2 laser in dermatology. Laser Ther 23(1):49–60
10. Ross EV, McKinlay JR, Anderson RR (1999) Why does carbon dioxide resurfacing work? A review. Arch Dermatol 135(4):444–454
11. Issa MCA, Tamura B (2018) Lasers, lights and other technologies. Springer
12. Jeong JY (2015) CO2 laser in dermatology (Koean). MDworld, Seoul
13. Fitzpatrick RE, Smith SR, Sriprachya-anunt S (1999) Depth of vaporization and the effect of pulse stacking with a high-energy, pulsed carbon dioxide laser. J Am Acad Dermatol 40(4):615–622
14. Baba M, Bal N (2006) Efficacy and safety of the short-pulse erbium:YAG laser in the treatment of acquired melanocytic nevi. Dermatol Surg 32(2): 256–260
15. Riggs K, Keller M, Humphreys TR (2007) Ablative laser resurfacing: high-energy pulsed carbon dioxide and erbium:yttrium-aluminum-garnet. Clin Dermatol 25(5):462–473
16. Fulton JE, Shitabata PK (1999) CO2 laser physics and tissue interactions in skin. Lasers Surg Med 24(2):113–121
17. Kim YJ, Whang KU, Choi WB, Kim HJ, Hwang JY, Lee JH et al (2012) Efficacy and safety of 1,064 nm Q-switched Nd:YAG laser treatment for removing melanocytic nevi. Ann Dermatol 24(2):162–167
18. Ortiz AE, Goldman MP, Fitzpatrick RE (2014) Ablative CO2 lasers for skin tightening: traditional versus fractional. Dermatol Surg 40(Suppl 12):S147–S151
19. Sriprachya-anunt S, Marchell NL, Fitzpatrick RE, Goldman MP, Rostan EF (2002) Facial resurfacing in patients with Fitzpatrick skin type IV. Lasers Surg Med 30(2):86–92
20. Goldsmith LA, Katz SI, Gilchrest BA, Paller AS, Leffell DJ, Wolff K et al (2012) Fitzpatrick's dermatology in general medicine. McGraw-Hill Professional, New York
21. Ogawa R (2020) Total scar management. Springer, Singapore
22. You HJ, Kim DW, Yoon ES, Park SH (2016) Comparison of four different lasers for acne scars: resurfacing and fractional lasers. J Plast Reconstr Aesthet Surg 69(4):e87–e95
23. Bogdan Allemann I, Kaufman J (2010) Fractional photothermolysis—an update. Lasers Med Sci 25(1):137–144
24. Keyvan N (2012) Lasers in dermatology and medicine. Springer-Verlag, London
25. Goldman MP (2013) Lasers and energy devices for the skin. [S.I.]. Taylor & Francis
26. Hruza GJ, Tanzi EL (2018) Lasers and lights. Elsevier, Edinburgh
27. Jung JY, Lee JH, Ryu DJ, Lee SJ, Bang D, Cho SB (2010) Lower-fluence, higher-density versus higher-fluence, lower-density treatment with a 10,600-nm carbon dioxide fractional laser system: a split-face, evaluator-blinded study. Dermatol Surg 36(12):2022–2029
28. Helou J, Maatouk I, Obeid G, Moutran R, Stephan F, Tomb R (2014) Fractional laser for vitiligo treated by 10,600 nm ablative fractional carbon dioxide laser followed by sun exposure. Lasers Surg Med 46(6):443–448
29. Yang YJ, Lee GY (2011) Treatment of Striae Distensae with nonablative fractional laser versus ablative CO(2) fractional laser: a randomized controlled trial. Ann Dermatol 23(4):481–489

Part IV

Treatment of Scar and Melasma

11 Various Treatments of Scar

11.1 Types of Scars

There are many types of scars. They vary according to the shape of the scar surface, shape of the scar itself, color, and chronology. Scars may be classified by scar surface (flat, elevated, depressed, or irregular) by morphology (atrophic, normorophic, hypertrophic, or keloid) by color (depigmented, hypopigmented, hyperpigmented, or discolored) or by chronology (acute, chronic, immature, or mature) [1].

Scars also have different origins that give them unique characteristics, such as injury (e.g., accidental trauma, contusion, laceration, burn, or surgery), infection (e.g., bacterial (e.g., *Propionibacterium acnes*), fungal, or viral (e.g., chickenpox, smallpox, herpetic)) or inflammation (e.g., acne lesions, poor post-wound management, striae (after obesity or pregnancy)) [1]. For example, burn scars are usually wide and deep partial-thickness (second-degree) and full-thickness (third-degree) burns require skin grafts because other procedures are not sufficient. Striae distensae appear red at first (striae rubra) and later turn white (striae alba).

Scars can be divided into two types by shape of the scar surface, namely (1) depressed atrophic scars, and (2) elevated hypertrophic scars and keloids (Figs. 11.1 and 11.2) [2]. In this chapter, we will focus on the treatment of atrophic acne scars, the most common scar treated in private clinics.

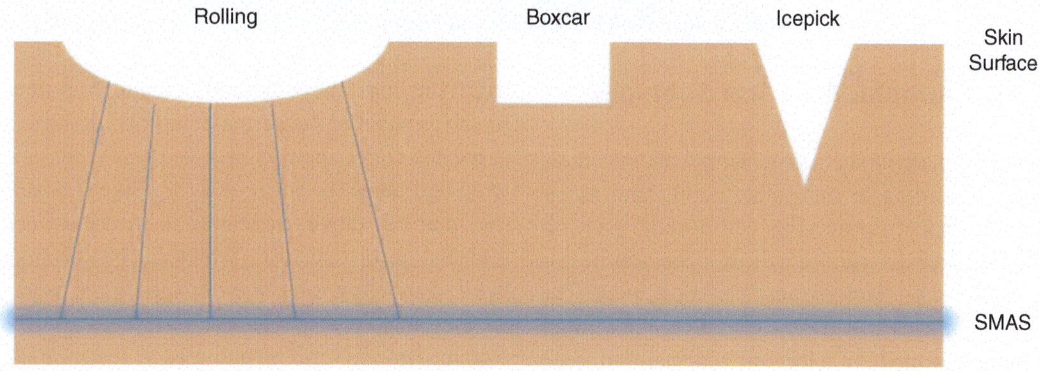

Fig. 11.1 Atrophic acne scar subtypes. (Reproduced from [3])

J. D. Lee et al., *Principles and Choice of Laser Treatment in Dermatology*,
https://doi.org/10.1007/978-981-15-6556-4_11

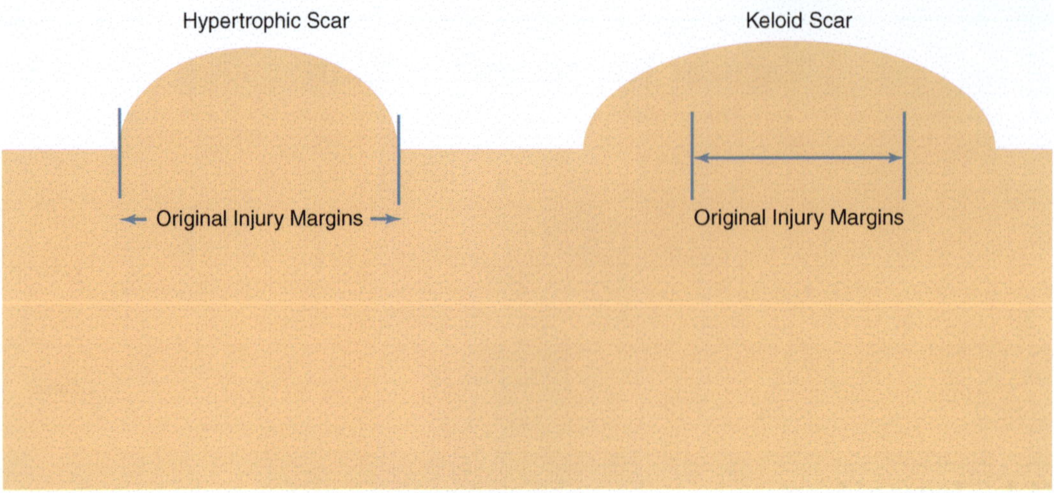

Fig. 11.2 Hypertrophic and keloidal acne scars. (Reproduced from [3])

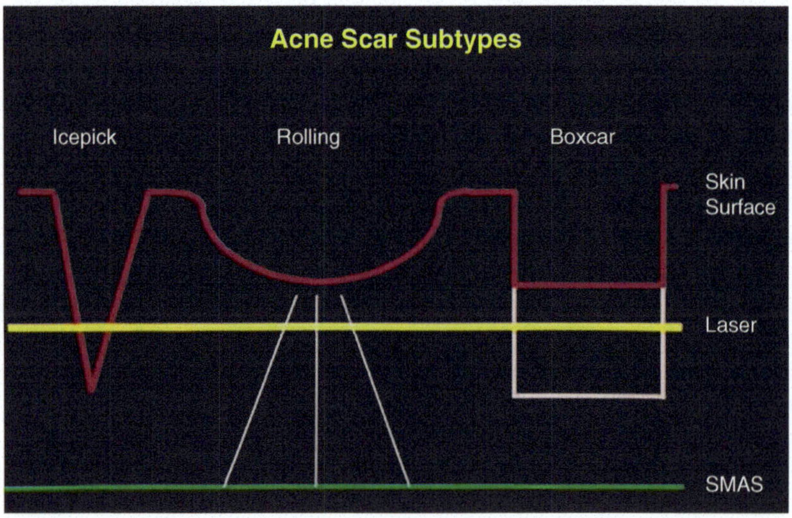

Fig. 11.3 Novel classification system of three basic scar types: icepick, rolling, and boxcar (superficial and deep). *Yellow reference line* denotes the depth of ablation and resurfacing capability of the carbon-dioxide laser. *Green line* represents the superficial musculoaponeurotic system (*SMAS*) to which fibrous bands adhere, creating rolling scars. (Reproduced from [4])

11.1.1 Atrophic Acne Scar Subtypes

Jacob et al. divided atrophic acne scars into three types according to their size, depth, and three-dimensional structure (Figs. 11.3 and 11.4) [4]. First, an icepick scar is a narrow, deep scar of less than 2 mm in diameter, just like an icepick. The opening in the surface is wider, taking the form of a funnel-shaped "V." Icepick scars are so deep that they are difficult to treat with laser resurfacing. Second, rolling scars are caused by dermal tethers that connect the dermis to the subcutaneous layer. They have an undulating form with shallow, rounded bases and take the form of an "M." The diameter is 4–5 mm. Treatment is done by the removal of the dermal tether. Third, boxcar scars are wider than icepick scars. The base is wide and takes the form of a "U," like a boxcar that is upside down. Boxcar scars can be divided into shallow boxcar scars, which can benefit from laser resurfacing, and deep boxcar scars, where the bottom is so deep that laser resurfacing is ineffective. However, all atrophic acne scars cannot be classified into these three types of scars, because they may have more than one characteristic. Thus, the classification of atrophic acne scars by Jacob et al. should be understood as a rough classification concept for approaching treatment.

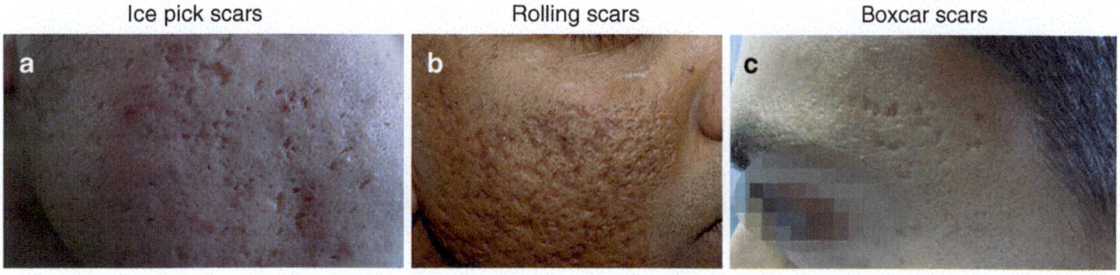

Fig. 11.4 Atrophic acne scars. (**a**) ice pick, (**b**) rolling and boxcar, (**c**) boxcar. All three subcategories can be deep and coexist, making a singular clinical identification difficult. Reproduced from [5]

In real practice, we usually see all of the three atrophic acne scars in a single patient. Most patients have more than one type of atrophic acne scar. I have never seen any patient with only rolling scars or only boxcar scars. Different types of atrophic acne scars coexist in a single patient, with a difference in proportions. Why is this so? I think this because acne itself has various acne symptoms caused by various inflammations. Acne is divided into comedonal lesions such as closed comedones (whitehead) and open comedones (blackhead), and inflammatory lesions such as papules, pustules, nodules, and cysts. Comedonal lesions and inflammatory lesions are not different disease entities but are descriptive definitions that describe the various skin changes observed in the progress of disease from closed comedones to inflammatory lesions. Inflammatory lesions, especially papules, pustules, nodules, and cysts, are the same lesions that appear different depending on the severity of inflammation. As a result, all these lesions are found in a single patient (pleomorphism). This is why atrophic acne scars caused by inflammation also show various types of scars. Therefore, in the treatment of acne scars, combination therapy using an effective treatment method for each atrophic acne scar is needed.

11.2 Wound Healing Process

To understand the cause of atrophic acne scars, let's first look at the wound healing process (Fig. 11.5).

When the skin is injured, the wound heals through three stages: the inflammatory phase, the proliferative phase, and the maturational phase [7, 8]. First, the inflammatory phase occurs within 1–3 days after the wound. The skin becomes pale as the blood vessels contract (vasoconstriction) for hemostasis. After hemostasis, the blood vessels widen (vasodilatation), causing erythema. In addition, melanin production may be increased at this time. Therefore, this stage is an important time for the development of postacne erythema and postacne hyperpigmentation. Since the severity and duration of inflammation are closely correlated with the occurrence of scars, the best way to treat acne scars is by actively treating acne lesions early, thus preventing acne scars. At this stage, granulation tissue is produced by various inflammatory mediators that are secreted by various cells such as granulocytes, macrophages, neutrophils, lymphocytes, fibroblasts, and platelets.

Second, the proliferative phase occurs between 4 and 21 days after the wound and is also called the granulation tissue formation phase. The damaged tissue is repaired and new blood vessels are made. Neutrophils are replaced by monocytes and macrophage thus secreting platelet-derived factor (PDGF), fibroblast growth factor (FGF), and transforming growth factor-α, β (TGF-α, β) to induce the migration and proliferation of fibroblasts (Fig. 11.6). Fibroblasts make new collagen, initially made of type III collagen, and only 20% of type I collagen. Later, much type I collagen is made, and it may take up as much as 80% of the total collagen just like normal tissues (Fig. 11.7).

Third, the maturational phase refers to the period from 21 days to 6 months or 1 year after the injury. This phase is also called the matrix

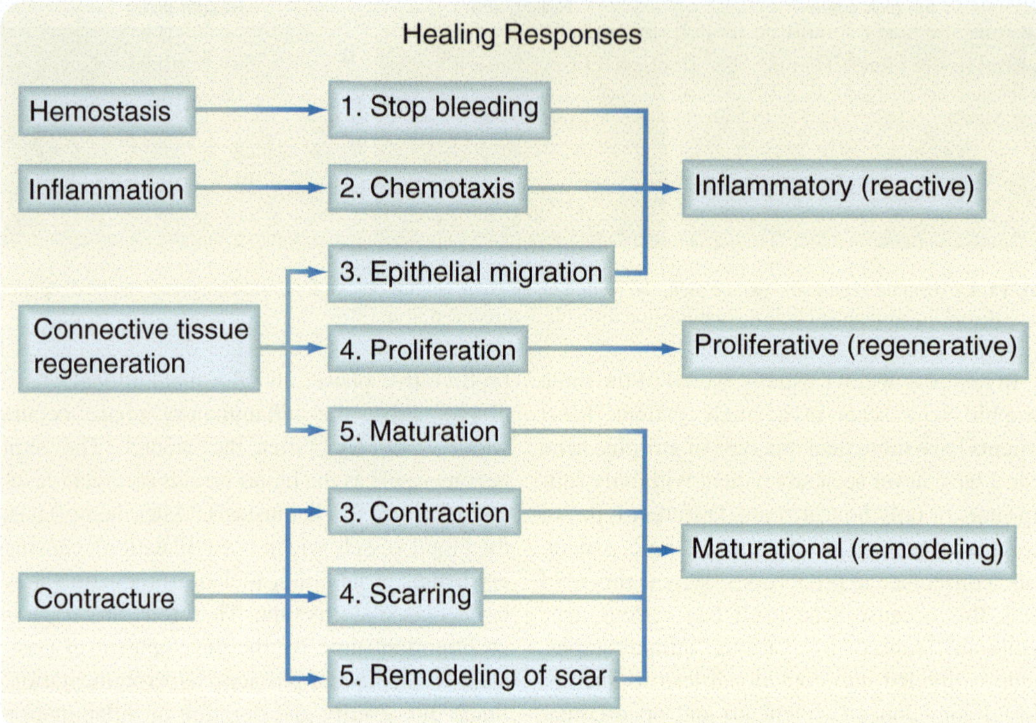

Fig. 11.5 Schematic diagram of the wound healing process. (Reproduced from [6])

Fig. 11.6 Time course of the appearance of different cells in the wound during healing. Macrophages and neutrophils are predominant during the inflammatory phase (peak at days 3 and 2, respectively). Lymphocytes appear later and peak at day 7. Fibroblasts are the predominant cells during the proliferative phase. (Reproduced from [6])

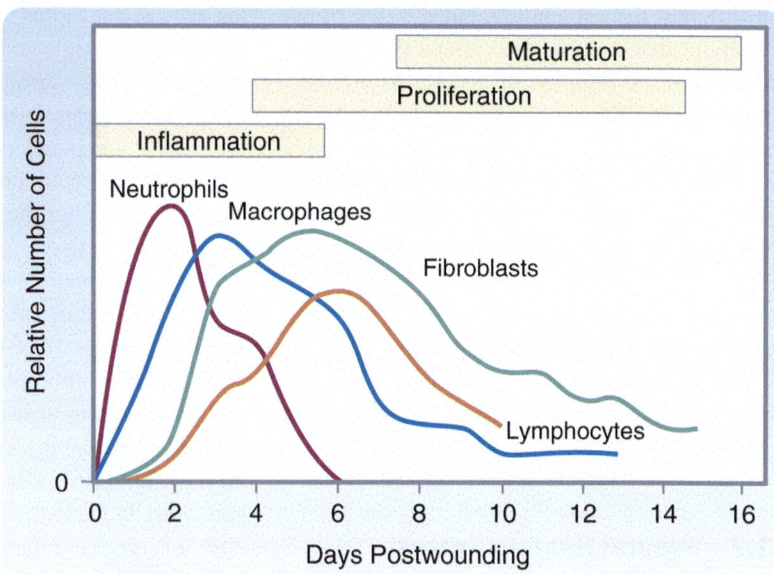

remodeling phase, fibroblasts and keratinocytes secrete matrix metalloproteinases (MMPs) and tissue inhibitors of MMPs. MMPs are enzymes that destroy the extracellular matrix (ECM). Wound healing occurs through balancing MMPs and MMPs inhibitors. If the ratio of MMPs/MMPs inhibitors is high, atrophic scars form. In contrast, if the ratio is low,

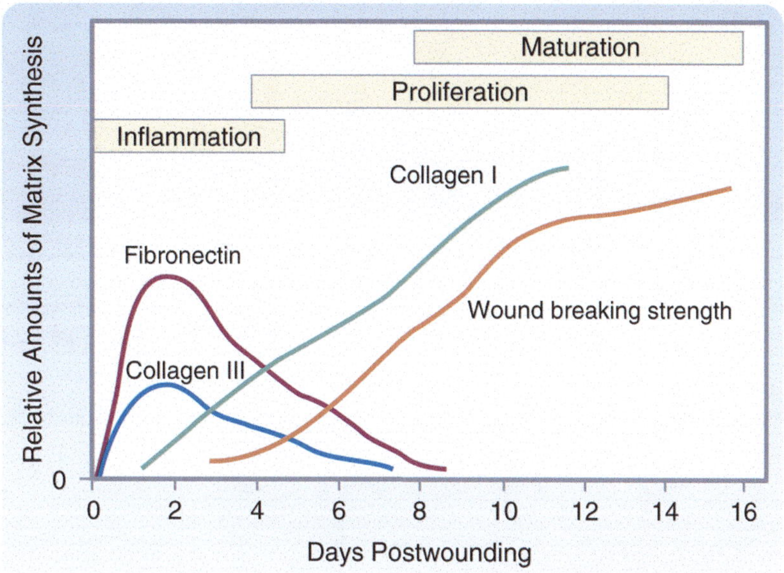

Fig. 11.7 Wound matrix deposition over time. Fibronectin and type III collagen constitute the early matrix. Type I collagen accumulates later and corresponds to the increase in wound-breaking strength. (Reproduced from [6])

hypertrophic scars form. Since the maturational phase is the final stage that affects scar development, various efforts have been made at this stage to prevent scars such as silicone gel sheets.

11.3 Histology of Scar Tissue

11.3.1 Histology of Mature Scar Tissue

What are the histological findings of scar tissue, i.e., granulation tissue made by the wound healing process? First, the collagen array in the shape of basketweave seen in normal tissue is changed into an array parallel to the epidermis in a mature scar. Newly formed blood vessels in the dermis are perpendicular to the epidermis, unlike normal blood vessels which are both horizontal and vertical to the epidermis. Mature scar tissue often shows the loss of elastic fibers and thinning of the epidermis, resulting in decreased skin tension. Epidermal appendages, such as hair follicles and sweat glands are completely destroyed and the rete ridge and papillary dermis are incompletely regenerated (Fig. 11.8) [5]. Thus, the skin regeneration procedure is less effective in mature scar tissue.

11.3.2 Histology of Atrophic Acne Scar Tissue

A detailed explanation or picture of the histology of atrophic acne scar tissue could not be found in books or papers, but histology of mature scar tissue and one paper [9] taken together led to this conclusion. Atrophic acne scars show dermal depression due to reduced collagen, which results in atrophic skin. Histopathologic findings are similar to mature scar tissue, with the loss of epidermal appendages and loss of elastic fibers. Irregular arrays of collagen fibers are observed in the dermal layer and fibrotic tissue is observed in the deep layer.

In view of the findings earlier, atrophic acne scar skin regenerated as granulation tissue has the following characteristics. First, they have decreased skin tension due to the loss of elastic fibers and irregular arrangement of collagen. Second, reepithelialization after an injury is poor due to the loss of skin appendages. Third, fibrous tissue forms in the deeper layers to compensate for decreased skin tension. The problem here is that the fibrous tissue prevents collagen remodeling.

Therefore, the following is required for scar treatments. First, normal collagen tissue must be remodeled. Procedures that remodel collagen as

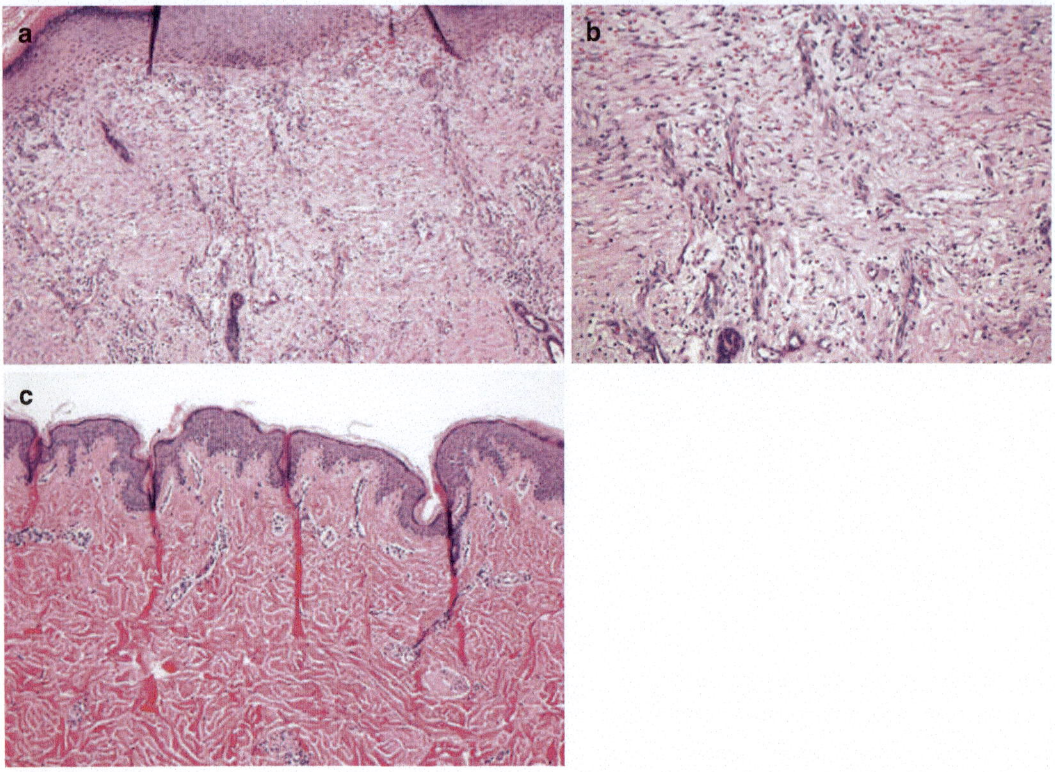

Fig. 11.8 The histologic comparison of an early and a late scar. (**a**) Low-power image of a newly forming scar demonstrating the cellular reticular dermis, increased vasculature, and absence of rete ridges and papillary dermis. (**b**) Higher power image of a newly forming scar with fine, horizontally oriented collagen bundles and increased vasculature with vessels oriented vertically. (**c**) An established scar with horizontally oriented thicker and more densely packed collagen bundles and loss of all skin appendages. (Reproduced from [5])

much as possible are optimal. Second, procedures that are problematic for regeneration should be avoided because reepithelialization after injury in scar tissue is poor. As reviewed in the Sect. 7.2.3 in "Chap. 7", injuries to the scar tissue should neither be too wide nor too deep. On the contrary, narrower and deeper injury (e.g., fractional laser or pinhole method) is safer. A narrow, deep injury may also remove the fibrous tissue in the deeper layers. There is also a need for knowledge of wet dressings to help reepithelialization. Third, fibrous tissues that interfere with collagen remodeling should be removed. But if all the fibrous tissues are removed at once, the same fibrous tissue form to fill the empty space. Thus, partial and multiple removal of fibrous tissue is recommended (Fig. 11.9).

11.4 Treatments for Atrophic Acne Scars

There are many ways to treat atrophic acne scars. As shown in the Table 11.1, it can be classified into five treatment methods according to mechanism [10]. It can also be classified into two types: surgical methods and methods using laser or energy. But I think that the classification of atrophic acne scar treatment is less important and it is more important to select the treatment method that is suitable by checking the principles and pros and cons of each treatment method.

There is one thing to note here. Scars are not easily treated, and there is no 100% in scar treatment [11]. Patients also understand this, so if having to choose between "efficacy" and "safety," efficacy should come before safety (See Sect.

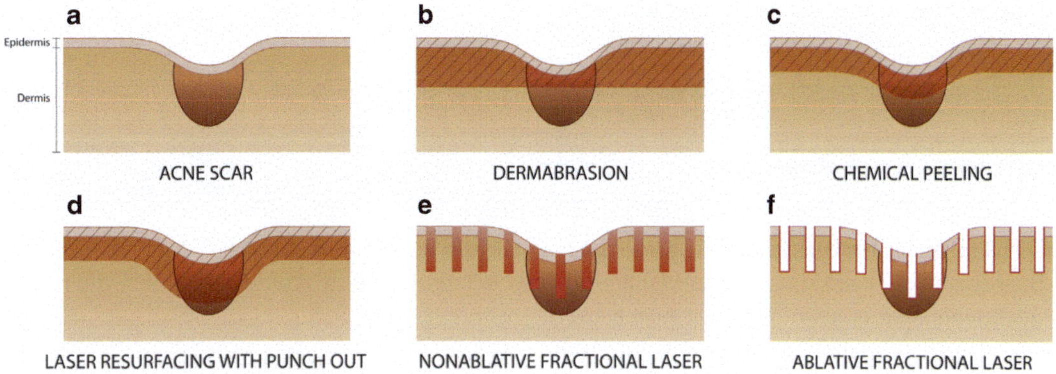

Fig. 11.9 (**a**) The appearance and thickness of the epidermis of the acne scar are similar to that of the surrounding tissue, but a thick collagen bundle of scars exists deep in the dermis. (**b**) Dermabrasion (**c**) Chemical peeling (**d**) Laser resurfacing (**e**) Nonablative fractional laser; NAFL (**f**) Ablative fractional laser; AFL. Reproduced from [9]

Table 11.1 Treatments for atrophic acne scars by mechanism [10]

Mechanisms	Modalities
Surgery/movement-related modalities	Punch techniques (punch elevation, punch excision), elliptical excision Botulinum toxin Facelift
Lifting-related modalities	Subcision
Volume-related modalities	Soft tissue augmentation, dermal grafting, fat transplant, platelet-rich plasma
Resurfacing modalities	Microdermabrasion, dermabrasion, chemical peeling Chemical reconstruction of skin scars (CROSS) Skin needling (percutaneous collagen induction therapy) Laser resurfacing
Skin-tightening modalities	Lasers (fractional lasers, nonfractional, nonablative lasers, picosecond 755-nm alexandrite laser) Fractional radiofrequency

Table 11.2 Hierarchy of therapy for atrophic acne scars, in descending order of efficacy

1. CO_2 ablative laser
2. 1450-nm diode laser/Nd:YAG laser
3. Long-pulsed/combined 585/1064-nm laser
4. Glycolic acid/biweekly peels
5. Percutaneous collagen induction/TCA peels
6. Subcision
7. Autologous fat transfer
8. Injectables
9. Dermabrasion
10. Topical retinoids

Based on the Clinical Evidence GRADE scores assigned to categorize all interventions according to their likely effectiveness based on the type of study, quality, dose response, consistency of results, and significance of results. Treatments listed on the same lines were both equally effective. Reproduced from [5]

3.2.2 in "Chap. 3"). For example, temporary scabs, bruises, swellings, etc., that occur immediately after the procedure, and erythema or postinflammatory hyperpigmentation (PIH) that occur after the procedure are visually undesirable side effects but are not permanent, which makes energy levels or procedures that induce these side effects acceptable in scar treatments. But, informed consent will be needed from the patients prior to the procedure. However, energy levels or procedures that cause permanent side effects such as blisters or scars should be avoided. Therefore, it is important to know what scar treatments are effective, and in what order they are effective. It is also important to know which treatments are effective without significant side effects in ethnic skin. Table 11.2 shows the effectiveness of the treatments used in atrophic acne scars in The Scar Book [5]. I do not agree with all the order, but I also concur that CO_2 ablative lasers are the most effective.

In the following, we will discuss the principles and advantages and disadvantages of each treatment.

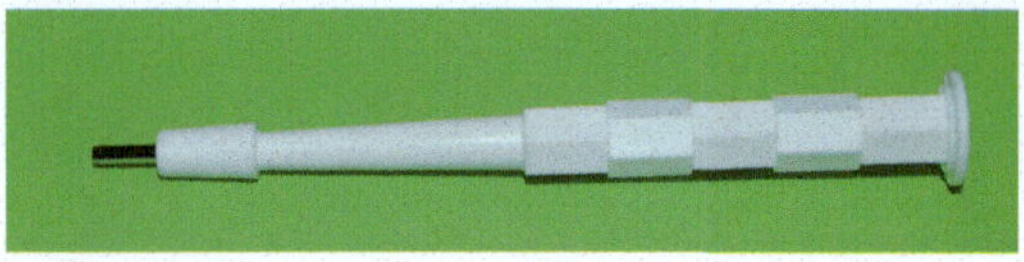

Fig. 11.10 Punch for a punch biopsy

11.4.1 Punch Techniques

Punch technique is also known as punch excision, punch elevation, and punch grafting. Indications are deep boxcar scars less than 3–4 mm in diameter or big icepick scars. Because these scars are difficult to treat with laser resurfacing, the punch technique is performed together with laser resurfacing. Fractional laser after the punching technique softens the edges of the scar, bringing out better results.

The punch excision treatment uses a punch (Fig. 11.10) to remove the entire skin including scar tissue and afterward suture the defect vertically to the relaxed skin tension line (RSTL) (Fig. 11.11) [12]. Indications are boxcar scars less than 3 mm in diameter or big icepick scars. Scars larger than 3.5 mm in diameter should be subjected to elliptical excision or punch elevation, not punch excision [10].

Punch elevation, like punch excision, first excises the skin, but unlike punch excision does not remove it. The punched skin is elevated and sutured or taped. Indications are boxcar scars with sharp edges and flat bases with larger than 3 mm in diameter. There are technical difficulties because it is necessary to make an exact excision matching the edges.

11.4.2 Botulinum Toxin and Facelift

Severe atrophic acne scars (grade 3) may seem deeper with normal facial muscle movements, making the scars more visible. Therefore, some authors recommend botulinum toxin injection for acne scars. It may be beneficial for atrophic acne scars on the forehead, glabella, and jaw [10]. Also, as patients age, soft tissue laxity makes atrophic acne scars more visible, especially in patients with multiple rolling scars. In this case, a

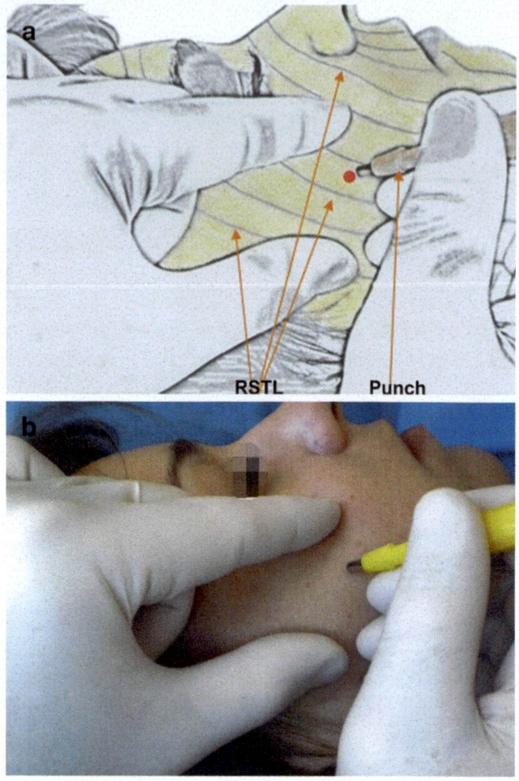

Fig. 11.11 Punch excision. (**a**) Scheme. (**b**) Photo. (Reproduced from [13])

facelift can be performed for scar reducing effect [14]. But both botulinum toxin and facelift do not treat scars themselves. They are both secondary treatments, preventing the scars from appearing deeper.

11.4.3 Subcision

Subcision is a treatment that breaks the dermal tether, a fibrous tissue that is connected to the scar, by inserting a needle under the scar (Fig. 11.12). If the fibrous tissue is broken the scars rise. In addition, injury to the dermis results in clot formation and neocollagenesis, filling the void and further enhancing scar treatment. Traditionally, 18G Nokor needles were used but due to the high price, I currently use 23G or 25G needles (Fig. 11.13). The target location of the needle inside the skin is the upper dermis and subcutaneous fat layers (bi-level subcision).

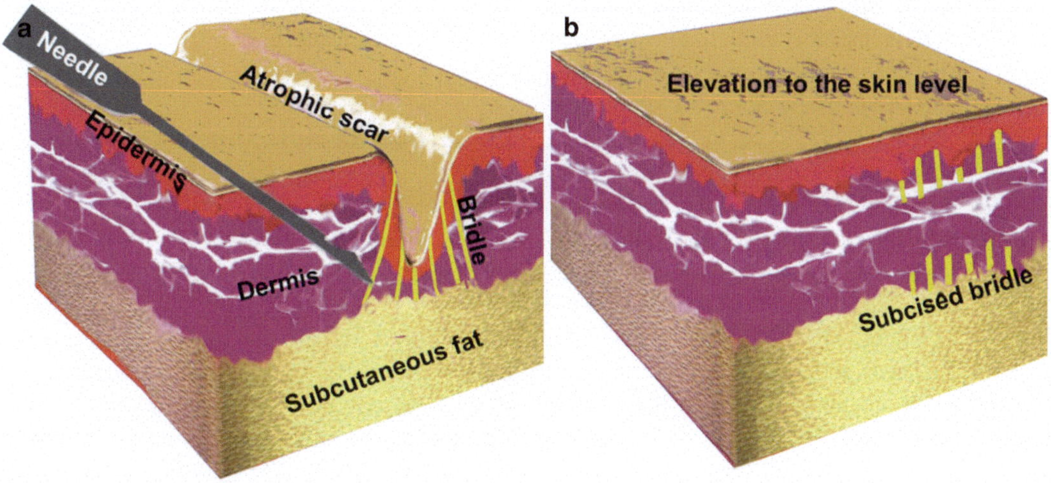

Fig. 11.12 Subcision procedure scheme. (**a**) Before procedure. (**b**) After procedure. (Reproduced from [13])

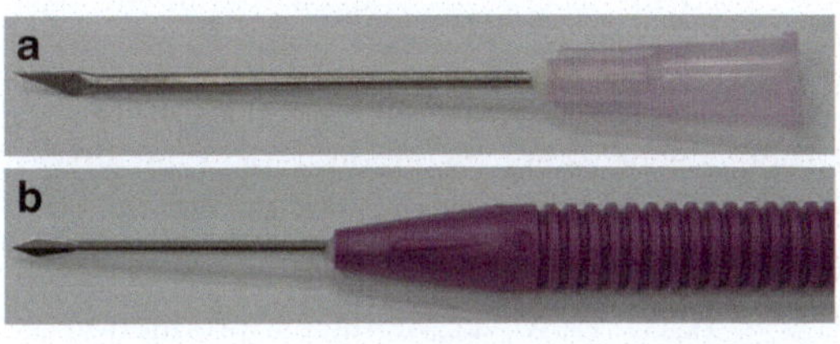

Fig. 11.13 Hypodermic needles used for subcision: (**a**) Nokor needle, (**b**) cataract blade. Reproduced from [15]

Indications for subcisions are rolling scars or scars with bands. It works best on deep, wide, prominent rolling scars. On the other hand, small or shallow boxcar scars, least benefit from subcision. Subcision can be combined with other scar procedures. Side effects include bleeding, bruising, infections, etc. Also, if the acne sinus tract is disturbed during the procedure it may worsen acne [10].

11.4.4 Volume-Related Modalities

Volume-related modalities are a way to improve scars by filling depressed areas of atrophic acne scars. They are classified into several types depending on the graft material: First, synthesized fillers. Fillers are indicated in rolling scars or boxcar scars. But they are not suitable for icepick scars or hard fibrotic scars. Although it can be performed independently, it is often performed together with subcision. There are various types of fillers such as hyaluronic acid fillers, calcium hydroxyapatite fillers, poly-L-lactic acid (PLLA) fillers, and polymethylmethacrylate (PMMA) fillers. Hyaluronic acid fillers are known to have an effect of inducing collagen production as well as filling the volume. The disadvantage is that the duration is short and must be repeated several times. I prefer hyaluronic acid fillers with fewer side effects than permanent or semi-permanent fillers and use BDDE-free hyaluronic acid usually used in the joint to achieve additional effects during subcision.

Second, there is a dermal grafting. Dermal transplantation is a treatment that is currently not popular. This treatment involves transplanting the dermis of normal tissue into the dermis after subcision. Dermal grafting is suitable for soft, round, or oval scars that are at least 4–5 mm in diameter and are not suitable for scars that are too large or uneven. But because of multiple incisions, it may create new scars, and ablative therapies may be further needed to smoothen the skin surface. There is also the possibility of granuloma. Because of these reasons, dermal grafts have recently been replaced by “combination therapy of post-filler fractional laser procedures.”

Third, there is fat transplantation. Fat transplantations are indicated in atrophic scars caused by the destruction of deep tissues such as fat layers. It is mainly applied to scars that develop after severe inflammatory acne lesions, such as nodular or cystic acne. As with other methods, subcision is first performed followed by fat transplantation. Fat transplantation is also effective for skin texture as well as atrophic scars. The drawback is that not all of the transplanted fat survives, and the results are operator-dependent. There is also a question about the duration of effect, in which some report that they only last 6–18 months. Moreover, there are no papers that advocate the use in the case of atrophic acne scars.

11.4.5 Dermabrasion

Mechanical dermabrasion is a method of physically grinding the skin using a dermabrader such as sandpaper or grinder (Fig. 11.14). Mechanical dermabrasion is very technique dependent and is currently not used because it has no advantages over laser resurfacing [11]. It is known to be effective against atrophic scars, but like laser resurfacing, it is not effective in icepick scars or deep boxcar scars. Disadvantages include severe pain and long recovery periods. Side effects can include pigmentation, hypertrophic scars, keloids, and milia formation. To avoid these side effects, microdermabrasion such as diamond peeling or crystal peeling has been developed. However, because this is superficial peeling, the effect is known to be insignificant compared to mechanical dermabrasion.

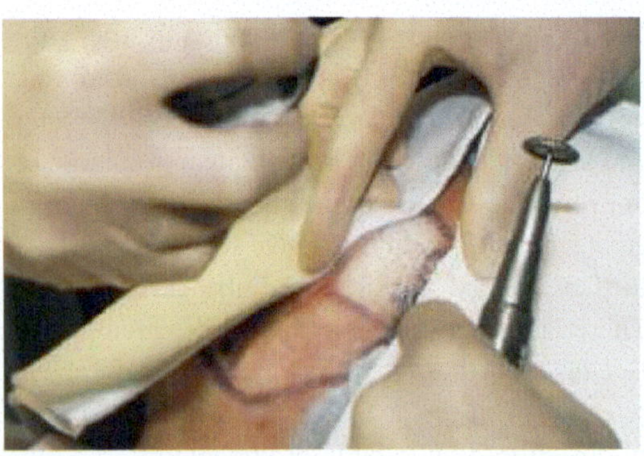

Fig. 11.14 Mechnical dermabrasion. This technique is performed with a diamond fraise over rigid skin cooled with a topical refrigerant spray. (Reproduced from [16])

11.4.6 Microneedle Therapy System

Microneedle therapy system (MTS) is also called microneedling and percutaneous collagen induction therapy (PCI). MTS is a method of creating microcleft in the dermis using several fine needles [10]. As the wound healing process progresses due to the dermal wounds caused by needles, it releases various cytokines which induce collagen production to improve atrophic acne scars (Fig. 11.15). Contraindications to MTS include people who have taken anticoagulants, have skin infections, have been injected with fillers or collagen within the past 6 months, and have a history or family history of hypertrophic scars or keloids. MTS improves atrophic acne scars by grade 1 or 2 in almost every patient (Fig. 11.16). One study found that it was as effective as the CROSS method with 100% TCA. However, collagen production is slow, and it takes 8–12 months to see the final result. Multiple procedures are also needed and it is more painful than other procedures. But the biggest advantage is that it is not related to skin

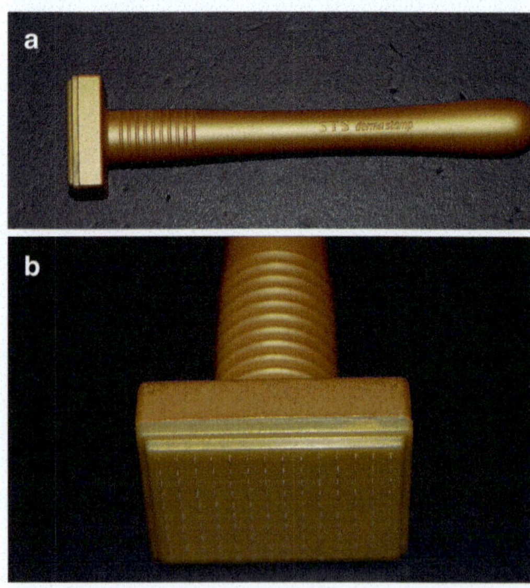

Fig. 11.15 Dermastamp, 'a type of MTS. (**a**) side view and (**b**) front view'

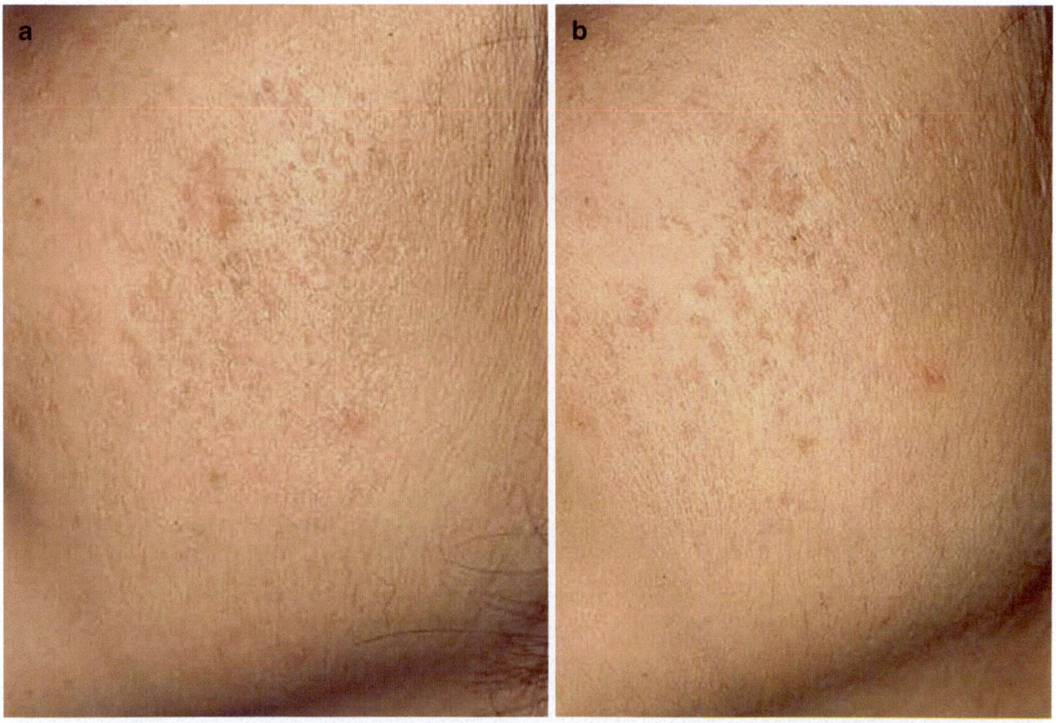

Fig. 11.16 Effect of microneedle array treatment on shallow boxcar acne scars. Before (**a**) and after (**b**) two sessions at 2-week intervals. (Reproduced from [4])

pigmentation and can be used safely in people with ethnic skin without side effects related to pigmentation. Combination therapy with platelet-rich plasma (PRP) can be synergistic.

11.4.7 Chemical Reconstruction of Skin Scars Method

Chemical reconstruction of skin scars (CROSS) method is a method of topically applying a 65–100% TCA solution to atrophic acne scars to regenerate new skin through deep chemical peeling [10]. A thin toothpick with 65–100% TCA or a 30G needle connected to a 1 cc syringe is applied or stabbed to the atrophic scar. No special pretreatment or anesthesia is needed and the procedure is performed five or more times at intervals of 4–6 weeks. Frosting usually occurs within 10 s after the procedure (Fig. 11.17). Frosting is a bleaching phenomenon that occurs when the skin is coagulated by TCA. There are some prickling and burning sensations, but patients usually tolerate the pain. After the procedure, the crust lasts for about a week and then erythema lasts for 1–3 months. Patients may wash their faces 24 h after the procedure, but makeup should be avoided for a week so that the crust does not fall off [17].

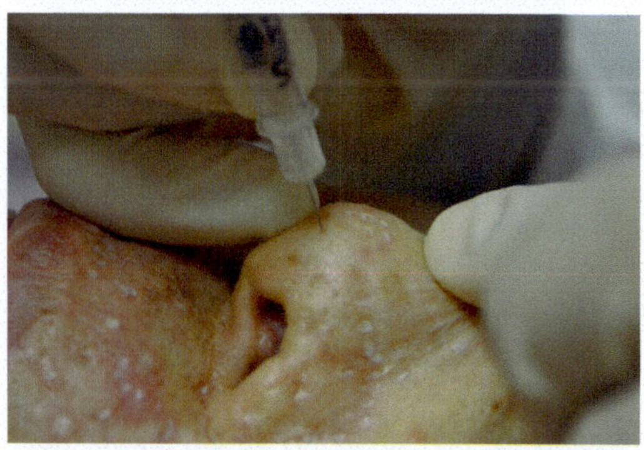

Fig. 11.17 Treatment of enlarged pores with the CROSS method by using a straight needle of an insulin syringe. (Reproduced from [17])

To reduce the inconvenient process of first, coating the needle with the TCA solution, and

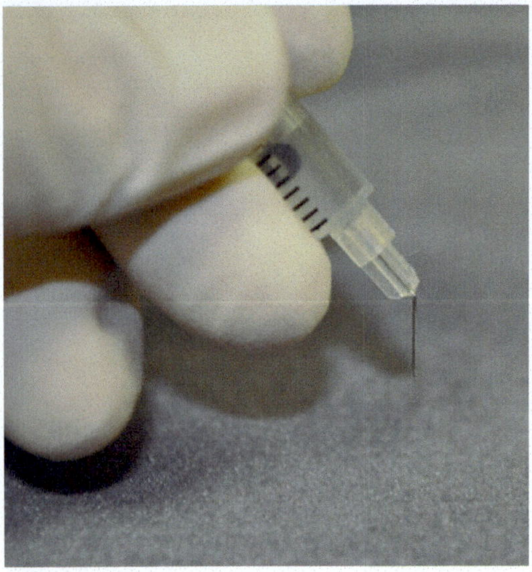

Fig. 11.18 Needle on an insulin syringe bent for CROSS. (Reproduced from [17])

second, applying the TCA coated needle to the skin, there is another method. The TCA solution is put inside the insulin syringe and the stopper is removed. The needle tip is bent at a 45° angle so that the TCA solution comes out at a constant speed (Fig. 11.18) [17]. However, I do not use this method because even if the needle was bent, the rate at which the TCA solution flowed out did not change, and if the needle could not move quickly to another scar, the TCA solution would fall on top of normal tissue, which could cause new scars.

The most important thing in the CROSS method is that the TCA solution should only be applied to the base of the scar and not to the surrounding normal tissue. If too much TCA solution is used, it may come in contact with surrounding normal tissues resulting in a wider scar [18]. In very small icepick scars, even 30G needles may cause TCA to come in contact with surrounding tissues. In this case, I think it is better not to administer the CROSS method.

Weber et al. performed the CROSS method on icepick scars and boxcar scars with 80% TCA in a 28-year-old white female patient [19]. One month after the second procedure, some of the scars became wider (Figs. 11.19 and 11.20). After 2 months of observation without treatment,

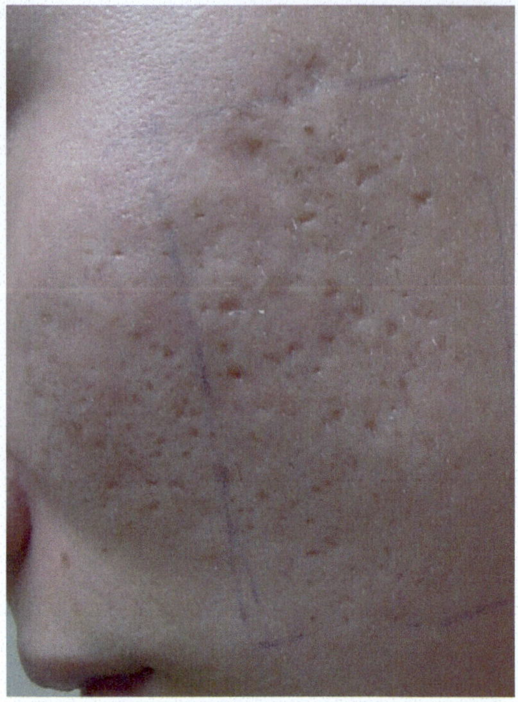

Fig. 11.19 Ice pick- and boxcar-type scars in the malar regions before treatment. (Reproduced from [19])

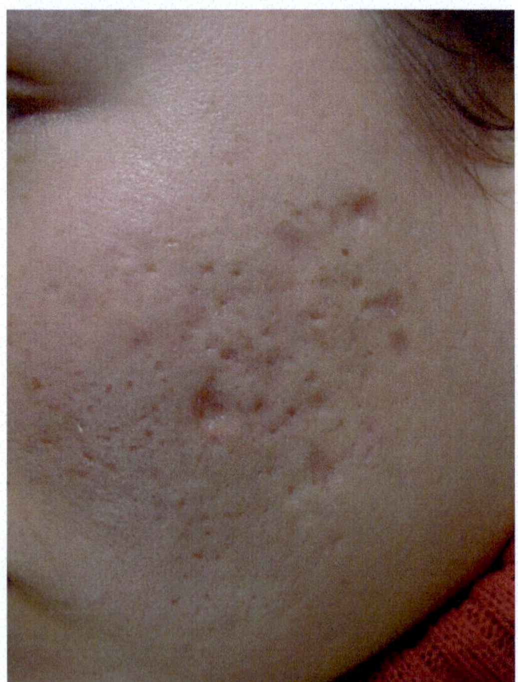

Fig. 11.20 Atrophy in some of the treated scars, after the second application. (Reproduced from [19])

the scars improved, making them inconspicuous. In this paper, the scars eventually improved, but because of the widening of the scars, the patient may complain. Therefore, only a small amount of TCA solution should be used only on the base of the scar.

The method of applying TCA to the bottom of the scar is called dot peeling, and the method of stabbing the bottom of the scar with TCA, resulting in better effect is called the CROSS method. Therefore, in the CROSS method, a slight stab is necessary. In my personal experience with the CROSS method, stabbing led to the spreading of TCA to the reticular dermis, resulting in two patients with larger scars. I currently apply the TCA solution rather than stabbing, i.e., use dot peeling rather than CROSS peeling.

In TCA peeling, the depth of peeling is determined by the concentration of TCA. What percentage of TCAs should be used for the CROSS method? Lee et al. analyzed 65 patients with atrophic acne scars who were treated with the CROSS method. Thirty-three patients were treated with 65% TCA and 32 patients were treated with 100% TCA [20]. All patients had Fitzpatrick skin types IV–V.

Patient treatment data indicated that 27 of 33 patients (82%) (the 65% TCA group) and 30 of 32 patients (94%) (the 100% TCA group) improved over 50%. All patients in the 100% TCA group who received five or six courses of treatment improved over 70%. There was mild erythema which disappeared within 2–8 weeks, and post-inflammatory pigmentation (PIH) which also disappeared within 6 weeks. Mild pustules occurred in four patients but disappeared within a week of taking antibiotics. There were no serious side effects.

This paper was first published by Professor Jeongbok Lee, as he named the method as CROSS. The results showed that there were no special side effects other than temporary erythema and PIH, and the effect was satisfactory. In addition, it is concluded that 100% TCA is superior to 65% because it has no difference in side effects but the effect is better. However, there are other papers that claim to use 70% TCA because of its side effects.

As mentioned earlier, the CROSS method is effective and has few side effects (Fig. 11.21). There are also articles that show scar improvement both clinically and histologically [21]. It

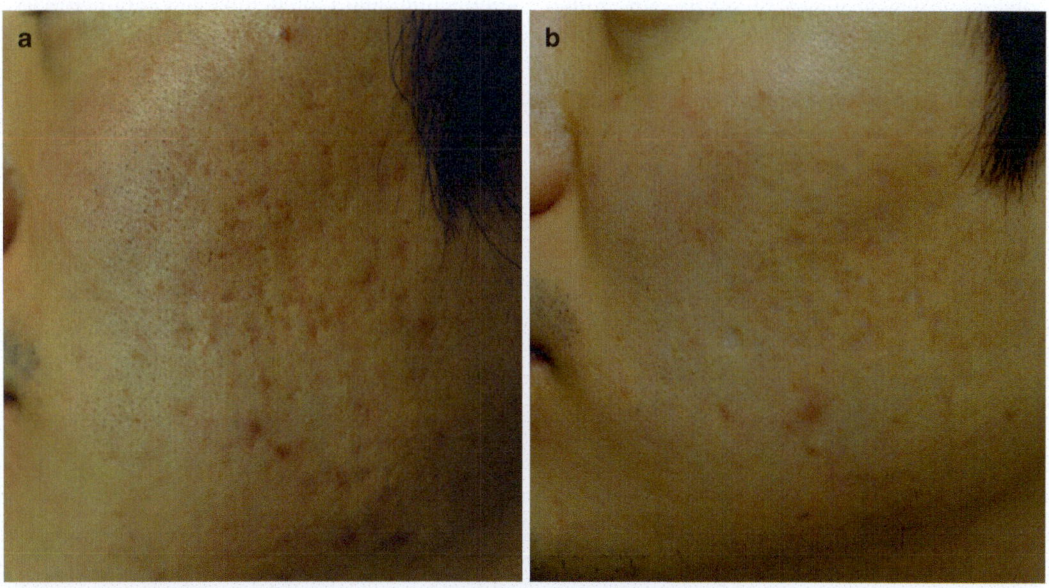

Fig. 11.21 CROSS with 100% TCA using a syringe with fine needle for acne scars on the cheek: (**a**) before and (**b**) after five courses and 5 months after the last treatment. Reproduced from [17]

can also be applied to all atrophic acne scars, including icepick scars as well as severe boxcar scars. Recently, however, a paper has been published that shows that the CO_2 laser pinhole method is more effective than the CROSS method for icepick scars.

Ahmed et al. assigned 28 patients with icepick scars to two groups: 14 patients received pinpoint irradiation by CO_2 laser (CO_2 laser pinhole method) and the other 14 patients received the TCA CROSS method [22]. In both treatments, there were four sessions at 3-week intervals and 3 months of follow up. The parameters of the CO_2 laser were 0.12 mm spot size, 1.0 ms pulse duration, 0.9 W, and focused at 99 Hz. There was a statistically significant difference in acne scar severity index (patients with 51–70% improvement was 36% in CO_2 pinhole vs. 21% in CROSS) and qualitative scarring grading system (CO_2 pinhole > CROSS) in the improvement results between the two groups. Complications included transient pigmentation and inflammation, which resulted less in CO_2 pinhole than in CROSS.

This paper describes that the CO_2 pinhole method is more effective than the CROSS method in icepick scars. CO_2 pinhole method, like the CROSS method, does not require anesthesia and is more convenient than CROSS therapy, which requires first taking the TCA solution and then administering it. However, the effects on scars other than icepick scars are not shown in this paper. The authors believe that the CO_2 pinhole method is more effective than the CROSS method because CO_2 pinhole method induces neocollagenesis by thermal damage, which is not present in the CROSS method. A technique tip for the CO_2 pinhole method is that the skin is pulled back to irradiate the scar base with the tip.

After reviewing this paper, I have attempted the CO_2 pinhole method on very small icepick scars that are difficult to treat with the CROSS method. Currently, I also use the CO_2 pinhole method for rolling scars and boxcar scars, in which only 1–2 procedures are necessary for a noticeable improvement in the scar.

11.4.8 Laser Resurfacing

Peeling the entire skin is called skin resurfacing or ablative rejuvenation. There are chemical, physical, and laser methods. Chemical methods include peeling using phenol, and physical methods include dermabrasion using sandpaper or grinder. Lasers include laser resurfacing using CO_2 lasers or Er:YAG lasers. Among the three methods, the easiest to control is laser resurfacing, and it is known that laser resurfacing is more effective than other methods due to neocollagenesis by thermal damage (Fig. 11.22) [9].

Laser resurfacing is not only effective for acne scars, but also facial tone, skin texture, collagen contraction, and remodeling, and skin elasticity, making the skin look 10 years younger. Laser resurfacing using a CO_2 laser improves atrophic acne scars by 50–80% [23], and scars are known to improve gradually up to 18 months after the procedure [11]. However, laser resurfacing requires general anesthesia and needs closed dressing such as a mask, which makes social life

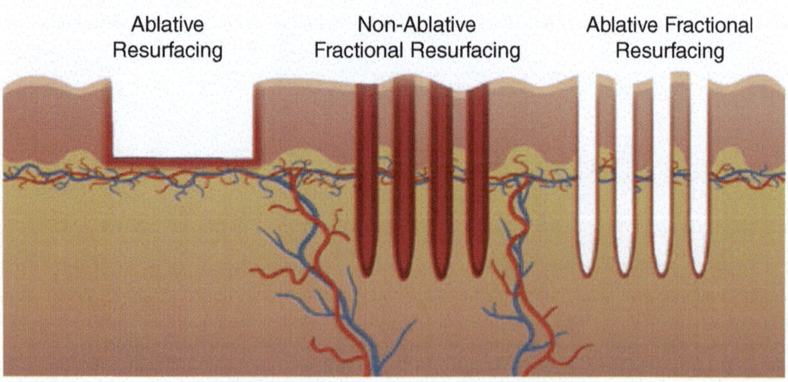

Fig. 11.22 Schematic figure for the zone of damage in ablative and fractional lasers. (Reproduced from [15])

difficult and requires hospitalization. In addition, side effects are so severe that erythema, edema, and oozing occurs, and complications such as inflammation, milia, and PIH are not uncommon. Erythema lasts from 1 month to 6 months. This is why laser resurfacing is seldom used these days.

11.4.8.1 Focal Acne Scar Treatment Method

Laser resurfacing is effective, but due to the recovery period, side effects, and complications, it is not popular these days. However, there are ways to apply the principle of laser resurfacing to scars with fewer side effects.

Schweiger et al. treated acne scars in a new way using a CO_2 fractional laser [24]. Only areas with scars were treated, normal areas were not treated. The authors of the paper define this method as "Focal Acne Scar Treatment" and call it the "FAST method." All six patients treated with the FAST method had significant improvement posttreatment ranging from 40–70% as estimated by the treating doctor and the patient at 4 weeks posttreatment. Patient satisfaction was high following the FAST method. Temporary post-inflammatory hyperpigmentation was seen in two patients but resolved after a single 1550-nm Erbium Glass fractional laser treatment. Schweiger et al. concluded that the FAST method is an effective method of improving the appearance of atrophic acne scars. Higher energy and density levels can be used when utilizing this technique, resulting in improved outcomes when compared with whole face fractional CO_2 laser resurfacing. Healing is improved and faster with this technique and no increased incidence of permanent adverse events was found.

This is the same method I currently use. In principle, the treatment density should be reduced in fractional lasers to reduce side effects, and energy should be increased to increase the effectiveness [25]. On the other hand, laser resurfacing is a way to increase treatment density. In my opinion, a more effective and safer treatment is possible if these two are combined: the treatment density and the energy must both be increased, but only the scars should be treated, leaving the normal tissue intact. That is, "The fractional laser should be used fractionally." The paper earlier defines this as the FAST method. I use the CO_2 fractional laser to increase energy and treatment density and treat only scars with a 5 × 5 mm area.

11.4.9 Fractional Laser

As we reviewed in "Chap. 10," a fractional laser is a treatment method between ablative rejuvenation that requires a long recovery period and has many side effects and nonablative rejuvenation that is less effective. Fractional laser has fewer complications but is much more effective than nonablative rejuvenation. It is a suitable treatment for ethnic skin and although combination treatments are possible, multiple treatments are needed.

The first fractional laser to be developed was 1550-nm Er:Glass fractional laser, a nonablative fractional rejuvenation. But now ablative fractional rejuvenation such as CO_2 fractional laser is considered the gold standard in skin resurfacing; 1550-nm Er:Glass fractional laser shows a 51–75% improvement in acne scars after three treatments [23]. Side effects included temporary erythema and edema and pain. CO_2 fractional lasers show 43–80% (average 66.8%) scar improvement [2].

11.4.10 Platelet-Rich Plasma and Polydeoxyribonucleotide

The main component of platelet-rich plasma (PRP) extracted from the patient's blood is the platelet. Platelets are the first cells that arrive when a wound occurs. Platelets have α-granules. α-granules have various growth factors for wound healing, such as PDGF, TGF-β, insulin-like growth factor, FGF, epithelial grow factor, keratinocyte growth factor, and many cytokines, chemokines, and metabolites. These factors stimulate stem cells to promote wound healing. It is also known to make new collagen fibers. Therefore, PRP can be applied in the treatment of scars.

Lee et al. evaluated the synergistic effects of autologous PRP with CO_2 fractional resurfacing for acne scars [26]. A split-face trial was conducted in 14 Korean participants with acne scars. All participants received one session of ablative CO_2 fractional resurfacing. Immediately after resurfacing, facial halves were randomly assigned to receive treatment with autologous PRP intradermal injections on one side and normal saline injections on the other side. Erythema and edema on the PRP side improved faster than the other side. Participants were also assessed for the duration of posttreatment crusting, with a mean of 6.8 ± 1.0 days on the normal saline side and 5.9 ± 1.1 days on the PRP side ($p = 0.04$). Four months after the final treatment, the clinical appearance of acne scarring was significantly better on the PRP side (2.7 ± 0.7) than on the control side (2.3 ± 0.5) ($p = 0.03$).

As mentioned in the paper earlier, PRP is thought to reduce side effects, shorten the recovery period, and improve scars by helping wound healing caused by other procedures. They are known to have synergy when used in combination with other treatments. On the other hand, Faghihi and Ibrahim, claim that adding PRP to CO_2 fractional lasers or MTS has no advantage over monotherapy.

Because I think that the main purpose of PRP is to promote wound healing, I use it to reduce side effects and shorten recovery time after CO_2 fractional lasers or MTS rather than use it to improve scars. However, because the process of obtaining PRP, taking the patient's blood and extracting PRP takes much time and money, i.e., is inconvenient compared to the scar improvement effect, these days I use PDRN instead.

Polydeoxyribonucleotide (PDRN) is known to promote wound healing and has a high proportion of low molecular weight DNA extracted from salmon trout sperm. When PDRN encounters enzymes in the cell wall, it breaks down into purine and pyrimidine DNA, which promotes the transport of vascular endothelial cells and act on adenosine A2A receptors to promote the growth of fibroblasts and osteoblasts. PDRN aids in wound healing by promoting angiogenesis and fibroblast growth. PDRN has been proven to heal wounds in ischemic skin flaps and graft donor sites and is known to increase blood flow and promote corneal epithelial regeneration in peripheral artery occlusive disease. It also has a regenerative effect that treats heat and UV damage. Clinically, it has been shown to be effective in the treatment of pressure ulcers, diabetic foot ulcers, and male genital lichen sclerosus [27].

Yu et al. induced wounds on 12 rats aged 8 weeks using a fractional ablative CO_2 laser [27]. The treatment group received daily injections of intraperitoneal PDRN and the control group received injections of normal saline. The process of wound healing was faster in the treatment group than in the control group. In the histopathological examination, the granulation tissue thickness score of the treatment group was significantly higher than that of the control group.

Although this study was conducted on rats, and it was a study in which PDRN was injected into the abdominal cavity, not the skin, and there is no information on collagen regeneration or scars, it suggests that PDRN after CO_2 fractional lasers can shorten the recovery period and promote wound healing.

11.4.11 Nonablative Laser

A nonablative laser promotes collagen production by penetrating deep into the dermis and giving thermal injury to the dermis while protecting the epidermis by epidermal cooling. Due to its collagen-producing effects, it may be used for atrophic acne scars. However, the efficacy is known to be less compared to the ablative laser or the fractional laser.

Examples of nonablative lasers are 1320-nm Nd:YAG lasers, 1450-m diode lasers, and 1554-nm Er:Glass lasers. Of these lasers, the 1450-nm diode laser is known to be more effective. Most of these lasers have been withdrawn from private practices due to severe pain and side effects. However, the 1450-nm diode laser is still used in private practices due to its acne treatment effect, rather than its skin rejuvenation effect. Also, the 585-nm PDL laser, a vascular laser, regenerates collagen and is effective in atrophic acne scars.

11.4.12 Fractional Microneedle Radiofrequency

Fractional microneedle radiofrequency (needle RF) is a method of improving the scars by inserting multiple microneedles into the skin and letting high-frequency flow through the needles, stimulating collagen production and improving scars. Needle RF is known to be more effective than bipolar RF. The improvement of the scar was 25–75% with needle RF performed three to four times at intervals of three or more weeks and after 3 months of follow-up [10]. Needle RF is very effective in post-inflammatory erythema. In addition, when used for the treatment of patients with acne scars and pores, needle RF improved skin roughness in more than 70% of patients. The advantage of Needle RF is that it is safe to use in Fitzpatrick skin types III and IV because of its lack of melanin absorption unlike lasers, and it may also be used in combinations with minimally invasive technologies such as the 1540-nm Er:Glass laser.

On the other hand, there are papers that show that the 1550-nm Er:Glass laser, a nonablational fractional laser, is more effective for atrophic acne scars than Needle RF [28]. However, many of these studies have different results depending on the patient group, evaluation method, and parameters, so it is difficult to conclude that the 1550-nm Er:Glass laser is more effective than Needle RF. More research is needed.

11.4.13 Picolasers

With the recent release of picolasers (subnanosecond laser), skin rejuvenation and scar treatment have been attempted using photodisruption effects through laser-induced optical breakdown (LIOB). Usually, a picolaser is equipped with a zoom handpiece to focus the beam like a CO_2 laser to increase the power density for skin rejuvenation and scar treatment [29].

One reason for focusing is to generate plasma, but I think the other reason is to increase the peak tensile stress through making the shock waves stronger. Higher tensile stress leads to stronger shock waves and cavitation in the dermis, leading to mechanical injury, which in turn may lead to the creation of new collagen as the wound healing process progresses. In particular, due to focusing, the epidermal layer remains intact, resulting in faster recovery time and fewer side effects. In addition, like fractional photothermolysis, a fraction of the skin is treated at one time, which increases safety.

After picolaser irradiation on ex-vivo skin tissue with a zoom handpiece, biopsy examination showed an oval cavity. Whereas 30 min after irradiation on in-vivo skin tissue, biopsy examination did not show oral cavities but showed distorted cavities [30]. This may be because when cavities form in living tissue, they may seem to disappear as the skin collapses. In both cases, we can see that due to picolaser, sufficient damage has occurred to the dermal layer.

Tanghetti et al. used a 755 nm picolaser (Picosure™, Cynosure, Westford, MA) with a zoom handpiece with three different energy settings (0.71 J/cm^2, 0.4 J/cm^2, 0.25 J/cm^2) and compared histological examinations (Fig. 11.23) [31].

Biopsy results showed that vacuoles including cellular debris were found in the stratum spinosum of the epidermis, and normal tissues without significant heat damage were observed in the stratum corneum or the tissues around the vacuoles. It is interesting to note that the lower the energy, the smaller the size of the vacuole and lower the depth.

The results of this paper are interesting. First, picolasers using zoom handpieces are known to be effective for scars and wrinkles, but biopsy results showed that vacuoles formed on the epidermis and not on the dermis. Because the wavelength of 755 nm has a high absorption coefficient for melanin, vacuole formation on the epidermis is natural. However, how does the vacuole formation on the epidermis improve the dermis, thus making it effective for scars and wrinkles? Tanghetti et al. speculated that dermal remodeling may occur due to changes in cell signaling and various cytokines. Second, why does the

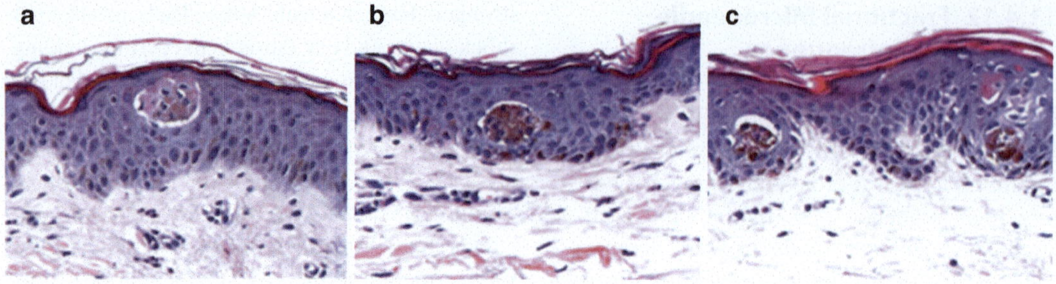

Fig. 11.23 Histology from a skin biopsy at 24 h post-treatment of skin type IV. MI = 31 demonstrating intraepidermal vacuoles created with F = (**a**) 0.71 J/cm^2, (**b**) 0.4 J/cm^2, and (**c**) 0.25 J/cm^2. The vacuoles contain cellular debris and the size and depth of the vacuole appear to diminish and increase, respectively, as the energy per micro-spot decreases. As we decrease the energy the vacuole diameter becomes smaller and the depth becomes deeper probably due to an increase in melanin density deeper in the epidermis (200×). Reproduced from [31]

vacuole form higher up on the epidermis as the energy increases? In the case of long-pulsed lasers or Q-switched lasers, photons pass from the epidermis to the dermis, and the highest temperature rises in the basal layer which has the highest melanin concentration, which induces the first changes. But in picolasers, when the energy is high, plasma is generated at the superficial layer rather than the basal layer due to the plasma shielding effect. After plasma formation, however, photons are unable to pass, resulting in superficial vacuole formation. Also, due to the high fluence large vacuoles form.

It is said that 755-nm picolasers are effective for treating scars and wrinkles, but they form vacuoles in the epidermis rather than the dermis, and the mechanism of dermal remodeling is thought to be because of cellular signals or cytokines. I think that 1064-nm picolasers which form vacuoles directly in the dermis may be more effective in treating scars and wrinkles.

Theoretically, we can speculate that picolasers are effective in treating scars. However, there are only two papers that used picolasers to treat scars. I will review both papers.

Brauer et al. treated 20 patients with acne scars using a 755-nm Alexandrite picosecond laser [32]. Patients received treatments with a spot size of 6 mm, fluence of 0.71 J/cm^2, a repetition rate of 5 Hz, and a pulse width of 750 ps in combination with a diffractive lens array. The procedure was undertaken six times at 4–8 week intervals. The mean pain score was 2.83 of 10, and the pain was not severe. Patients were satisfied to extremely satisfied with the improvement in appearance and texture, which was more than 2 points on the 4-point scale. (4-point scale—0, not satisfied; 1, dissatisfied; 2, satisfied; and 3, extremely satisfied) The assessment scores by the three evaluators were 1.5 and 1.4 at 1 and 3 months, showing 26% in improvement (4-point scale—0: 0–25%, 1: 26–50%, 3: 51–75%, 4: 76–100%). A three-dimensional analysis revealed a mean 24.3% improvement in scar volume. Histologic analysis revealed elongation and increased density of elastic fibers, with an increase in dermal collagen and mucin.

This paper shows that not only acne scars but also skin textures are improved with 755 nm picolasers and histological results show increased collagen. However, one study reported a 38% improvement in scar volume by ablative fractional lasers, by which we can evaluate that picolasers are less effective than ablative fractional lasers.

Bernstein et al. used 1064-nm and 532-nm Nd:YAG picolasers to treat rolling scars and boxcar scars [33]. A holographic optic was used for laser treatments. The system delivered a 10 × 10 array of 150-μm diameter microbeams arranged in a 6 × 6 mm^2. The parameters were 1.3–2.9 mJ/cm^2 at 1064 nm for 450 ps pulse duration and 6 Hz at 0.16–1.5 mJ/cm^2 for 532 nm for 375 ps pulse duration. The clinical endpoint was erythema and mild petechia. Two passes were done in a single treatment and each patient received four monthly treatments. Twenty-seven of 31 patients completed the study, 19 were treated using 1064 nm and 8 were treated at 532 nm. Posttreatment erythema, mild edema, and petechiae were the only side effects noted. Blinded reviewers revealed on a 10-point scale a mean improvement score of 1.4 for all patients, corresponding to a 14% improvement on average in the appearance of acne scars. No difference was noted in the mean improvement when comparing patients treated with 1064 nm to patients treated with 532 nm. The mean improvement score for the 16 patients whose baseline image was correctly identified by all three blinded reviewers was 2.8, corresponding to a 28% improvement on average in the appearance of acne scars.

This paper is about treating acne scars using the Nd:YAG picosecond laser. Evaluation was made by three blinded reviewers. If you look more closely at the results, blinded reviewers incorrectly identified the baseline image of 11 patients out of 29 patients and evaluated that the treatment was not effective or the scar aggravated. I believe that scars cannot be really aggravated by picolasers. Therefore, I think the results show that at least 37% (11 patients/29 patients) treated with picolasers can be judged to be ineffective.

Based on these two papers, I believe that picolasers are effective against atrophic acne scars but less effective than ablative fractional lasers. The advantage of picolasers, on the other hand, is that they do not damage the epidermis and therefore have fewer side effects and recovery periods than ablative fractional lasers. However, since the two papers are not comparison papers and there are only two papers on this subject, more study is needed.

11.4.14 Novel Therapeutic Modalities

Novel methods for scar treatment include intradermal injection of autologous bone marrow stem cells, autologous fibroblast intradermal injection, and topical epidermal growth factor (EGF) [10]. However, more research is needed. And even though it is proven to be effective, the technique and the cost may be a hurdle in private practice.

11.5 Combination Therapy

Kang et al. used a combination of dot peeling, subcision, and nonablational fractional laser treatment for atrophic acne scars [34]. Dot peeling was done by 100% TCA and subcision by 29G needle. The nonablative fractional laser was a 1550-nm Er:Glass laser and the parameters were four passes using 350–800 spots/cm^2 and 25 mJ per MTZ. Fractional laser was performed three to four times in 3–4 week intervals. Dot peeling and subcision were performed at the same time 2 weeks after the fractional laser, for a total of two times in 2–3 month intervals. The results showed that the acne scar severity score improved by 55.3%, and 80% of the patients had a "significant" or "marked improvement."

This paper used a combination of three treatments for acne scars. The reason for the combination therapy is described in the paper as follows: (1) Dot peeling is effective on individual atrophic acne scars but is limited to improving overall skin texture. (2) Fractional lasers are effective in improving overall skin texture and on shallow and small atrophic scars, but the effect is limited on icepick scars and boxcar scars. (3) Subcision is also effective for wide boxcar scars and rolling scars. Therefore, it is described that the effects and limitations of these three treatment methods can be complemented to each other by combination therapy, and the overall scar treatment effect can be enhanced.

Combination therapy is known to be more effective than single therapy in acne scars due to the complementary and synergetic effects described above. Acne scar treatment can be divided into (1) energy-based methods such as laser and radiofrequency and (2) energy-free procedures such as CROSS, subcision, filler, MTS, and punch techniques. What is important in combination therapy is that treatments with different mechanisms are needed to reduce side effects.

For example, laser and radiofrequency may be used in combination, but both procedures are "energy-based" methods and should be avoided. It would be better to combine treatments with different mechanisms, such as laser + subcision or laser + subcision + punch technique. Also, lasers are most effective for scars and should be included in combination therapy as the primary treatment for scars. Subcision is usually the first procedure of combination therapy.

11.5.1 Order of Combination Therapies

Let's think about the order of combination therapies. When several procedures are performed simultaneously on the same day, what is the principle in choosing the order of combination therapies? I believe that a deep procedure or laser with deep OPD should be performed first, followed by a shallow procedure or laser with shallow OPD. For example, in tattoo removals, CO_2 pinhole therapy first and 1064-nm Q-switched Nd:YAG lasers later, maybe more effective but may be more dangerous, considering the side effects. In other words, we must first put safety first, so "deep procedure → shallow procedure" should be one principle to follow when choosing the order of combination.

I perform the following procedures when treating scars: First, subcision is performed, followed by the CROSS method, CO_2 fractional laser, and MTS. Subcision is performed on the hypodermis, i.e., just below or to the dermis, the CROSS method aims to necrosis the entire dermis, and CO_2 fractional laser penetrates the epidermis and part of the dermis. But what about MTS? The clinical end point of the MTS is bleeding, which means that it is performed deep in the dermis, which is the same or deeper than the layer that CO_2 fractional laser targets. Then why is MTS performed last? Due to the bleeding of MTS, the CROSS method and CO_2 fractional laser may not be effective if they are performed after MTS. Thus, according to the principle of order of combination therapies, MTS should be done first, but because of the reasons mentioned earlier, I do it last. Although there are principles, the order of combination therapies may vary depending on the nature or characteristics of the laser or procedure.

11.6 Sculpting Technique

Dr. Yongsoo Lee, the author of "Scars and scarring" presented a new scar classification method and explained the sculpting technique in detail [35].

The sculpting technique usually involves using Er:YAG lasers to ablate atrophic scars, smoothing out the border between scar tissue and normal tissue. The reason why CO_2 lasers are not used for ablation is because CO_2 lasers cannot go deeper after four passes, and due to irregular residual thermal damage (RTD, I think "reversible thermal damage" is the more adequate term, rather than residual thermal damage), the surface becomes uneven. Er:YAG lasers, on the other hand, have a high absorption coefficient for water, which allows the skin to be finely ablated. However, since Er:YAG laser has less RTD, skin regeneration is not easy, Lee suggests using Er:YAG laser first, and the low-power CO_2 laser second to give additional RTD to the overall scar. RTD was considered important because it is thought to be the initial signal that makes keratinocytes migrate from the epidermis and hair follicles.

Lee's sculpting technique is as follows: First, acyclovir (400 mg tid) and cefaclor (375 mg bid) are prescribed for 5 days on the day of the procedure. Er:YAG laser is first used to shape the scar into a smooth concave wound with no sharp angles at the end of the scar. The CO_2 laser is then used to inflict nonfatal thermal damage on new skin to promote skin regeneration. The parameters of the CO_2 lasers were 1 mm spot size, 800 W, 0.1 ms, and 10 Hz. Because the deeper the RTD, the greater the regeneration, the CO_2 laser was aimed so that the RTD was deeper toward the center of the concave scar. CO_2 laser moved back and forth between the center of the concave scar and the end of the scar, just like drawing a flower. After sculpting the scar with the Er:YAG laser, dense white scar tissue (fibrotic tissue) is sometimes observed, which should be removed because it will interfere with skin regeneration. However, if all of the white scar tissue is removed, the same scar will reappear because the original wound made the current scar. Therefore, pinhole therapy using a CO_2 laser should remove only part of the white scar tissue. After the procedure, an ointment containing copper tripeptide-1, EFG, and bFGF is applied, next Vaseline and dry gauze are applied. The dressing should be maintained for 10–13 days. One week after the dressing is removed the nonablative laser and the fractional laser should be repeated in 2 week intervals.

Lee divided scars into four categories according to laser treatment effect and prognosis; nonhypertrophic scars (NHS), fibroproliferative scars (FPS, hypertrophic scars, and keloids), facial atrophic post-acne scars (FAPS), and burn scars. The difference of this classification from the existing scar classification is that the existing atrophic scars are classified as non-hypertrophic scars (NHS) and facial atrophic post-acne scars (FAPS). NHS refers to shallow atrophic scars with or without changes in texture, especially with acute-angled margins on the ends of the scar or irregular bottom of depressed areas. These scars are shallow, but cosmetics or sunscreen may accumulate inside the scar due to the sharp angle, and lights and shadows accentuate the scars, which is not cosmetically desirable. Lee saw NHS scars as the best indications for the sculpting technique.

On the other hand, FAPS is difficult to treat with the sculpting technique because they are clusters of small pleomorphic atrophic scars congregated closely and the openings are narrow in comparison to the depth. Sculpting technique is difficult in FAPS: First, when the sculpting technique is performed on densely congregated atrophic scars (FAPS), more epidermal cells are removed compared to sculpting single scars, and the distance from surrounding normal skin increases, resulting in a longer recovery period, and a higher risk of side effects. Also, large amounts of epidermal appendages disappear, increasing the risk of hypopigmentation and severe scarring.

Second, when performing a sculpting technique on the deep and narrow scar, the entrance should be sculpted widely. This also results in large amounts of epidermal appendages disappearing, increasing the risk of hypopigmentation and severe scarring. Therefore, FAPS should be first changed to NHS by the combination therapy of CROSS method, subcision, nonablational laser (1450-nm diode laser), and fractional laser. And then when it becomes NHS, the sculpting technique may be performed.

Lee retrospectively studied 24 Asians with 30 NHS who underwent sculpting technique [36]. The evaluators rated an average improvement of 86.8% (median 90%). Ten of 31 pairs of photographs were rated 100%, one of which was unanimous.

Lee also retrospectively studied 248 Asians who underwent a combination of scar procedures including sculpting technique, nonablative fractional laser, subcision, CROSS, and nonablative laser [37]. 248 pairs of pre and post photographs were evaluated by five evaluators. The results showed that the combination treatment with nonablative fractional laser was statistically significant. The optimal temporal treatment interval would be 3–4 weeks. The sculpting technique was more effective when it was performed after other procedures.

11.7 Conclusion

When treating atrophic acne scars, the following principles should be considered. First, a treatment that is more effective must be selected, unless it has a risk of permanent side effects. Second, because of various acne symptoms, various types of scars are present on the face at the same time. Therefore, only one procedure does not yield satisfactory results. Third, combination therapy is also more effective than monotherapy. Fourth, each treatment method has a different therapeutic effect for each type of scar. The first three criteria were reviewed earlier. Here, we will review the last principle.

Bhargava et al. reviewed 89 papers on the treatment of acne scars [10]. According to the quality of evidence, they were classified as level I-IV. The smaller the number, the higher the evidence. The result was as follows: First, there was no paper showing high evidence in the treatment of acne scars. Second, fractional lasers and radiofrequency waves were highly effective with most atrophic acne scars without serious side effects. Third, combination therapy is more effective than monotherapy.

Table 11.3 is important to note in this paper. This table shows the effect of each scar type according to various treatment methods. The effects vary depending on the type of treatment and the type of scar.

According to the four principles, the procedure should be selected as follows: First, the darkest blue that corresponds to "effective" must be selected. Second, because various types of acne scars are present on the face at the same time, four separate treatments for four types of scars must be selected for effective treatment. Third, because combination treatment is more effective, effective treatment for the four types of scars should be combined.

I use the Table 11.3 as follows:

(1) Ice pick scars.

The most effective methods for icepick scars are the CROSS method and punch excision. But I choose the CROSS method because patients are reluctant to have surgery, i.e., punch excision, and scars do not disappear, but somewhat recur after punch excision. (currently, I use CO_2 pinhole method rather than the CROSS method).

(2) Rolling scars and boxcar scars.

Subcision, MTS, fractional lasers, and needle RF are effective in rolling scars and boxcar scars. I prefer subcision, MTS, and fractional lasers.

(3) Deep boxcar scars.

Ablative lasers, punch elevation, and punch excision are effective in deep boxcar scars. But since punch elevation and punch excision are both surgical procedures, ablative lasers are preferred. However, ablative lasers have the possibility of serious side effects, so I use the FAST method by CO_2 fractional laser.

When combination therapies are performed on the same day, I perform in this order: Subcision, CROSS method, CO_2 fractional laser (FAST method), and MTS. And Finally, PDRN is applied to the skin to facilitate wound healing.

Next, we will review facial pores that are of great interest to Koreans and isotretinoin use during scar treatment.

11.8 Facial Pores

"Facial pores" are not a medical term. Like "spots," it is a term commonly used among the general public. In the dictionary, "pores" are defined as "enlargement of the entrance of the pilosebaceous follicles," but the word is usually used by the general public to indicate "holes in the face that are cannot be covered by makeup." One paper defines pores as "a hole of more than 0.02 mm^2," and another paper classifies pores into three types by Robo Skin Analyzer CS50: 0.1–0.6 mm^2 holes as "visible skin pores," 0.3–0.6 mm^2 holes as "enlarged skin pores" and open holes with open comedones as "blackhead embedded skin pores." However, pores are not fixed in size but vary in size depending on sebum secretion and aging, so there is a problem in applying this definition [38].

Skin pores result due to three major causes: First, increased sebum secretion, second, decreased elasticity around the pores, and third, hair volume, such as thick hair. Other causes may include chronic recurrent acne, sex hormones, improper use of cosmetics, poor skincare habits such as incorrect facial cleansing habits, and UV exposure [38]. Treatment should target these causes: First, sebum secretion should be reduced. The most powerful medication is the isotretinoin, an oral sebum inhibitor. Patients with severe acne should consider using isotretinoin, but in patients with few acne, I sometimes consider the use of dermal injections of botulinum toxin.

Rose et al. measured sebum secretion after injecting botulinum toxin into the forehead of 25 patients with oily skin [39]. A total of 30–45 U of botulinum toxin (Dysport, Medicis, Scottsdale, AZ) was used and ten injections were made on

Table 11.3 Efficacy of modalities per atrophic scar type. CROSS; chemical reconstruction of skin scars. [a]Modalities with substantial quality of evidence data are included. [b]Used as an adjunct to other procedures. (Reproduced from [10])

Type of Treatment	Modality[a]	Icepick Scars	Rolling Scars	Shallow Boxcar Scars	Deep Boxcar Scars
Resurfacing	Microdermabrasion	Less effective	Ineffective	Less effective	Ineffective
	Dermabrasion	Less effective	Ineffective	Less effective	Less effective
	Peels	Less effective	Ineffective	Less effective	Ineffective
	CROSS	Effective	Ineffective	Effective	Ineffective
	Needling	Ineffective	Effective	Effective	Effective
	Ablative laser	Less effective	Effective	Effective	Effective
Lifting-related	Subcision	Less effective	Effective	Less effective	Less effective
Volume-related	Filler	Ineffective	Effective	Less effective	Less effective
	Platelet rich plasma[b]	Ineffective	Less effective	Less effective	Less effective
Skin Tightening	Fractional/nonablative lasers	Less effective	Effective	Effective	Less effective
	Fractional radiofrequency	Less effective	Effective	Effective	Less effective
Surgery/movement-related	Punch elevation	Ineffective	Ineffective	Effective	Effective
	Punch excision	Effective	Ineffective	Less effective	Effective

Effective Less effective Ineffective

the forehead with 3–5 U per injection. Baseline and posttreatment sebum production were measured using a sebometer. Patients were also asked to rate their satisfaction with the treatment in terms of improvement in their oily skin. Treatment with botulinum toxin resulted in significantly lower sebum production at 1 week and 1, 2, and 3 months after injection ($p < 0.001$). Twenty-one patients (91%) reported that they were satisfied (50–75% improvement) with intradermal botulinum toxin as a treatment for oily skin. The mechanism by which botulinum toxin reduces sebum secretion is not yet proven, but the authors believe that botulinum toxin reduces sebum secretion by acting on muscarinic receptors in the arrector pili muscle and sebaceous gland.

Second, to increase skin elasticity, I use the most safe and effective fractional laser. Third, a hair removal laser is used to remove hair. For hairs inside the pores or trichostasis spinulosa, lasers with short pulse duration must be used, such as the 755-nm-long-pulsed alexandrite laser [40, 41].

However, the most important thing to remember is that because the main cause of the pores differs from each patient, it is necessary to choose the appropriate method tailored for each patient's pores [38].

11.9 Isotretinoin

In the 1980s and 1990s, there were reports of keloid formation after mechanical resurfacing, argon laser, and PDL for cosmetic purposes in patients who took isotretinoin for 6 months to 1 year prior to the procedure. The underlying mechanism is thought to be alterations in the pilosebaceous unit and inhibition of collagenase, resulting in delayed or change in epithelialization. Therefore, patients who took isotretinoin between 6 months and 1 year prior to laser treatment were contraindications in laser treatment [42].

However, there are patients who want acne scar treatment, but are on isotretinoin medication or have been in the past. Should we delay scar treatment at least 6 months to 1 year for these patients?

Kim et al. evaluated wound healing after ablative CO_2 fractional resurfacing for acne scars conducted during and/or within 1–3 months of oral isotretinoin (10–40 mg/day) treatment [42]. The parameters were 30–50 mJ, 0.96–1.67 ms pulse duration, 30 W, treatment density 100–200 MTZ/cm^2, coverage rate was 6.4–12.7%. The patients received the treatment one to six times, at least 1 month apart. All patients showed normal reepithelialization and were satisfied with the results of the laser treatments. All adverse events were minor and there were no hypertrophic scars or keloids.

Papers that reported complications related to scar treatment during isotretinoin use is as follows [43]: Rubenstein et al. first reported the development of keloids in the cheeks, jaw, and face of patients who underwent mechanical dermabrasion during (three cases) and before (three cases) isotretinoin use. Zachariae reported that keloids developed on the face of three patients who took isotretinoin; two patients received mechanical dermabrasion, and one patient received argon laser. Katz and McFarlane have reported atypical atrophic scars after mechanical dermabrasion in patients taking isotretinoin. Goihman-Yar has reported a case of natural keloids caused by isotretinoin alone.

However, most of these papers are case reports and are not papers that prove causality through statistics. And through these papers, we can see that scar formation cases after isotretinoin use are rare. Also, the treatment method used in most papers was mechanical dermabrasion, which is a more aggressive method than laser resurfacing and is currently not used well.

Spring et al. reviewed articles that underwent a number of laser or surgical procedures in patients who are or were taking isotretinoin from 1982 to 2017 [43]. A total of 32 relevant papers were found and the results were summarized according to five procedures: mechanical dermabrasion, chemical peel, cutaneous surgery, laser hair removal, and fractional ablative/nonablative laser. In conclusion, there was insufficient evidence to support delaying manual dermabrasion, superficial chemical peels, cutaneous surgery, laser hair removal, and fractional ablative and nonablative laser procedures for patients currently receiving or having recently completed isotretinoin therapy. Mechanical dermabrasion and fully ablative laser were not recommended in the setting of systemic isotretinoin treatment. In addition, full explanations of the risks to the patients and an earlier intervention may result in a better outcome.

Based on the earlier paper, I perform a variety of scar treatment procedures, including fractional lasers, even if the patient is taking isotretinoin or had taken isotretinoin for at least 6 months to 1 year, as long as the dose is low (10–20 mg/dL).

References

1. Committee C, Sl C, Kim IH, Kang JS, Park SH, Chung KY et al (2016) Laser and light treatment in Asian skin. Koonja, Paju
2. Sobanko JF, Alster TS (2012) Management of acne scarring, part I: a comparative review of laser surgical approaches. Am J Clin Dermatol 13(5):319–330
3. Zaleski-Larsen LA, Fabi SG, McGraw T, Taylor M (2016) Acne scar treatment: a multimodality approach tailored to scar type. Dermatol Surg 42(Suppl 2):S139–S149
4. Thiboutot D, Gollnick H, Bettoli V, Dreno B, Kang S, Leyden JJ et al (2009) New insights into the management of acne: an update from the global Alliance to improve outcomes in acne group. J Am Acad Dermatol 60(5 Suppl):S1–S50
5. Krakowski AC, Shumaker PR, Ovid Technologies I (2017) The scar book. Wolters Kluwer, Philadelphia, PA
6. Townsend CM, Beauchamp RD, Evers BM, Mattox KL (2016) Sabiston textbook of surgery E-book. Elsevier Health Sciences
7. Fabbrocini G, Annunziata MC, D'Arco V, De Vita V, Lodi G, Mauriello MC et al (2010) Acne scars: pathogenesis, classification and treatment. Dermatol Res Pract 2010:893080
8. Profyris C, Tziotzios C, Do VI (2012) Cutaneous scarring: pathophysiology, molecular mechanisms, and scar reduction therapeutics part I. the molecular basis of scar formation. J Am Acad Dermatol 66(1):1–10. quiz 1-2
9. You HJ, Kim DW, Yoon ES, Park SH (2016) Comparison of four different lasers for acne scars: resurfacing and fractional lasers. J Plast Reconstr Aesthet Surg 69(4):e87–e95
10. Bhargava S, Cunha PR, Lee J, Kroumpouzos G (2018) Acne scarring management: systematic review and evaluation of the evidence. Am J Clin Dermatol 19(4):459–477
11. Dreno B (2004) Acne: physical treatment. Clin Dermatol 22(5):429–433
12. Arndt KA, Dover JS, Alam M (2006) Scar revision. Elsevier/Saunders
13. Safonov I (2012) Atlas of scar treatment and correction. Springer Science & Business Media
14. Jemec GB, Jemec B (2004) Acne: treatment of scars. Clin Dermatol 22(5):434–438
15. Ogawa R (2020) Total scar management. Springer, Singapore
16. Bolognia J, Schaffer JV, Cerroni L (2018) Dermatology. Elsevier
17. Tung R, Rubin MG (2010) Procedures in cosmetic dermatology series: chemical peels E-book. Elsevier Health Sciences
18. Monheit GD (2011) Commentary: complication of CROSS technique on boxcar acne scars: atrophy. Dermatol Surg 37(1):95–96
19. Weber MB, Machado RB, Hoefel IR, Manzoni AP, Da Silva Bastos Geler A (2011) Complication of CROSS-technique on boxcar acne scars: atrophy. Dermatol Surg 37(1):93–95
20. Lee JB, Chung WG, Kwahck H, Lee KH (2002) Focal treatment of acne scars with trichloroacetic acid: chemical reconstruction of skin scars method. Dermatol Surg 28(11):1017–1021. discussion 21
21. Yug A, Lane JE, Howard MS, Kent DE (2006) Histologic study of depressed acne scars treated with serial high-concentration (95%) trichloroacetic acid. Dermatol Surg 32(8):985–990. discussion 90
22. Ahmed R, Mohammed G, Ismail N, Elakhras A (2014) Randomized clinical trial of CO(2) LASER pinpoint irradiation technique versus chemical reconstruction of skin scars (CROSS) in treating ice pick acne scars. J Cosmet Laser Ther 16(1):8–13
23. Raulin C, Karsai S (2011) Laser and IPL technology in dermatology and aesthetic medicine. Heidelberg: New York
24. Schweiger ES, Sundick L (2013) Focal acne scar treatment (FAST), a new approach to atrophic acne scars: a case series. J Drugs Dermatol 12(10):1163–1167
25. Hruza GJ, Tanzi EL (2018) Lasers and lights. Elsevier, Edinburgh
26. Lee JW, Kim BJ, Kim MN, Mun SK (2011) The efficacy of autologous platelet rich plasma combined with ablative carbon dioxide fractional resurfacing for acne scars: a simultaneous split-face trial. Dermatol Surg 37(7):931–938
27. Yu M, Lee JY (2017) Polydeoxyribonucleotide improves wound healing of fractional laser resurfacing in rat model. J Cosmet Laser Ther 19(1):43–48
28. Chae WS, Seong JY, Jung HN, Kong SH, Kim MH, Suh HS et al (2015) Comparative study on efficacy and safety of 1550 nm Er: glass fractional laser and fractional radiofrequency microneedle device for facial atrophic acne scar. J Cosmet Dermatol 14(2):100–106
29. Schomacker K, Bhawalkar JD. Mechanisms of Action of Fractionated 532nm and 1064nm Picosecond Laser for Skin Rejuvenation. https://www.semanticscholar.org/paper/Mechanisms-of-Action-of-Fractionated-532-nm-and-nm/9634c2b994648ecdc63b2576bd6223b0af0ac056#related-papers

30. Habbema L, Verhagen R, Van Hal R, Liu Y, Varghese B (2012) Minimally invasive non-thermal laser technology using laser-induced optical breakdown for skin rejuvenation. J Biophotonics 5(2):194–199
31. Tanghetti EA (2016) The histology of skin treated with a picosecond alexandrite laser and a fractional lens array. Lasers Surg Med 48(7):646–652
32. Brauer JA, Kazlouskaya V, Alabdulrazzaq H, Bae YS, Bernstein LJ, Anolik R et al (2015) Use of a picosecond pulse duration laser with specialized optic for treatment of facial acne scarring. JAMA Dermatol 151(3):278–284
33. Bernstein EF, Schomacker KT, Basilavecchio LD, Plugis JM, Bhawalkar JD (2017) Treatment of acne scarring with a novel fractionated, dual-wavelength, picosecond-domain laser incorporating a novel holographic beam-splitter. Lasers Surg Med 49(9):796–802
34. Kang WH, Kim YJ, Pyo WS, Park SJ, Kim JH (2009) Atrophic acne scar treatment using triple combination therapy: dot peeling, subcision and fractional laser. J Cosmet Laser Ther 11(4):212–215
35. Lee Y (2013) Scars and scarring: causes, types and treatment options. Nova Science Publishers, Inc.
36. Lee Y (2009) Combination treatment of surgical, post-traumatic and post-herpetic scars with ablative lasers followed by fractional laser and non-ablative laser in Asians. Lasers Surg Med 41(2):131–140
37. Lee Y (2018) Combination treatments of facial atrophic post-acne scars: retrospective analysis of 248 pairs of pre- and post-treatment photographs. J Dermatol Forecast 1(1):1–10
38. Lee SJ, Seok J, Jeong SY, Park KY, Li K, Seo SJ (2016) Facial pores: definition, causes, and treatment options. Dermatol Surg 42(3):277–285
39. Rose AE, Goldberg DJ (2013) Safety and efficacy of intradermal injection of botulinum toxin for the treatment of oily skin. Dermatol Surg 39(3 Pt 1):443–448
40. Toosi S, Ehsani AH, Noormohammadpoor P, Esmaili N, Mirshams-Shahshahani M, Moineddin F (2010) Treatment of trichostasis spinulosa with a 755-nm long-pulsed alexandrite laser. J Eur Acad Dermatol Venereol 24(4):470–473
41. Badawi A, Kashmar M (2011) Treatment of trichostasis spinulosa with 0.5-millisecond pulsed 755-nm alexandrite laser. Lasers Med Sci 26(6):825–829
42. Kim HW, Chang SE, Kim JE, Ko JY, Ro YS (2014) The safe delivery of fractional ablative carbon dioxide laser treatment for acne scars in Asian patients receiving oral isotretinoin. Dermatol Surg 40(12):1361–1366
43. Spring LK, Krakowski AC, Alam M, Bhatia A, Brauer J, Cohen J et al (2017) Isotretinoin and timing of procedural interventions: a systematic review with consensus recommendations. JAMA Dermatol 153(8):802–809

12 Etiology and Treatments of Melasma

12.1 Introduction

12.1.1 Definition of Melasma

Melasma is a common hypermelanosis that occurs in areas exposed to sunlight, especially the face. It occurs rarely before puberty and is commonly observed in women, especially women of childbearing age. It is also observed in 10% of men. New melasma often arises and existing melasma may worsen during pregnancy. Symptoms appear as brown macules with irregular borders and occur symmetrically in the photodistribution of sunlight on the face. They are often fused in a reticular pattern. They are darkened by sunlight, which makes them worse during summer and improves during winter, i.e., there is a seasonal change. Melasma is common among Asian and Hispanic women who live in areas with strong sunlight. It occurs frequently in patients with Fitzpatrick skin types IV, V, and VI [1].

Melasma may be classified into three types by facial patterns: centrofacial, malar, and mandibular (Fig. 12.1). The centrofacial pattern accounts for 63% of melasma and affects the forehead,

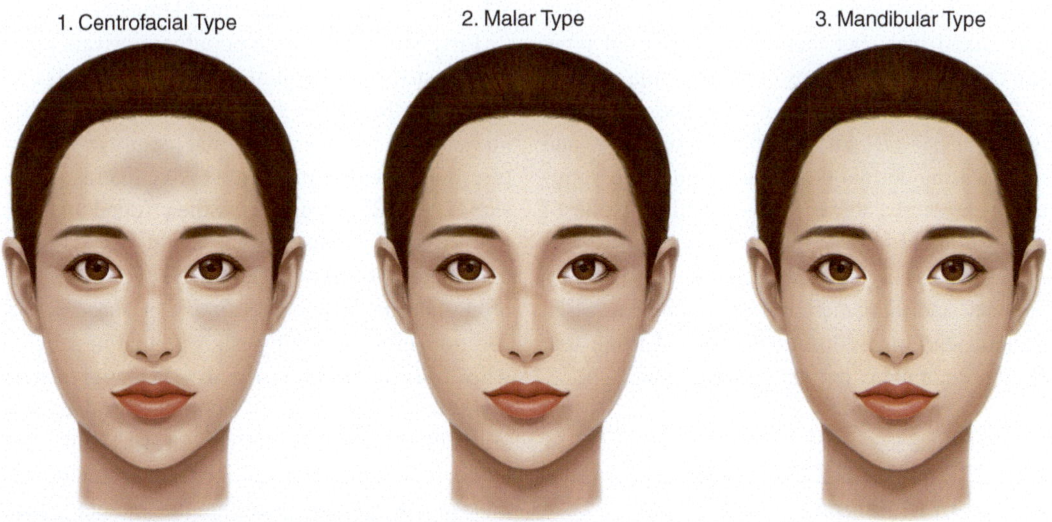

Fig. 12.1 Types of melasma according to its distribution. (Reproduced from [2])

J. D. Lee et al., *Principles and Choice of Laser Treatment in Dermatology*,
https://doi.org/10.1007/978-981-15-6556-4_12

nose, chin, and upper lip. The malar pattern accounts for 21% of melasma and is restricted to the nose and malar cheeks on the face. The mandibular melasma accounts for 16% of melasma and occurs along the mandibular ramus. A newer pattern termed extra-facial melasma can occur on non-facial body parts, including the neck, sternum, forearms, and upper extremities [1]. But, classifying melasma by distribution does not seem clinically meaningful. However, we know empirically that melasma under the eyes are treatment-resistant.

Melasma may also be classified into three types histologically, by the depth of melanin pigments: epidermal, dermal, and mixed. Wood's lamp is used to distinguish between epidermal and dermal melasma. Epidermal melasma is accentuated while dermal melasma is not. Epidermal melasma responds better to topical treatment compared to dermal melasma [1].

Lee et al. studied 411 melasma patients at five university hospitals in Korea [3]. Melasma was classified into three types. Regular borders with brownish color were classified as epidermal type. Irregular border with bluish color was classified as the dermal type. When both epidermal and dermal types were seen, they were classified as a mixed type. According to this study, 36% (145 patients) had epidermal type, 64% (235 patients) had mixed type, but there was no dermal type. Kar et al. performed biopsies on melasma patients in India [4]; 51.66% (31 patients) had epidermal type, 48.33% (29 patients) had mixed type, and there was no dermal type. The results were similar to the study above. Based on the results of both studies, I believe that mixed-type melasma makes up a high percentage of all melasma patients, and thus, melasma treatments are often difficult and time-consuming. Also, I think that there are not many dermal type melasma.

12.1.2 Differential Diagnosis of Melasma

The differential diagnosis for melasma includes nevus of Ota, abnormal bilateral nevus of Ota like macule (ABNOM, Hori's macules), medication-induced hyperpigmentation, erythema dyschromicum perstans (EDP), Lichen planus pigmentosus, abrupti dermacation between sideburn and the lighter skin posteriorly, lichenoid drug eruption, Riel's melanosis, post-inflammatory hyperpigmentation (PIH), maturational dyschromia, periorbital hyperpigmentation, acanthosis nigricans, ephelides, lentigines, exogenous ochronosis, etc. [5].

Rodriques et al. mentioned two features of melasma that are helpful in differentiating from other pigmentation disorders [5]. First, melasma occurs in the orbital rim and rarely in the mandible. Second, melasma is neither dark, such as pigmentation by medication-induced hyperpigmentation or erythema dyschromicum perstans (EDP) nor gray like cement. In practice, however, it is often difficult to differently diagnose melasma.

12.2 Issues of Melasma

Laser treatment of melasma may cause three problems. First, latent melasma may convert to actual melasma. Second, existing melasma may get worse. Third, after laser treatment, melasma can occur even in areas not irradiated by laser. We will review these three problems one by one.

First, when IPLs were popular in private practice, post-IPL pigmentations similar to melasma were often found. Negishi et al. studied this phenomenon by comparing normal pictures with pictures taken with ultraviolet (UV) cameras [6]. A survey of 223 Japanese women found that 63 (28.3%) had melasma that could not be seen under normal light but could be seen with UV light. That is, latent melasma was observed. In addition, clinical findings showed that in patients who had latent melasma by UV light, new melasma occurred in the clinically same area after IPL. During laser treatment, it is important to keep in mind that although we cannot see melasma when we examine the patient's face with our bare eyes, there is always a possibility of latent melasma.

Second, when treating melasma with laser parameters known to be effective in other pigmentation disorders, melasma may seem to disappear at first but becomes darker with time, and then with another laser treatment, it may seem to disappear again, only to become darker again. Thus, the vicious cycle. If melasma is not diagnosed accurately and treated like another pigmentation disorder, melasma can get worse. Therefore, accurate diagnosis is important in melasma.

Third, after laser treatment, melasma can occur even in areas not irradiated by laser. Lee et al. treated a 37-year-old female patient with ABNOM with 1064-nm Q-switched Nd:YAG laser five times at 4-week intervals [7]. A month later melasma was observed around the ABNOM. Melasma occurred in areas not irradiated by laser (Fig. 12.2).

The three problems reviewed above—Latent melasma converting to actual melasma. Existing melasma getting worse. Newfound melasma after treating other pigmentation disorders such as ABNOM—may happen during laser treatment in private practice. These situations gave both the doctor and the patients a hard time. So, in the past, lasers were contraindicated in treating melasma.

Although not explicitly mentioned in papers and books, I believe that activated melanocytes are the fundamental issue for these causes.

12.3 Causes and Theories of Melasma

Why does this happen? The pathogenesis of melasma is not well known, but biologically active melanocytes, genetic causes, hormonal effects, and UV light are known to be important [8]. I especially believe that activated melanocytes are the fundamental issue. Other causes may include birth control pills, estrogen replacement therapy, mild ovarian or thyroid dysfunction, ovarian tumors, cosmetics, nutrition, phototoxicity, photoallergic drugs, and epilepsy drugs [8].

However, recent papers have been published that are contrary to the causes of existing melasma. First, a study of 324 patients at 12 medical facilities in nine countries found that only about 50% of melasma patients had a family history [9]. Melasma occurred usually in the 20s and 30s, but some occurred in the 40s (14%) and 50s (6%). Melasma occurred early in brighter skin while it occurred late in darker skin type (Fitzpatrick skin type V, VI), some even after menopause. Thus, it is likely that racial causes are more likely to be a cause of melasma than familial causes. In terms of hormonal effects, only 20% of melasma patients developed melasma during pregnancy and contraceptives

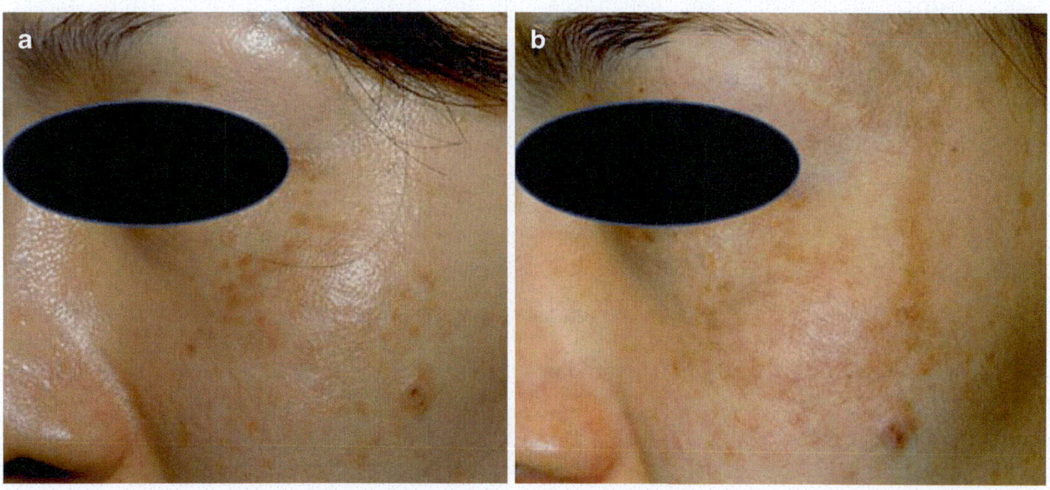

Fig. 12.2 (**a**) Clinical photography of ABNOM before the laser treatment. Small, bilateral, blue-brown discrete patches on both cheeks and periorbital area. (**b**) Newly developed melasma lesion on the left periorbital area. Irregular brownish confluenting patches are noted. (Reproduced from [7])

had a minor effect on melasma occurrence. And although UV radiation is known to be a major cause of melasma recurrence, melasma recurrence has been reported in many of the melasma patients who applied sunscreen thoroughly. Recently there are reports that visible light rather than ultraviolet light (UVB) is another cause of increased skin pigmentation, especially in Fitzpatrick skin types IV–VI. Thus, there are arguments that sunscreens have limited preventive effects and colored sunscreens (such as BB creams) that block visible lights may be more effective in preventing melasma from recurring.

It is interesting that cosmetics are among the causes of melasma. Kenichirou Kasai, the author of the "Skin spots treatment clinics," suggested that the cause of melasma was due to "breakdown of barriers caused by chronic hyperstimulation (too much rubbing)" [10]. In other words, it is hypothesized that melasma occurs by the same mechanism as PIH to protect the skin as the skin barrier is broken due to the chronic hyperstimulation caused by cosmetics. Kasai, a Japanese medical doctor in private practice, examined melasma patients, and found interesting trends (chronic hyperstimulation) in melasma patients. He observed that there was always "barrier destruction" in the melasma lesion area and no "barrier destruction" in areas without melasma. In addition, it was observed that when measures to reduce barrier breakdown were undertaken melasma was alleviated and when measures to worsen the barrier were undertaken melasma also worsened. Also, the age at which melasma occurs coincides with the age at which one "wears cosmetics." There was no melasma in children or the elderly, who did not wear cosmetics.

Kasai believes that daily makeup and makeup removal are the main causes of skin barrier destruction. In addition, applying and removing various cosmetic products to hide the melasma, further destroys the skin barrier and makes the melasma worse. Therefore, the reason that many skin problems (e.g., poison ivy allergic contact dermatitis, erythema, flaking, etc.) are common in melasma patients could be explained by skin barrier destruction. For this reason, Kasai speculates that melasma topical treatments may cause irritation symptoms and frequent side effects.

However, since these speculations are only hypotheses based on simple observations, Kasai says he has published a book called "Skin spots treatment clinics" in the hope that future generations will confirm that the hypothesis is correct. Now we will review various papers to see whether Kasai's hypothesis is true, i.e., whether skin barrier destruction by chronic hyperstimulation may be a cause of melasma.

12.3.1 Pathology of Melasma

In order to investigate the causes of melasma, we will review the histological characteristics of melasma in various papers.

Grimes et al. compared the histological examination of melasma skin and surrounding normal skin in 21 melasma patients [11]. The results showed that mild lymphohistiocytic infiltrates were present in 75% of the hyperpigmented areas. The areas of hyperpigmentation showed increased deposition of melanin in the epidermis and dermis of all cases. There was a statistically significant increase in the content of epidermal melanin. There were no quantitative increases in melanocytes in the hyperpigmented areas of skin. However, the melanocytes in the hyperpigmented areas were larger, intensely stained cells with very prominent dendrites. Electron microscopy revealed more melanosomes in keratinocytes, melanocytes, and dendrites in the involved skin in comparison to the uninvolved skin. The number of dendrites per melanocyte was increased in comparison with normal skin (normal skin 5.28 ± 1.85, melasma skin 7.55 ± 2.53, $p < 0.05$). The results of this study suggest that melasma is a consequence of specific "hyperactive" melanocytes with increased melanogenesis, resulting in increased epidermal melanin and dermal melanophages.

Kang et al. compared the histological examination of melasma skin and surrounding normal skin in 56 Korean melasma patients [12]. The results showed that melanin was significantly increased in the epidermis, especially in the basal layer. In addition, a statistically significant increase in solar elastosis was observed in melasma skin compared to normal skin. Electron microscopic findings revealed that melanocytes in melasma skin had more mitochondria, Golgi apparatus, rough endoplasmic reticulum, and ribosomes than normal melanocytes (Fig. 12.3). In other words, melanocytes in the melasma skin are "activated melanocytes" which are more activated than normal to make melanin, and actually make more melanosomes.

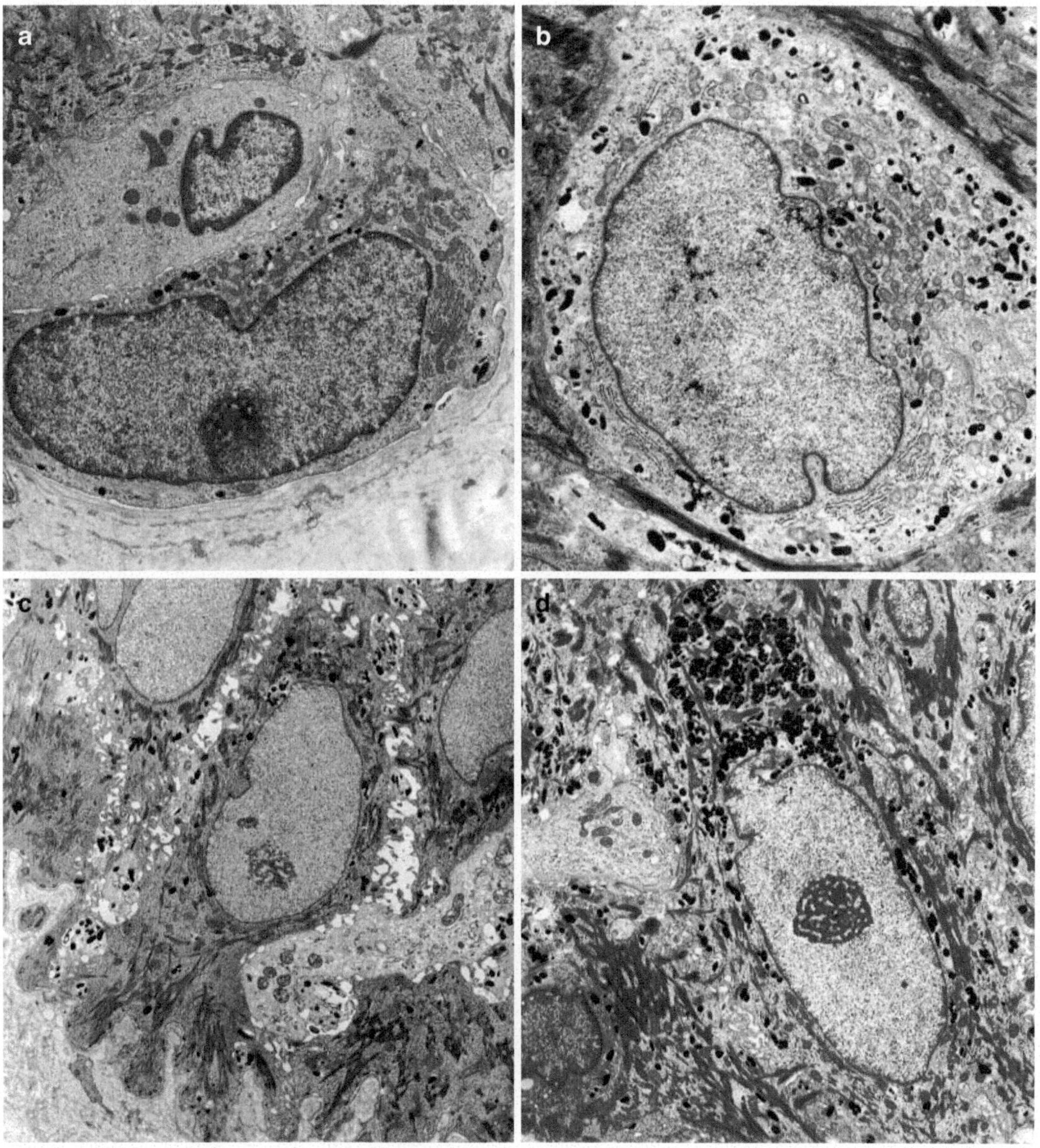

Fig. 12.3 Electron microscopy of perilesional skin and melasma skin. Melanocytes in (**a**) perilesional skin and (**b**) melasma skin. Lesional melanocytes were filled with more mitochondria, Golgi apparatus, rough endoplasmic reticulum, and ribosomes in the perikaryon than were normal skin melanocytes. Basal keratinocytes in (**c**) perilesional skin and (**d**) melasma skin. More melanosomes were seen in membrane-bound clusters and were more densely packed in the basal keratinocytes in melasma skin than in normal facial skin (original magnification: **a**,**b**, ×7000; **c**,**d**, ×4400). (Reproduced from [12])

Kang et al. observed melasma through equipment called reflectance confocal microscopy (RCM) and compared the results with histology [13]. The results are as follows. First, compared to normal skin, melasma skin has an increased melanin pigment and flattened rete ridge. Flattened rete ridges are phenomena that are observed when the skin ages. Second, the number of dendrites per melanocyte was increased in activated melanocytes. Third, melanocytes were seen as dropping cells from the epidermis to the dermis (protruded melanocytes). Fourth, melanophages were observed in the dermis. Fifth, there was a significant increase in solar elastosis and blood vessels in the dermis, which is a sign of aging and inflammation. Finally, melanophages were found in the dermis, but only in a portion of melasma skin. The distribution was very heterogenous when observed by a microscope.

12.3.2 Recent Papers on Melasma

Now we will look at some papers that suggest the causes of melasma.

Noh et al. investigated the inflammatory features of melasma [14]. Hundred and ninety-seven women with melasma completed a questionnaire concerning triggering or aggravating factors. These cases were divided into "non-inflammatory" and "inflammatory" groups. The questionnaire examined 31 factors including aggravating factors and inflammatory response factors. Inflammatory responses were classified into seven categories: itching/tingling sensation, dryness, erythema/telangiectasia (Table 12.1). If the patient had more than five out of seven responses, they were classified as the "inflammatory" group.

Table 12.1 Inflammatory response item in the questionnaire. (Modified from [14])

Itching/ tingling sensation	1. Aggravation of melasma after itching 2. Sensitivity or itching in response to cosmetics
Dryness	3. Aggravation of melasma after dryness 4. Severe dryness after washing 5. Misuse of strong soap or moisturizer
Erythema/ telangiectasia	6. Aggravation of melasma after erythema 7. Facial flushing

Among the 197 subjects, 50 patients (25.4%) were categorized into the inflammatory group. Biopsy showed that the inflammatory group had statistically significant basement membrane disruption, rete ridge flattening, basal hyperpigmentation, inflammatory cell infiltration, and solar elastosis compared to the non-inflammatory group. Immunohistochemistry showed that $CD68^+$ melanophages and $CD117^+$ mast cells (inflammatory cells) and LCA^+ leukocytes were significantly increased in the inflammatory group. Therefore, Noh et al. suggested that inflammation should be considered as a major cause of melasma, such as UV rays and hormones, which are already known as major causes of melasma. Noh et al. also suggest that melasma should be divided into inflammatory melasma and non-inflammatory melasma, and treatment should be different for these two melasmas.

Kang et al. obtained skin samples of lesional and nonlesional facial skin of 52 Korean women with melasma [15]. Immunohistochemistry and reverse transcriptase-polymerase chain reaction (RT-PCR) analysis was performed to determine the expression of stem cell factor (SCF) and c-kit in melasma. SCF is known as a cytokine for melanogenesis. SCF is observed in keratinocytes in the epidermis and in fibroblasts in the dermis.

1. The SCF of the dermis was 0.014 ± 0.012 in melasma skin and 0.005 ± 0.004 in normal skin. That is, the SCF of the dermis was increased in melasma skin ($p < 0.001$). The SCF of the epidermis was 0.48 ± 0.11 in melasma skin and 0.43 ± 0.19 in normal skin, which was statistically not significant ($p = 0.5$).
2. C-kit of the epidermis was 0.14 ± 0.017 in melasma skin and 0.08 ± 0.06 in normal skin. That is, c-kit increased in the epidermis of melasma skin ($p < 0.005$). Also, c-kit concentration per unit area of the epidermis was 25,375 ± 1023 in melasma skin and 18,124 ± 1044 in normal skin. That is, c-kit concentration was statistically significantly increased in the epidermis of melasma skin

($p < 0.005$). However, there was no difference in the concentration of c-kit in the dermis of melasma and normal skin, which were 3.13 ± 6.0 and 2.75 ± 4.8 cm^{-1}, in melasma and normal skin respectively.

In other words, SCF-producing melanin was observed in dermal fibroblasts. The discovery of SCF in the dermis is related to inflammation. Dermal fibroblasts are known to secrete SCF in response to inflammation. In contrast, c-kit, the receptor for SCF, was found only in the epidermis, not the dermis. In conclusion, it can be assumed that SCF increased in the dermis due to dermal inflammation and binds to c-kit of epidermal keratinocytes and causes melanogenesis in the epidermis.

Recently, senescent fibroblasts have been reported to be associated with melasma as well as solar lentigo. Fibroblasts are known to secrete more skin aging-associated secreted proteins (SAAP) than normal fibroblasts as they age. SAAP not only includes secreted factors that regulate the extracellular matrix but also includes melanogenic cytokine that makes pigments such as stem cell factors (SCF), keratinocyte growth factors (KGF), and hepatocyte growth factors (HGF). Kim et al. obtained skin samples of the lesional and nonlesional facial skin of 38 women with melasma and investigated cells with the senescent maker $p16^{INK4A}$ [16]. The results showed that there was no difference in the number of $p16^{INK4A}$ cells in the epidermis of melasma and normal skin, whereas the number of cells in the melasma dermis was higher than that of normal skin (5.58 ± 4.55 vs. 2.05 ± 1.71, $p < 0.001$). In particular, most of the cells were congregated in the superficial dermis near dermo-epidermal junction rather than the deep dermis. That is, in melasma, we can see that aging cells are accumulated in the dermis. To remove aged fibroblasts, Kim et al. performed invasive bipolar radiofrequency needle RF (SYLFIRM™, Viol, Gyeonggi, Korea) on three patients by repeat method (in the original paper, this was expressed as "pulsed type") and compared the results. The patients were treated five times at 2 weeks intervals with level 2, needle penetration depth 1.5 mm, using 25 insulated needles at 2 MHz. The results showed clinically improved melasma and improved lightness value (54.67 ± 6.20 vs. 60.87 ± 4.32). Histologically, the number of $p16^{INK4A}$ cells was reduced and procollagen-1 associated with epidermal pigment reduction was increased. Epidermal pigmentation by Fontana-Masson stain was also reduced.

Based on the results of these two papers, it can be assumed that dermal inflammation and aged fibroblasts make epidermal pigmentations. It can also be assumed that epidermal and dermal tissues are both involved in the production of epidermal pigmentations.

Kim et al. investigated vascular endothelial growth factor (VEGF), the major angiogenic factor of the skin in melasma patients [17]. First, the a* value indicating the degree of erythema was measured using a colorimeter. Second, the melasma and normal areas were compared by biopsy in 50 Korean female patients with melasma. Third, factor VIIIa-related antigen and VEGF were measured by immunohistochemistry. The results were as follows. The a* values of the right and left cheeks of normal skin were 10.24 ± 1.35 and 10.53 ± 1.73, respectively, and the a* values of right and left cheeks of melasma skin were 12.92 ± 1.96 and 12.78 ± 2.19, respectively. The a* value was higher in melasma skin ($p < 001$). Also compared to normal skin, melasma skin had higher blood vessel thickness (16.28%), blood vessel density (33.89%), and blood vessel area (68.75%). The number of blood vessels and the degree of melasma pigmentation showed a statistically significant correlation. Finally, a comparison of the staining area per unit epidermal area of VEGF showed that normal skin was 0.137 ± 0.132 and melasma skin was 0.270 ± 0.237, indicating higher VEGF concentration ($p = 0.034$). Kim et al. suggested the following opinions by analyzing the above results. Increased vascularization is a characteristic feature of the aging process, so melasma can be thought of not only as an epidermal pigmentation disorder but also as a unique phenotype due to photodamaging [17]. Thus, melasma treatment requires not only pigmentation treatments but also anti-aging and anti-angiogenic treatment.

Hernadez-Barrera et al. evaluated mast cells and solar elastosis areas in biopsies of 27 melasma patients using a computer-assisted image-analysis [18]. Melasma skin had abundant elastotic material compared with normal skin (13.3 ± 2.8% vs. 10.2 ± 2.9%, $p < 0.001$). Mast cells were more prominent in the elastotic areas of melasma skin (173 ± 57% vs. 145 ± 57%, $p = 0.04$). This paper shows that solar elastosis is observed in the dermis and mast cells are also increased, as seen in the Sect. 12.3.1. Solar elastosis is known to be mainly caused by photoaging, so it can be considered that photoaging plays an important role in the occurrence of melasma. In the paper above, the phenomenon of increased blood vessels was also thought to be caused by photoaging. However, I think that solar elastosis and increased blood vessels in melasma are not only caused by UV light but is also due to damage to the dermis by various irritation and inflammation.

The role of mast cells in melasma is not yet known, but some studies have shown that histamine plays a role in melanogenesis [19, 20]. In other words, UV rays increase histamine secretion in mast cells and histamine promotes melanocyte proliferation and migration. There is also a paper on the relationship between mast cells and photoaging, suggesting that there is a significant increase in mast cells in photoaged skin. Therefore, some papers consider the role of mast cells important in melasma, like the Fig. 12.4 [20].

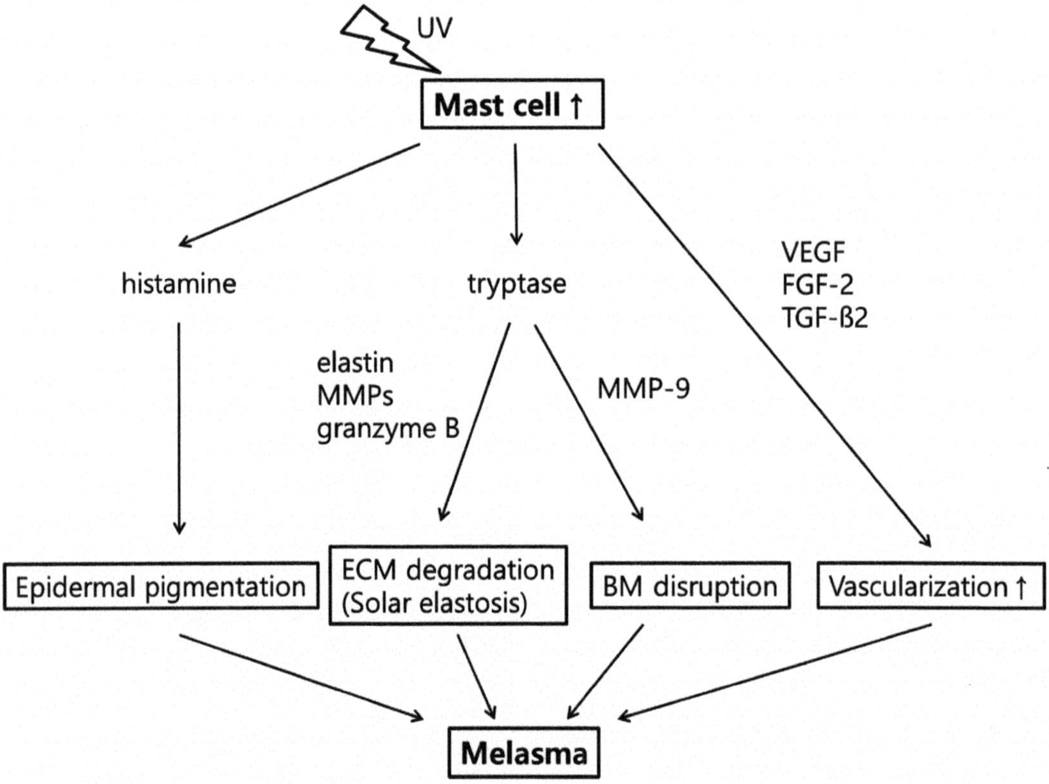

Fig. 12.4 The role of mast cells in melanogenesis and photoaging. *UV* ultraviolet, *MMPs* matrix metalloproteases, *VEGF* vascular endothelial growth factor, *FGF-2* fibroblast growth factor-2, *TGF-β* transforming growth factor-β, *ECM* extracellular matrix, *BM* basement membrane. (Reproduced from [20])

12.3.3 Defective Barrier Function and Pigment Incontinence

Lee et al. compared the lesional and perilesional normal skin of 16 melasma patients [21]. The stratum corneum hydration was significantly higher in lesional skin than in perilesional normal skin. No significant difference was found between lesional and normal skin in terms of basal transepidermal water loss (TEWL) level. However, the rate of TEWL after barrier perturbation was significantly higher for lesional skin and the barrier recovery rate was significantly delayed (Fig. 12.5). Biopsy was performed on 11 of the 16 patients, and the stratum corneum was thinner at the melasma area than in normal skin (melasma, 10.4 ± 2.9 μm; normal, 14.5 ± 5.5 μm, $p = 0.052$). Furthermore, this was correlated with the barrier recovery rate (correlation coefficient, 0.721). Six of the 11 patients who underwent biopsy showed lower peroxisome proliferator-activated receptor alpha (PPAR-α), an important factor for lipid metabolism.

The papers earlier show that the barrier function of melasma skin is decreased, especially the barrier recovery rate.

Shin et al. reported a case report of two patients with unusual histological findings [22].

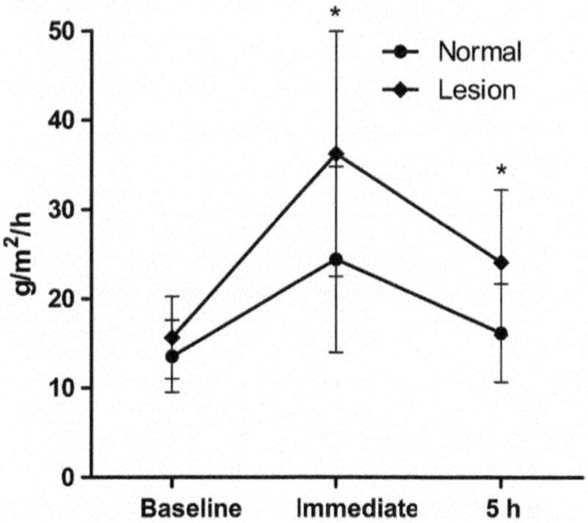

Fig. 12.5 Epidermal permeability barrier function. TEWL was significantly higher after barrier perturbation in lesional skin. A significantly delayed barrier recovery rate was demonstrated in lesional skin 5 h after repeated tape stripping. *$P < 0.05$. (Reproduced from [21])

The first patient showed histological findings of melanocytes or keratinocytes protruding into the dermis. The second patient showed dermal melanocytosis, i.e., melanocytes present in the dermal layer, such as Ota's nevus or ABNOM. However, unlike the melanocytes which are located at a depth of 1.3 ± 0.1 mm in the Ota's nevus, the melanocytes of this patient were located at 0.35 mm, which was very shallower in comparison. The combined histological findings of the two patients showed that prolonged sun exposure turns epidermal melanocytes into pendulous melanocytes, which eventually fall into the dermis, resulting in dermal melanocytosis. Therefore, the authors of this paper concluded that considering these histological findings, different treatments for epidermis, dermis, and basement membrane are needed.

Torres-Alvarez et al. evaluated melasma lesions and compared them with perilesional skin and photo-protected skin [23]. They took samples from lesional and photo-protected nonlesional (buttocks) skin in 24 patients (group A). In the other 24 patients, they took biopsies of lesional and perilesional (10 mm away from melasma) skin (group B). In group A, histologic examination of Periodic acid–Schiff (PAS) staining revealed the total absence of basement membrane in three of 24 patients (12.5%) and in 87.5%, the basement membrane was missing or partially broken. The loss rate of the basement membrane per biopsy was 25.85 ± 11%. In group B, the total absence of the basement membrane was observed in three patients (12.5%). In melasma skin, 95.8% of the tissues showed basement membrane loss, higher than the surrounding skin (58.3%). In addition, basement membrane loss per tissue was 23 ± 2%, which was statistically significantly higher than that of the surrounding normal skin (15 ± 7%) ($p < 0.002$) (Fig. 12.6). Immunohistochemistry of anti-collagen IV showed that the basement membrane loss in melasma skin was 83%, which was higher than normal skin (66%) (Fig. 12.7). In addition, basement membrane loss per tissue in melasma skin was 19.3 ± 14.4%, which was statistically significantly higher than that of normal skin (10 ± 14.8%) ($p < 0.054$).

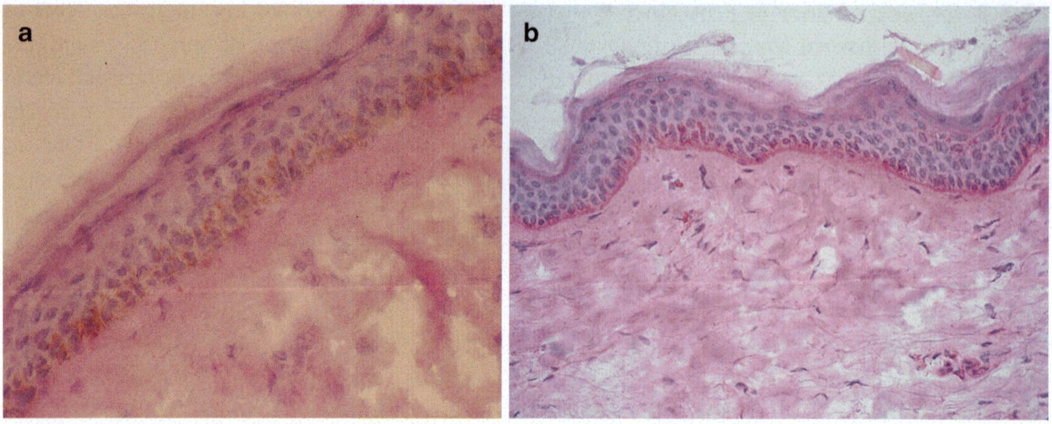

Fig. 12.6 PAS stain sections showing an absence of basal membrane in melasma skin (**a**), the integrity of the basal membrane in the perilesional skin of the same patient (**b**). Original magnification ×400. (Reproduced from [23])

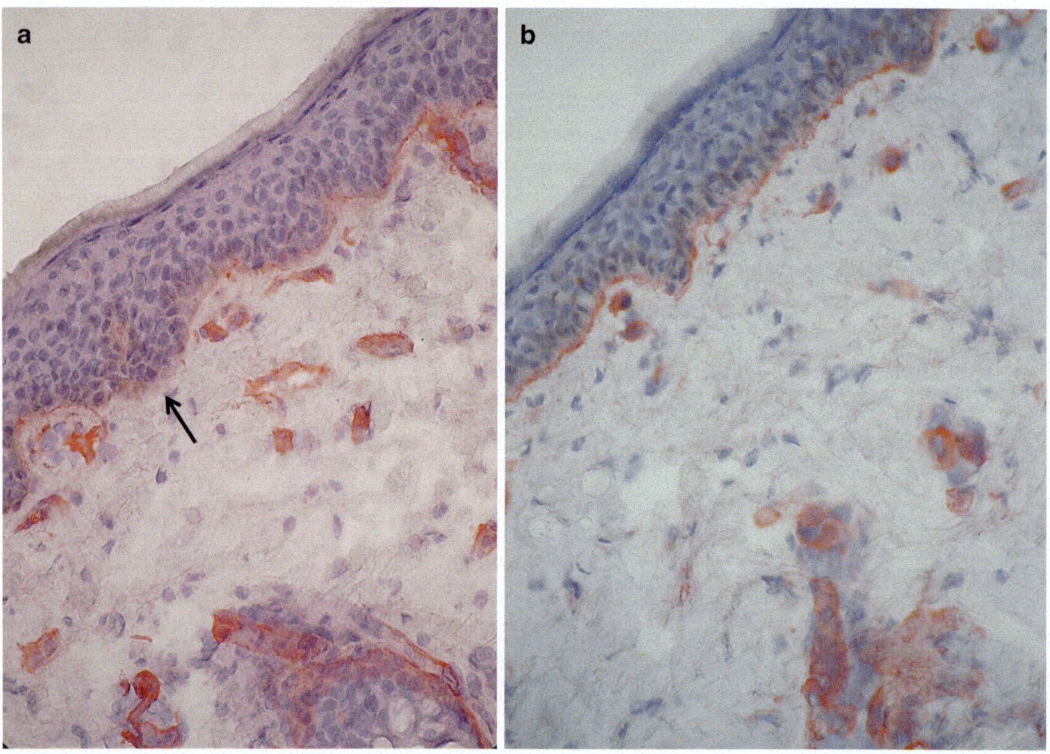

Fig. 12.7 Immunohistochemistry with antibody to collagen type IV showing disruption (arrow pointing) of basal membrane in melasma skin (**a**), integrity of the basal membrane in perilesional skin of the same patient (**b**). Original magnification ×400. (Reproduced from [23])

Pigment incontinence is a histological phenomenon of melanin accumulation in the upper dermis [24]. Normally, there should be no pigmentations in the dermis. The reason for melanin accumulation in the dermis is related to the damage to the basal layer of the epidermis and basement membrane. Due to the inflammation of the basal layer, the basal layer and the basement membrane becomes damaged and keratinocytes or melanocytes with melanin fall into the dermal layer. Histologically, melanocytes and melanophages (melanosomes phagocytosed by macrophages) are observed in the dermal layer.

In the papers earlier, pigment incontinence is also observed in melasma. Melasma may be classified into three types histologically, by the depth of melanin pigments: epidermal, dermal, and mixed. Considering pigment incontinence seen in melasma, I speculate that original melasma may have been present only in the epidermal type and then progressed to mixed or dermal type due to pigment incontinence. This is probably the reason why epidermal and mixed melasma is more common than dermal melasma. Also due to damage to the basement membrane and pigment incontinence, melasma treatment is challenging and melasma relapse is common. Therefore, there is a need for procedures that can restore the basement membrane to prevent recurrence and improve long-term results.

12.3.4 Sensitive Skin

In one laser book, melasma is explained as follows [25]. "Melasma is characterized by asymptomatic inflammation, i.e., subclinical, invisible, mild inflammation. In other words, melasma is sensitive skin." I have also observed that melasma patients had more sensitive skin than other patients. And among those with melasma, patients with sensitive skin did not respond well to treatment. In addition, I have experienced melasma occurrence in patients with sensitive skin, and thus treat patients with sensitive skin as if they have melasma, although they do not have melasma.

12.4 Probable Causes of Melasma

I summarized the histological findings in melasma, in the Table 12.2. Probable causes and mechanisms of melasma are summarized in the Table 12.3. Based on the contents so far, I think the probable mechanism of melasma is as follows. "In patients with genetically or hormonally sensitive skin, inflammation may be caused by chronic irritation, such as UV rays or cosmetics, this may break the epidermal barrier, resulting in the damaged basement membrane and inflammation in the dermis. In order to protect the damaged skin, pigmentations appear on the epidermal layer, thus melasma occurs."

Then how should we treat melasma? First, we can't change the genetic factor, but since melasma is associated with estrogen, low-dose estrogen contraceptives (e.g., Yaz®) should be recommended for patients taking birth control pills. In addition, UV protection should be thorough, and the skin should not be irritated. Second, the epidermis, basement membrane, and the dermis should all be regenerated to repair damaged skin. The inflammation of the dermis should be reduced as well. That is, the whole skin needs to be improved. Finally, the activity of the melanocytes should be reduced, new pigmentation should not be made and already formed pigmentation should be removed. The specifics will be reviewed later.

Table 12.2 Histological findings in melasma

Histological findings in melasma
1. Epidermal thinning, rete ridge flattening
2. Increased epidermal pigment. Melanocytosis?
3. Activated melanocytes in the epidermis.
4. Damage in the basement membrane. Protruded melanocytes.
5. Melanophages in the dermis. Very heterogeneous.
6. A significant increase in solar elastosis and blood vessels in the dermis.
7. Perivascular lymphohistiocytic infiltrate, mast cell infiltration

Table 12.3 Probable causes and mechanisms of melasma

Probable causes of melasma	Probable mechanism of melasma
Active melanocyte Genetics, hormone, UV, cosmetics, etc. Inflammation	1. Epidermal barrier dysfunction 2. Basement membrane disruption 3. Dermal inflammation 4. Epidermal hyperpigmentation

Like Kenichirou Kasai, I also see the "breakdown of barriers caused by chronic hyperstimulation (too much rubbing)" as the main cause of melasma. In addition to Kasai's hypothesis, I attached papers that studied the histological findings of the melasma and papers that suggest the causes of the melasma. But these are all still hypotheses. It is just one step further from Kasai. Like Kasai, I am also in private practice, and there are difficulties performing clinical or experimental studies. I also look forward to seeing the exact mechanism of melasma unfold through future studies.

12.5 Treatment of Melasma

12.5.1 Consensus on Melasma Treatment

The three major treatment options for melasma are as follows [1]. First, UV protection and topical whitening medications such as hydroquinone (HQ), tretinoin, azelaic acid, rucinol, and kojic acid. Triple combination therapy (Kligman formula) is a combination of hydroquinone, tretinoin, and steroid, and is the mainstay of topical treatment. Second, chemical peeling. Third, laser treatment may be helpful, but hyperpigmentation may occur. But sometimes avoidance of aggravating factors like UV exposure and hormonal stimulation may be sufficient for melasma treatment.

As shown in Table 12.4, it can be seen that various whitening drugs including triple combination therapy are effective for melasma. Chemical peeling and oral medications are also effective. There is a paper that acknowledges the so-called laser toning and CO_2 fractional laser as effective treatments for melasma. Interestingly, there are controversies over the effectiveness of the Er:Glass laser, a nonablational fractional laser approved by the US FDA for the treatment of melasma. There are both papers that support or do not support the efficacy of Er:Glass laser for melasma. There is also a paper that supports IPL for the treatment of melasma, which is known as a contraindication in private practice [27].

From these various treatments, what is the most effective treatment? In a review paper by Trivedi et al. the following treatments were recommended for melasma [28]. First-line therapy should be topical medications that include HQ. For second-line therapy, chemical peeling was recommended. And for third-line therapy, laser and light therapy including IPL was recommended. Rivas et al. published a review article on melasma treatment [29]. Laser treatments produced mixed results, with increased

Table 12.4 Melasma treatments, mechanisms of action, and adverse effects

Modality	Treatment	Mechanism of action	Adverse effects (AE)
Topical	Iron oxide	Block visible and ultraviolet light	Irritation
	Hydroquinone (HQ), Azelaic acid, ascorbic acid, Kojic acid	Tyrosinase inhibitor	Irritation, exogenous ochronosis (with HQ)
	Tretinoin	Increased keratinocyte turnover	Irritation, redness
	Corticosteroids	Anti-inflammatory with non-selective inhibition of melanogenesis	Telangiectasias, epidermal atrophy, steroid-induced acne, striae, hypopigmentation
	Ascorbic acid	Inhibition of reactive oxygen species	No significant AE
	Niacinamide	Inhibition of melanosome transfer	Irritation
Oral	Tranexamic acid	Inhibits plasminogen/plasmin pathway → inhibition of melanin synthesis Decreases vascular proliferation	Abdominal bloating, menstrual irregularities, headache, deep venous thrombosis
	Polypodium leucotomos, glutathione	Inhibition of reactive oxygen species	No significant AE

Table 12.4 (continued)

Procedural	Q-switch ruby laser, Q-switch Nd:Yag laser	Melanosome destruction	Burn, post-inflammatory pigment alteration (PIPA)
	Nonablative Fractional lasers	Fractional photothermolysis leading to melanin extrusion	Burn, PIPA
	Chemical peels	Increased keratinocyte turnover	Burn, peeling, PIPA
	Microneedling	Transdermal drug delivery	Erythema, edema, tram-track marks, PIPA
	Intense pulsed light	Extrusion of melanosomes	Burn, PIPA
	Radiofrequency	Cellular biostimulation Transdermal drug delivery	Burn

AE adverse effects, *HQ* hydroquinone, *PIPA* post-inflammatory pigment alteration, *Nd:YAG* neodymium-doped yttrium aluminum garnet. (Reproduced from [26])

risk of irritation and subsequent hyperpigmentation, particularly in darker-skinned individuals. Hence, lasers should be considered as a third-line therapy when treating melasma in darker-skinned individuals.

From the papers earlier, we can see that many papers are doubtful about laser treatment for melasma. But are these conclusions reliable? In the past decades, melasma treatment has evolved. Before the onset of laser, only medication and chemical peeling were available as treatment options for melasma. And through many studies, we now know the optimal dose and type of medication for melasma. Since laser treatment for melasma is relatively recent, maybe the problem is that we do not know the optimal energy and type of laser for the treatment of melasma.

I think that the greatest advantage of lasers is their specificity. Only melasma or pigmentations can be treated selectively. On the other hand, medication or chemical peeling is not selective. But I do not think that laser treatment is the most effective treatment for melasma. There is no single treatment that is most effective for melasma. I think a combination treatment of effective medication, chemical peel, and laser according to mechanism is most important in melasma treatment.

12.5.2 Consensus on Medical and Chemical Peeling Treatment for Melasma

Medication and chemical peeling have been used for a long time for melasma treatments. Thus, the optimal dose and type of medication and treatment methods for melasma have already been established. Then what are the most effective medication and chemical peel for melasma?

In 2006, the Pigmentary Disorders Academy (PDA) reviewed papers concerning melasma treatment over the past two decades and classified them from I to IV by quality of evidence (indicating that the paper is objectively well designed, the smaller the number, the higher the quality) and from A to E by level of evidence (the closer to A, the higher the evidence) [30] (Table 12.5).

The results show that among topical agents, the only agent with quality of evidence I and level of evidence A is the Kligman formula. 4% hydroquinone, 0.1% tretinoin, a combination of 4% hydroquinone and GA 10%, and 20% azelaic acid has a quality of evidence I and level of evidence B. There was no quality of evidence I papers concerning chemical peeling. The highest quality of evidence was II-i with a level of evidence B, which was a combination of 20–30% GA peeling and 4% hydroquinone, and 70% GA peeling. The quality of evidence and level of evidence for both laser treatment and dermabrasion were low.

In 2014, Shankar et al. analyzed several papers related to chemical peeling [31]. The results showed that there were no randomized controlled trials (RCTs) and GA peeling had the highest strength of recommendation (Table 12.6).

There are various medications and chemical peels, but in this book, I will briefly discuss the following: the triple combination therapy, tranexamic acid, and GA peeling.

Table 12.5 Level and quality of evidence for melasma therapies

Therapy	Quality of evidence	Level of evidence
Topical		
2% HQ	II-ii	C
4% HQ	I	B
0.1% tretinoin (RA)	I	B
0.05% RA	I	C
0.05% isotretinoin	II-ii	C
4% N-acetyl-4-S-cysteaminylphenol	III	C
5% HQ + 0.1–0.4% RA + 7% lactic acide/10% ascorbic acid	III	C
3% HQ + 0.1% RA	III	C
4% HQ + 0.05% RA + 0.01% fluocinolone acetonide	I	A
2% HQ + 0.05% RA + 0.01% dexamethasone (modified kligman)	III	C
2% HQ + 0.05% RA + 0.01% dexamethasone (modified kligman) + 30% ~ 40% GA peel	III	B
5% HQ + 0.1% RA, and 1% hydrocortisone	III	C
4% HQ + 5% RA	II-ii	B
4% KA + 5% RA	II-ii	B
2% KA + 2% HQ + 10% GA	II-iii	C
2% HQ + 10% GA	II-iii	C
4% HQ + 10% GA	I	B
20% Azelaic acid	I	B
20% Azelaic acid +0.05% RA	III	C
Vitamin C iontophoresis	II-i	C
Adapalene	II-ii	B
Chemical peels		
10–50% GA	II-ii/III	C
10% GA + 2% HQ + 20–70% GA	II-ii	C
20–30% GA + 4% HQ	II-i	B
70% GA	II-i	B
Jessner's solution	II-i	C
20–30% salicylic acid	III	C
1–5% RA	III	C
50% GA + 10% KA	III	C
Laser therapy (+ chemical peels and topical therapies)		
Q-switched ruby	IV	C
Pulsed CO2 + Q-switched alexandrite	IV	C
Q-switched alexandrite	IV	C
Q-switched alexandrite laser +15–25% TCA peel + Jessner's solution	III	C
Erbium:YAG	III	D
Dermabrasion	II-iii	E

GA Glycolic acid, *HQ* hydroquinone, *KA* kojic acid, *KF* Kligman's formula, *RA* retinoic acid, *TCA* trichloroacetic acid. (Modified from [30])

Table 12.6 Levels of evidence and strength of recommendation for various peeling agents in ethnic skin

Classification	Peeling agent	Level of evidence	Strength of recommendation
Superficial peel	Phytic acid	Expert opinion	C
	Lactic acid	Uncontrolled trial	B
	Glycolic acid	Non-randomized controlled study	A
	Salicylic acid	Uncontrolled trial	B
	Jessner's solution	Uncontrolled trial	B
Superficial-medium peel	Pyruvic acid	Expert opinion	C
Medium-depth peel	Trichloro-acetic acid	Uncontrolled trial	B

A: There is good evidence to support the use of the procedure, B: There is fair evidence to support the use of the procedure, C: There is poor evidence to support the use of the procedure. (Reproduced from [31])

12.5.3 Triple Combination Therapy

The triple combination therapy (TCT) was made by Dr. Albert M. Kligman (1916–2010) in 1975 [2]. Also called the Kligman formula, this original formula employed dexamethasone 0.1% in combination with 0.1% tretinoin, and 5% hydroquinone (HQ). Kligman formula has been modified in a number of ways over the years (Fig. 12.8).

The drug with the main mechanism of action is thought to be HQ, which inhibits tyrosinase, which is the most important enzyme in melanin synthesis. This is why the TCT shows a strong whitening effect. HQ is an oxidant that binds and reacts rapidly with oxygen, making it difficult to

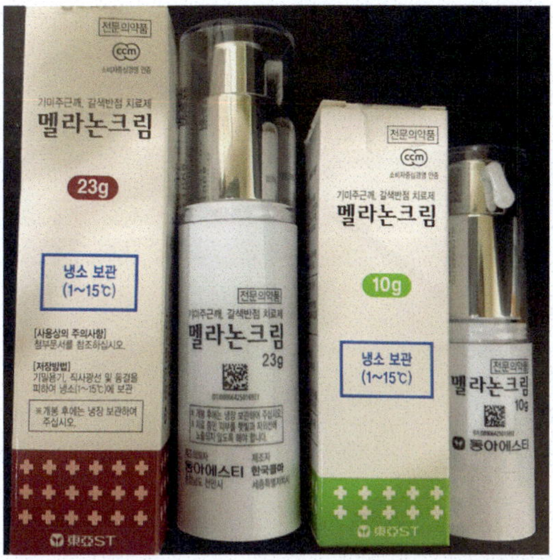

Fig. 12.8 Triple combination therapy. (Reproduced from [2])

make a stable form. Tretinoin prevents the oxidation of hydroquinone, enhances epidermal penetration, removes pigmentations, and proliferates keratinocytes. Finally, topical steroids act to reduce cell metabolism, inhibit melanin synthesis, and reduce medication-induced irritation.

Chan et al. compared the efficacy and safety of a TCT (fluocinolone acetonide 0.01%, HQ 4%, tretinoin 0.05%) versus HQ 4% after 8 weeks of treatment of moderate to severe facial melasma in 240 Asian patients [32]. TCT had superior efficacy to HQ in the melasma global severity score (64.2% vs. 39.4%), but there was no 100%. More patients had related adverse events on TCT than on HQ (48.8% vs. 13.7%). The most common side effects were erythema (24.0% vs. 4.6%), skin irritation (10.9% vs. 3.8%), skin exfoliation (5.4% vs. 0.8%), skin discomfort (6.2% vs. 1.5%), but most were mild and not severe.

TCT should be used once a day for the first 12 weeks and twice a week for the next 12 weeks while closely monitoring the patient's compliance and side effects.

TCT is a medication that has been used for a long time and has been proven effective, but as shown in the Sect. 5.2.8 in "Chap. 5," although the possibility is low, it may cause exogenous ochronosis. And through animal experiments using rodents, it has been suggested that HQ may be a carcinogen. Above all, it may cause skin irritation and erythema and cause PIH. In particular, the patient's compliance is low and is often applied incorrectly. This is why I prescribe tranexamic acid, rather than TCT.

12.5.4 Tranexamic Acid

Tranexamic acid (TA) began to gain attention in 1979 after Nijo Sadako (Japan) used it to treat chronic urticaria and incidentally found that the melasma severity of that patient was significantly reduced [33]. Since then, TA has been widely used for melasma in Japan and various papers on TA have been published.

TA is a plasmin inhibitor and has been used as a medication to control bleeding by inhibiting plasminogen activator (PA). Keratinocytes produce PA and plasminogen, and plasminogen induces melanin synthesis by UV light (Fig. 12.9). Plasmin is also involved in the secretion of fibroblast growth factor (FGF), a growth factor for melanocytes. TA reversibly blocks the lysine binding site of plasminogen and inhibits the conversion of plasminogen to plasmin by inhibiting PA [33]. In animal experiments, TA reduced the pigmentation caused by UV light by binding plasminogen to keratinocytes and reducing tyrosinase activation in melanocytes. In one study, TA interferes with the catalysis of tyrosinase, which in turn inhibits pigmentation [34]. Other studies have shown that TA reduces α-melanocyte-stimulating hormone (α-MSH), which stimulates melanin synthesis.

The recommended dose of oral TA is as follows: 250 mg two to three times a day. At least 1 month of medication is needed for it to take effect. Longer duration of medication is known to be more effective than higher doses of medication. Besides oral TA, there are intradermal injection methods, but the efficacy is not yet proven. Topical application is difficult because of irritation symptoms and lack of commercialized products. TA may penetrate the skin by iontophoresis, but the efficacy is not yet proven. In 2007 Taiwan, intravenous (IV) injection of 500 mg of tranexamic acid with ascorbic acid at intervals of

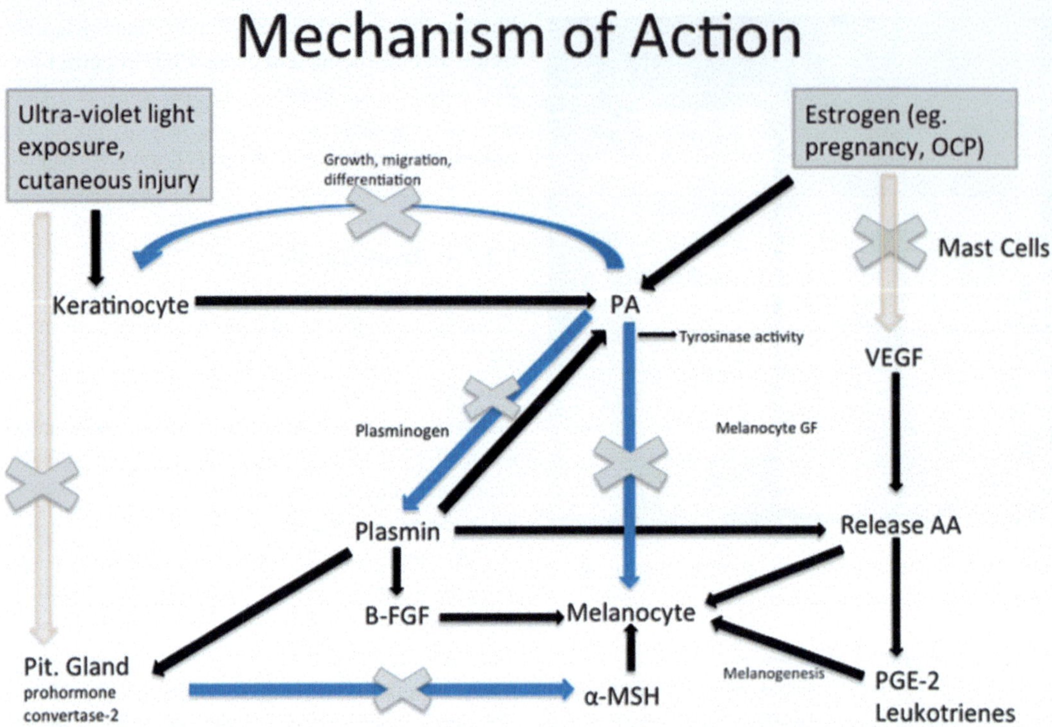

Fig. 12.9 Tranexamic acid, mode of action. Plasminogen (PA) resides in keratinocytes and basal cells. Ultraviolet (UV) radiation stimulates the keratinocyte–PA pathway and thus melanogenesis. Hormones also stimulate the keratinocyte–PA pathway. Tranexamic acid inhibits pigmentation induced by ultraviolet radiation by various mechanisms including the following: plasmin increases single-chain urokinase PA (Sc-uPA), which increases tyrosinase activity and keratinocyte growth. Tranexamic acid is thought to inhibit this pathway and thus decrease the activity of tyrosinase. Tranexamic acid prevents the binding of plasminogen to the 'keratinocyte' Tranexamic acid reduces the production of prohormone covertase (PC2). PC2 is involved in the proopiomelanocortin system (PMOC) in producing α-melanocyte–stimulating hormone (α-MSH). This subsequent decrease in α-MSH despite UV stimulation of the PMOC gene results in the lightening of the skin. Via blocking plasminogen to plasmin, inflammatory mediators such as AA, prostaglandin E2 (PGE2), leukotriene, and fibroblast growth factor (FGF) are reduced decreasing melanogenesis. *AA* arachondonic acid, *VEGF* vascular endothelial growth factor, *UV* ultraviolet. (Reproduced from [34])

2–4 weeks was popular under the trade name "whitening of skin." But there were no studies concerning the injection, and the concentrations were very low which also raised questions about its effectiveness. In addition, due to IV injections, there is a risk of phlebitis or cardiac diseases.

TA dose for bleeding control is 0.5–1.5 g, three times a day. Even at high doses like this, changes in coagulation factors are not seen and the incidence of thrombosis does not increase. Therefore, I think that the dose used for melasma, 0.5–0.75 g/day, is a very safe dose. It does not affect the fetus or fetal malformation because it does not cross the blood-brain barrier (BBB) and placenta but is still contraindicated during pregnancy or lactation. In addition, patients with coronary artery disease or coagulation disorder, patients taking thrombolytics such as aspirin, and patients with too high expectations for treatment outcomes are also contraindications [33].

Wu et al. evaluated the improvement of pigmentation and reduction in melasma size in 74 female patients who took 250 mg of TA twice a day for 6 months [35]. The results showed a significant improvement of pigmentation of 82.4% in the first month, which increased to 94.6% in 2 months and 95.9% in 6 months (10.8% excellent, 54% good, 31.1% fair, 4.1% poor). Adverse events included nausea, diarrhea, abdominal pain, hypomenorrhea, skin rash, hair loss, drowsiness, and decreased libido, but they were mild and the incidence was low. Interestingly, melasma improved during the treatment period, but there was no difference in other pigmentations such as lentigines and ephelides. Karn et al. compared the efficacy of oral TA for the treatment of melasma by comparing two groups [36]. The first group (A) was given oral TA (a dose of 250 mg twice a day) and local HQ for 3 months while the second group (B) was treated only with local HQ for 3 months. Melasma Area Severity Index (MASI) score and patient satisfaction index were measured at 8 and 12 weeks. Group A showed a statistically significant decrease in the melasma index at 8 and 12 weeks. There was a statistically significant decrease in the melasma index at 8 weeks in group B, but not at 12 weeks. The patient satisfaction index was 82.3% in group A and 40.8% in group B. Side effects included mild oligomenorrhea, belching, abdominal cramps, palpitations, and urticarial rashes. Interestingly there was a significant improvement in exogenous ochronosis in two patients taking TA.

I only prescribe oral TA 250 mg bid to melasma patients (Figs. 12.10 and 12.11) and penetrate TA through the skin by iontophoresis. Occasionally, I use "injectable glow." I combine TA with hyaluronic acid and inject it into the dermis.

12.5.5 Glycolic Acid Peeling

Alpha-hydroxy acid (AHA) is an organic acid that is found in fruits and milk in nature and causes moisturization and exfoliation. Glycolic acid (GA) is a representative medication of AHA peeling and is extracted from sugar cane. GA is known to have the smallest molecular weight and can penetrate deeper into the epidermis [37].

GA peeling has been widely used as a peeling agent since the late 1980s. GA peeling does not dissolve keratinocytes like TCA peeling but changes the binding of corneocytes to remove the stratum corneum. It also stimulates the germinative layer and fibroblasts and is known to show anti-inflammatory and antioxidant effects. GA peeling is known to be effective both in the epidermis and the dermis.

The advantages of GA peeling are as follows. First, it does not impair the skin barrier function. Transepidermal water loss (TEWL) does not increase as compared with normal skin and there is no indication of inflammation. Second, no

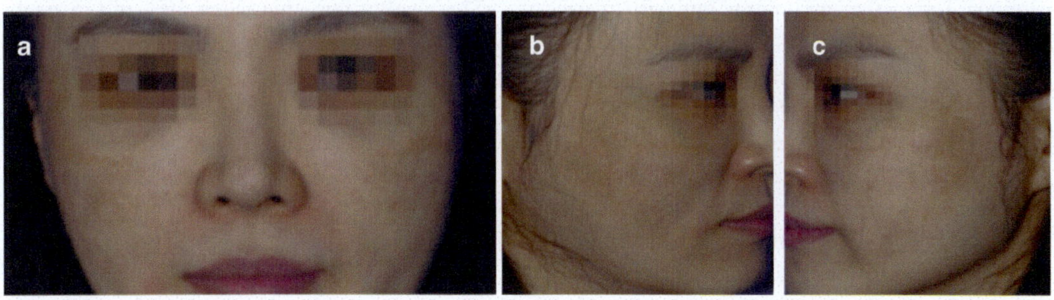

Fig. 12.10 Thirty-eight-year-old woman with melasma, which occurred after pregnancy. Symmetrical brown melasma is seen on both side malar cheeks

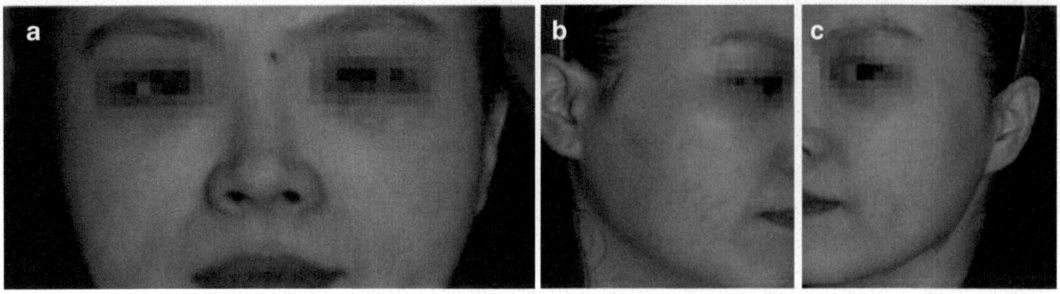

Fig. 12.11 Symptom improvement after behavioral therapy and TA for 3 months

necrosis or degeneration of tissues is found, and barrier recovery functions are observed, such as increased secretion of lamellar bodies. Third, irrespective of the depth, GA peeling affects the dermis and stimulates the fibroblasts of the dermis, resulting in the synthesis and proliferation of collagen, elastin, glycosaminoglycans, etc. Fourth, the recovery time is short, which is good in terms of cosmetic treatment. Fifth, it is applicable to all skin types and can also be used in sensitive skin.

The advantages of GA peeling may be helpful for melasma. GA peeling can restore skin barrier function, which is thought to be a problem of melasma. It does not cause inflammation and improves the dermis. It is also applicable to sensitive skin, which a lot of melasma patients have. Finally, there is no downtime. These are the reason why I use GA peeling for melasma.

However, there are many disadvantages of GA peeling. First, the treatment intensity varies depending on multiple variables such as concentration, pH, and application time. Thus, GA peeling must be made with caution and the procedure should be unified. Second, because the depth of penetration is not homogeneous and may vary depending on the condition or the site of the skin, it is important to educate estheticians to neutralize GA peeling immediately if an adverse reaction occurs. Third, GA peeling requires neutralization [38].

Several papers evaluated GA peeling effectively in ethnic skin [37]. Javaheri et al. performed 50% GA peeling on 25 Indian women with melasma at a monthly interval for a total of 3 months. It was shown to be effective in 91%. Besides one woman with hyperpigmentation on the eyebrows, there were no side effects. GA peeling is considered effective and safe. The advantage that GA peeling has over other peelings is that it is safe for people with ethnic skin, who have sensitive skin. GA peeling is also known to be effective for rosacea because it prevents the attachment of demodex mites to hair follicles.

Erbil et al. enrolled 28 patients with recalcitrant melasma and divided them into two groups [39]. The chemical peel group received GA peeling in combination with topical azelaic acid and adapalene while the control group received only topical azelaic acid and adapalene. GA peeling was performed every 2 weeks, and the concentration was increased little by little once a month.

The results show that when 50% of GA peeling is used, the decrease in the MASI score is more prominent compared to the control group (Fig. 12.12). This is the reason why I choose to use a 50% concentration in GA peeling.

Next, we will review the laser treatments of melasma. In particular, we will review laser toning, which is widely used in private practice. We will also review the principle and choice of laser in pigmentation disorders and review the pigmentation treatment strategy. Finally, we will review the principle and choice of laser in melasma treatment.

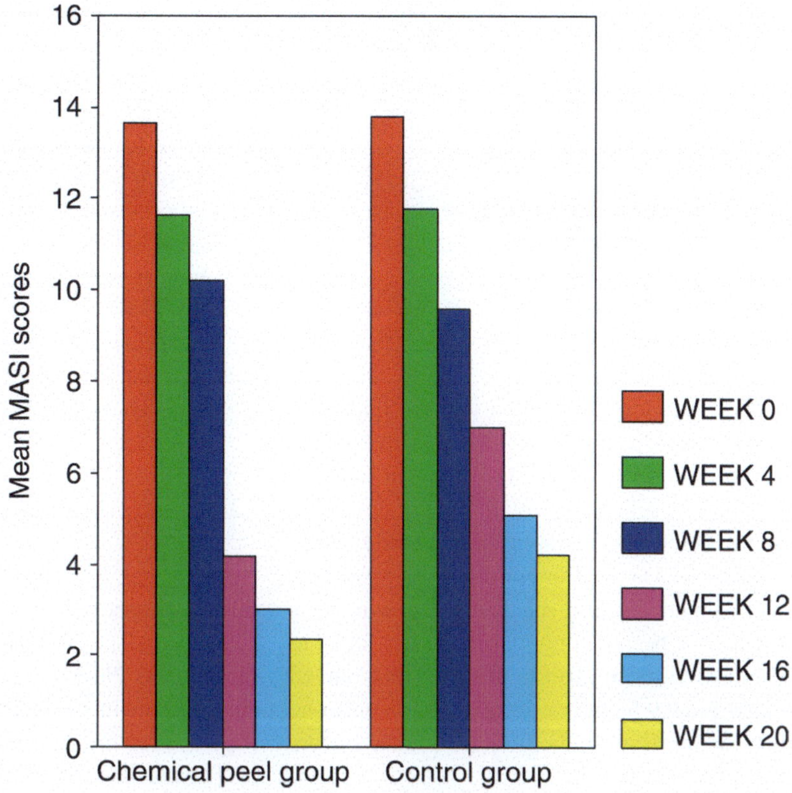

Fig. 12.12 Changes in Melasma Area Severity Index (MASI) scores during monthly follow-ups. (Reproduced from [39])

12.6 Laser Toning

12.6.1 Conventional Laser Toning

Before laser toning, lasers were not used to treat melasma. Laser was contraindicated in the treatment of melasma due to side effects such as rebound hyperpigmentation and hypopigmentation [40]. However, since 2005, private clinics in East Asia found 1064-nm Q-switched Nd:YAG lasers ("laser toning") effective in melasma treatment. Thus "laser toning" first started in private practice and was later researched in the university hospital.

Chung et al. used low-fluence 1064-nm Q-switched Nd:YAG laser in 27 melasma patients. Seventeen patients (58.8%) showed over 50–75% improvement in pigmentation [40]. This paper is the first paper on "laser toning." The parameter was different from what was used for conventional pigmentation treatment: Large spot size, low energy, multiple passes, weekly procedures, multiple times. This treatment method was called "laser toning." In the paper it is referred to as "low-fluence Q-switched Nd:YAG laser" or "low-dose Q-switched Nd:YAG laser." However, I will use the term "laser toning" in this book.

The parameters of conventional laser toning used in private practice and written in papers are as follows. First, 1064-nm Q-switched Nd:YAG laser is used. Second, relatively low energy of 1.6–3.5 J/cm^2 is used. Third, a relatively large spot size of 6–8 mm is used. Fourth, multiple passes are performed at 10 Hz resulting in more than 1000 shots. Fifth, treatment is performed with a very short interval of every 1–2 weeks. Sixth, 5–10 sessions of treatment are needed instead of just once. Seventh, the clinical end point is erythema.

Are these parameters correct? We will now review the general aspects of laser toning, and later, I will comment on the seven parameters of laser toning.

12.6.2 Subcellular Selective Photothermolysis

In the Sect. 3.1.3 in "Chap. 3" we reviewed papers on "subcellular selective photothermolysis" the basis of laser toning.

The following is a summary of the important points in the paper on subcellular selective photothermolysis (Table 12.7) [41]. First, in order to meet the subcellular selective photothermolysis theory, the fluence should be relatively lower than the fluence used in conventional pigmentation treatment. Second, the therapeutic window is very narrow because only 0.4 J/cm^2 was found to be effective from various fluences that ranged from 0.3 to 0.9 J/cm^2 in zebrafish. Third, only one shot was performed. Fourth, recurrence occurs even with laser toning.

Here are my thoughts regarding the four points above. First, we do not know the exact fluence of the "relatively low fluence." Therefore, the appropriate energy must be found for the conventional laser toning with multiple passes and multiple shots. The energy of the one-shot toning that I currently use is mentioned in the Sect. 3.1.3 in "Chap. 3" in And there is no absolute parameter. The energy must be adjusted according to the patient. The energy should be adjusted so that the energy is "dark lesion weak, light lesion strong."

Table 12.7 Important points and countermeasures of subcellular selective photothermolysis

Important points of subcellular selective photothermolysis	Countermeasures
Relatively low fluence	Find the therapeutic fluence
Very narrow therapeutic window	Fluence < therapeutic window
Only one shot	One-shot toning
Recurrence	Behavior change, suppress melanin synthesis, dermal improvement, repeat laser toning?

Second, the therapeutic range is very narrow. Even if the appropriate energy is found, it is still very dangerous. It is safer to use less than adequate energy because it is better to be less effective than to have side effects. Third, in the "subcellular selective photothermolysis" paper, the authors used just one shot [42]. Even if the "One shot toning" that I mentioned is not used, it is better to predetermine how many shots you want to shoot on one site. Fourth, measures to prevent recurrence are needed. This part requires an understanding of the underlying causes of melasma. This will be explained again below.

12.6.3 Effects of Laser Toning

Next, we will look at two papers that studied the effects of laser toning.

Mun et al. performed laser toning by 1064-nm Q-switched Nd:YAG laser in 16 patients and observed the melasma lesion by electron microscopy and reconstructed it into 3D images [43].

The results were as follows. First, the volume of the melanocytes was reduced and the number of melanosomes was reduced (Fig. 12.13). Second, the "dendrectomy" phenomenon, in which the melanocyte dendrite was reduced, was observed (Fig. 12.14). Third, mature melanosomes of stage IV decreased, and fourth, degraded melanosomes and traces were observed. Fifth, immature melanosomes in stages I and II were unchanged (Fig. 12.15).

What is interesting about this paper is the "dendrectomy" phenomenon, which is the reduction of the dendrites of melanocytes. The authors of this paper assume that the reason for this is because stage IV melanosomes are located more on the dendrite than any other parts of the melanocyte, so due to the thermolytic effect of laser, the dendrite disappears [43]. I think this phenomenon is due to "inactivation of melanocyte." The most important role of melanocytes is to make melanosomes and deliver them to keratinocytes. Thus, the reduced dendrites imply that the role of melanocytes has ceased. I think that laser toning induces melanocyte inactivation. In addition, after laser toning, melanosomes in the melano-

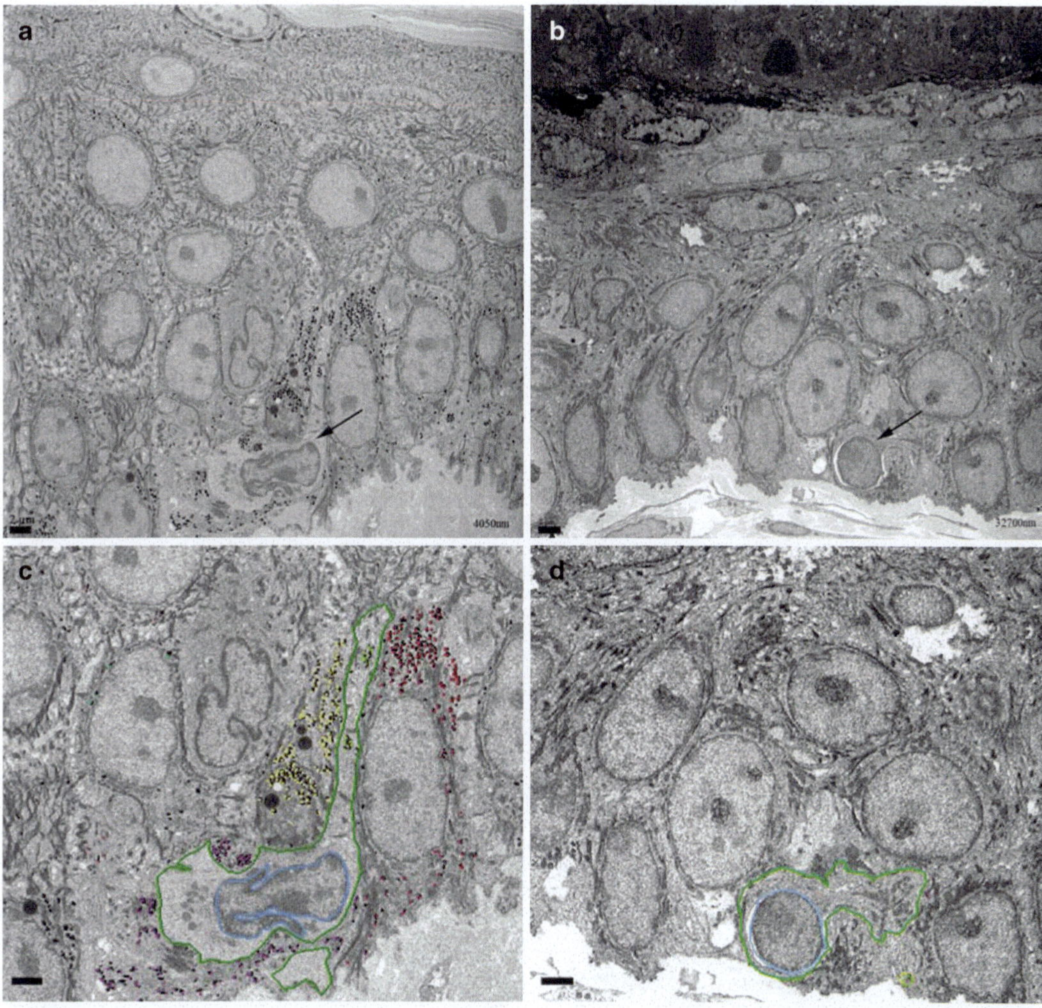

Fig. 12.13 SBF-SEM images of the epidermis layer. (**a**, **c**) Images of prelaser treatment. (**b**, **d**) Images of postlaser treatment. The images (**a**) and (**b**) show one section among over 500 serial sections. Arrows in (**a**) and (**b**) represent melanocytes. In (**c**) and (**d**), dark green represents melanocytes and light blue shows nucleus. Yellow, purple, red, and cyan dots show melanosomes. The images (**c**) and (**d**) show a decrease in the volume of melanocyte and the number of melanosomes after laser treatment (size bar is 2 μm). (Reproduced from [43])

cytes disappear, the volume of melanocytes become smaller, and nuclear fission is reduced as shown in Fig. 12.13, which I believe are all signs of melanocyte inactivation.

I also believe that the mechanism of the brightening of melasma by laser toning is due to dendrectomy rather than by breaking the melanosome. In the "subcellular selective photothermolysis" paper, the melanosomes of the zebrafish were broken by laser toning. But if the melanosome breaks inside the cell, does this result in making the overall melasma tone brighter? Melanosomes broken by laser toning do not disappear out of the cell but remain broken inside the keratinocytes or melanocytes. When the melanin breaks up and spreads, it appears bright microscopically, but the overall amount of melanin remains unchanged. In other words, there is no big difference when seen with eyes. This is the reason we cannot clinically observe immediate brightening after laser toning. I think dendrectomy prevents melanocytes from delivering

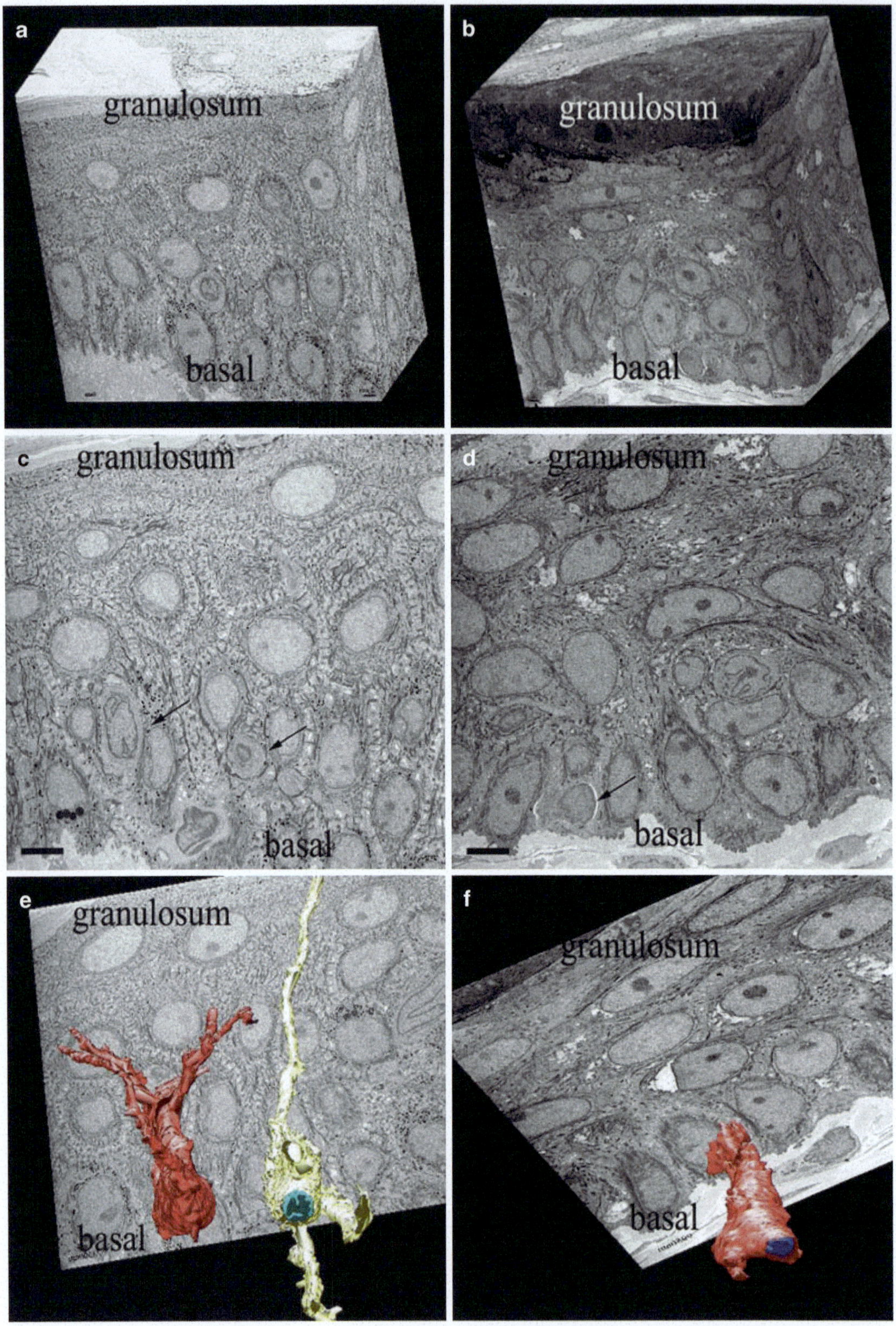
a
granulosum
basal
b
granulosum
basal
c
granulosum
basal
d
granulosum
basal
e
granulosum
basal
f
granulosum
basal

Fig. 12.14 3D structures of melanocytes in the epidermis layer of melasma patients. (**a**, **c**, **e**) Images of prelaser treatment and (**b**, **d**, **f**) images of postlaser treatment. 3D volume of over 500 serial images using 3VIEW was showed by IMOD (**a**, **b**). (**c**, **d**) One of the serial images for 3D reconstruction of (**e**) and (**f**). Arrows of (**c**) and (**d**) show the reconstructed melanocytes in (**e**) and (**f**). The size bar of (**c**) and (**d**) is 5 μm. The images (**e**) and (**f**) show the surface model of melanocytes showing the cell body and their dendrites. Each nucleus was assigned a separate color (**e**, cyan blue; **f**, blue). Melanocytes in melasma patients have many dendrites and stretch from basal layer to granulosum layer (**e**). After laser toning treatment, the 3D structure of melanocytes contained fewer dendrites (**f**). Reproduced from [43]

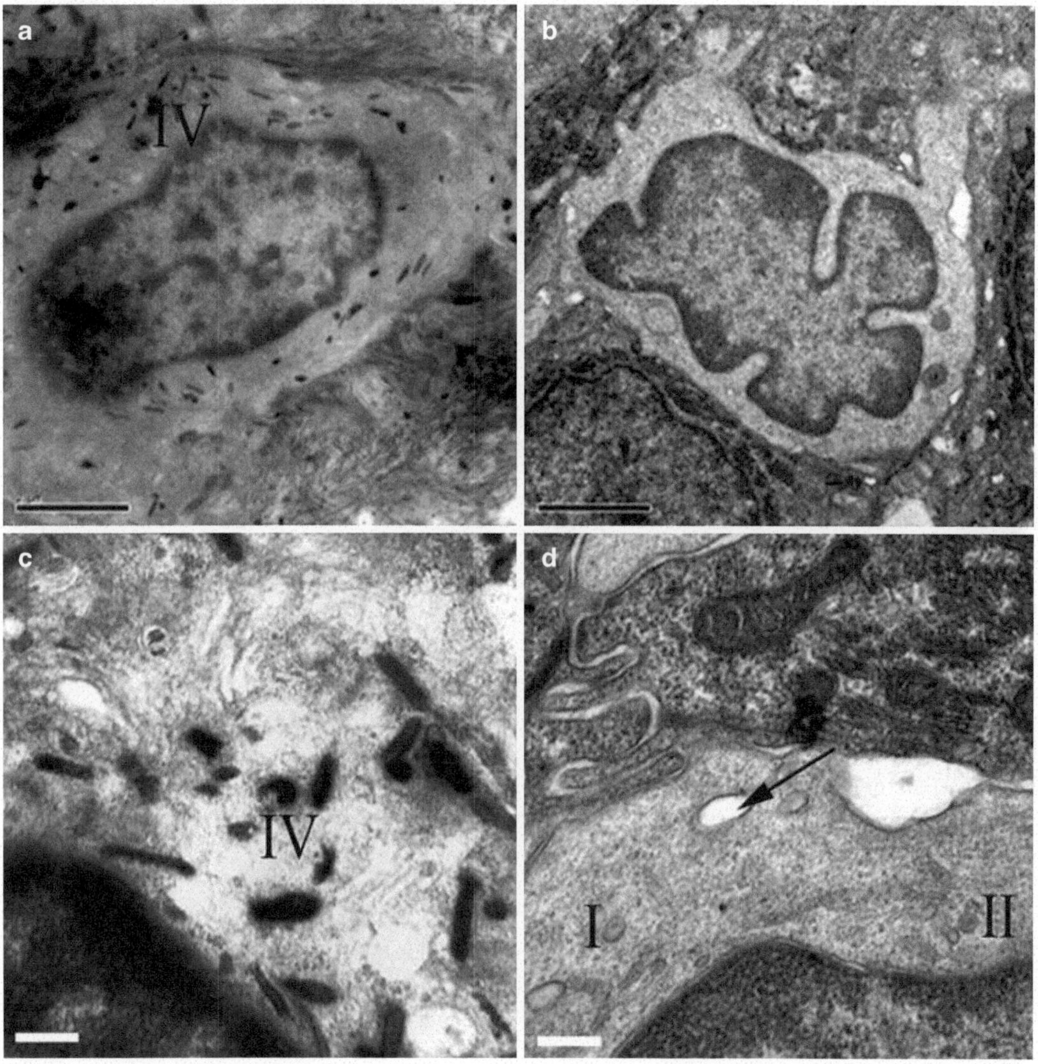

Fig. 12.15 Transmission electron microscopy images of melamosomes in melanocytes of melasma patients. The image of melanocyte from a melasma patient (**a**, **c**, and **e**) and that after postlaser treatment (**b**, **d**, **f**) were compared for investigation of the ultrastructural change of melanosome after laser treatment. Melanocytes in melasma patients without laser treatment have many melanosomes (**a**, **c**, **e**). After laser toning treatment, the melanocytes had far fewer melanosomes (**b**, **d**, **f**) and remnant (**d**), and lysed form (**f**) of Stage IV melamosome in melanocyte was observed. Arrow of (**d**) shows the remnant of Stage IV melanosome. Lysed Stage IV melanosome was represented as a circle in (**f**). However, melanosomes in the early stage like Stages I and II were observed without any change (**d**, **f**). The size bar of (**a**) and (**b**) is 2 μm and that of (**c**–**f**) is 0.2 μm. (Reproduced from [43])

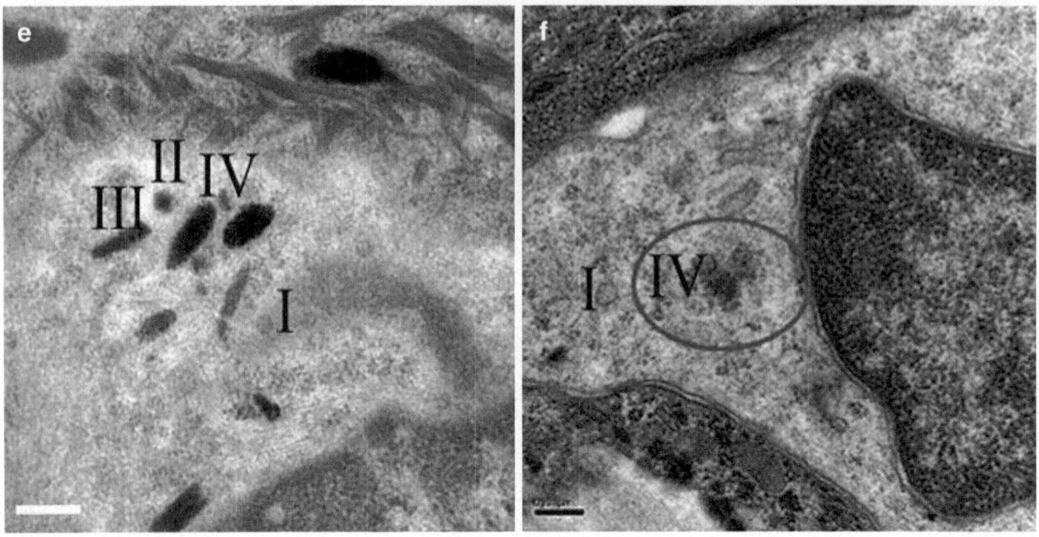

Fig. 12.15 (continued)

melanosomes to the keratinocytes for at least 2 weeks, so during the epidermal turnover, melanosome-free keratinocytes develop and the face brightens. This is the reason why laser toning doesn't immediately improves melasma, but brightens the face after 4 weeks, after an epidermal turnover.

One more thing to mention is that many think that laser toning only damages melanosomes in melanocytes. However, most melanosomes are in keratinocytes, and melanocytes have mature melanosomes in their dendrites, which disappear after dendrectomy while immature melanosomes (stage I, II) are not affected by laser toning, i.e., the melanocytes do not become brighter or disappear. Therefore, laser toning not only improves the appearance of melasma but also brightens the overall tone of the face.

Kim et al. observed changes before and after laser toning through histopathological examination [44]. Compared with nonlesional skin, samples from melasma lesions showed increased reactivity in melanin and melanogenesis-associated proteins, including α-melanocyte-stimulating hormone (α-MSH), tyrosinase, tyrosinase-related protein (TRP)-1, TRP-2, nerve growth factor (NGF) and stem cell factor (SCF). After laser treatment, the melasma skin showed a decrease in the number of melanosomes and reduced expression of melanogenesis-associated proteins.

This paper shows that laser toning reduces the proteins involved in melanogenesis. In other words, laser toning does not simply break melanosomes, but inhibits melanin synthesis, which is not permanent, but melanin production temporarily stops, resulting in brightening.

Based on the two papers earlier, the brightening effect of laser toning is due to first, inhibition of melanin synthesis, and second, by blocking the transmission of melanosome.

12.6.4 Prognosis of Laser Toning

Zhou et al. recruited 55 patients and performed 1064-nm Q-switched Nd:YAG laser at low energy levels weekly for nine sessions [45]. Patient satisfaction, melanin index (MI), and melasma area and severity index (MASI) were measured. The results were as follows: First, patient satisfaction was 84% and not all patients were satisfied. Second, mean MASI scores decreased by 61.3%, and only 10% had 100% clearance. Most patients still had melasma after laser toning (Fig. 12.16). Third, melasma does not improve immediately after laser toning, but is improved after 4–6 weeks, and is gradually improved as the laser toning is repeated. Fourth, minor side effects such as erythema, heat sensation, tingling, swelling, and purpura occurred, but no serious side effects were observed. Fifth, when treatment was discontinued, recurrence occurred in 64% after 3 months, which was quite high.

Although the fluence of this paper is slightly higher than that of conventional laser toning (2.5–3.4 J/cm^2), this paper shows the typical effect and progress of laser toning.

12.6.5 Side Effects of Laser Toning

As the effects of subcellular selective photothermolysis and laser toning have been demonstrated, laser toning has become popular in private practice. However, many laser toning procedures resulted in frequent side effects of laser toning. The side effects of laser toning are summarized in Table 12.8 [46].

The side effects listed on the left side of Table 12.8 are temporary and are not usually a big problem, but the side effects on the right are serious permanent side effects.

If we look through the mild side effects, the first is skin dryness. This is thought to be related to the reduction of sebum, one phenomenon of laser toning [47]. Milium formation or herpes simplex reactivation is thought to be very rare as I have never observed it. Acneiform eruption is often found, but after I applied laser hair removal

Table 12.8 Side effects in laser toning

Side effects of laser toning	
Mild side effects	Severe side effects
Skin dryness	Nonresponse (10–20%)
Milium formation	Relapse
Physical urticaria	Rebound hyperpigmentation
Acneiform eruption	Leukoderma (=vitiligo)
Minute petechia	Mottled hypopigmentation (1.6%)
Whitening of fine facial hair	
Herpes simplex reactivation	

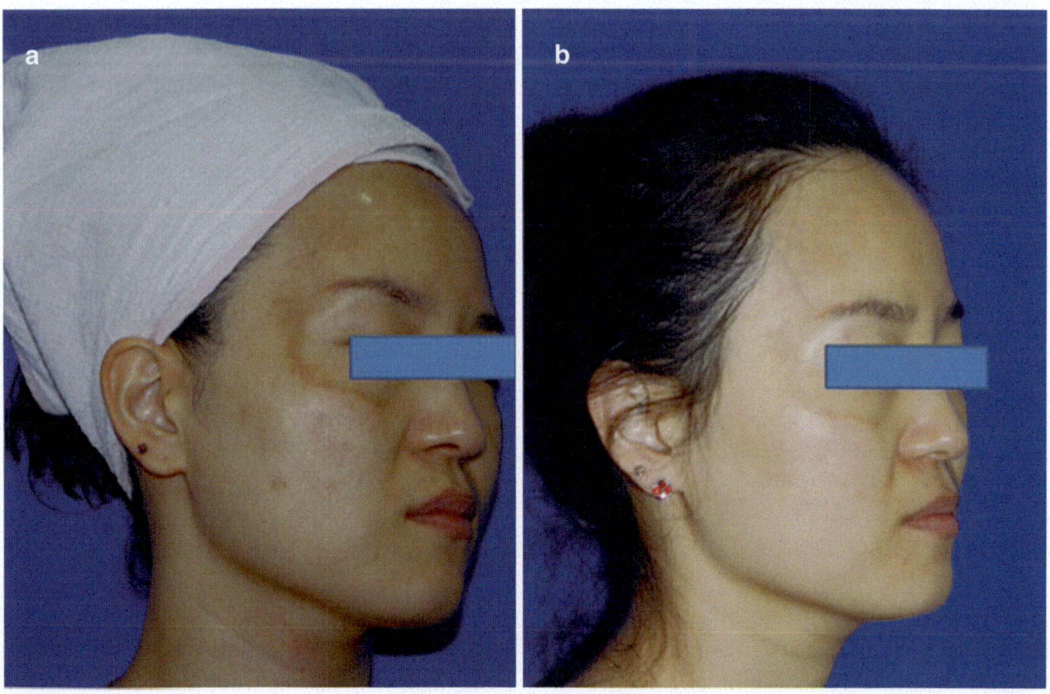

Fig. 12.16 Melasma improvement can be seen after the laser toning 10 times. Left: before treatment, right: after treatment

with a 755-nm long-pulsed alexandrite laser the frequency has been reduced. I think acneiform eruption is caused by the burning of hair by laser toning. In some cases, wheals were observed after laser toning without any particular history. In this case, urticaria of other causes was unlikely by history taking and physical examination. Most subsided within several minutes. The exact cause is unknown, but I think this may be due to the breakdown of mast cells and the release of histamine (physical urticaria). If petechia occurs after laser toning, the energy is considered to be too high. I have not observed this either since I perform laser toning with relatively low energy.

The severe side effects of laser toning are as follows. Non-response (10–20%), relapse, rebound hyperpigmentation and hypopigmentation. In particular, mottled hypopigmentation (punctate leukoderma) is a serious side effect and is found in about 1.6% [48]. Next, let's take a closer look at these serious side effects.

12.6.5.1 Recurrence

Zhou et al. performed laser toning in 55 melasma patients for 9 weeks and after a 3-month follow-up found that 64% had recurrences [45]. Gokalp et al. performed laser toning in 34 melasma patients for six to ten times (mean eight times) at 2-week intervals, and after a 1-year of follow-up, 58.8% (20 patients) showed recurrence, which is similar to the study by Zhou et al. [49]. Thus, Gokalp et al. concluded that while new treatments have appeared in the treatment of melasma there is no golden standard in laser treatment that has long-term effects, hence "once melasma, always melasma."

The cause of melasma must be known in order to prevent melasma. However, since the exact cause of the melasma is not yet known, there is no certain way to prevent a recurrence. However, taking certain causes of melasma into account, I think these measures may prevent the recurrence of melasma. First, behavioral therapy is needed to prevent UV rays and to protect the skin. Second, medications that inhibit melanosome production must be continued. Third, measures to recover the skin, especially improving the dermis must be taken. Fourth, laser toning should be repeated.

12.6.5.2 Rebound Hyperpigmentation

After laser toning, phenomenon such as melasma darkening may occur. This phenomenon was observed even before laser toning was introduced. Energy that is too high is thought to be the reason. Lower energy must be used and measures should be taken to find the appropriate energy. The appropriate energy will be discussed later, in the Sect. 12.6.6.

12.6.5.3 Mottled Hypopigmentation (Punctate Leukoderma)

Kim et al. performed laser toning on a total of 259 Korean women and mottled hypopigmentation occurred in three patients (1.6%) [48]. Interestingly, mottled hypopigmentation occurred after two laser toning in two patients and five laser toning in one patient.

The most serious side effect after laser toning is mottled hypopigmentation. Mottled hypopigmentation is a phenomenon in which multiple small circulars to oval hypopigmented plaques with clear boundaries are observed (Fig. 12.17).

It is difficult to consider mottled hypopigmentation as a side effect of laser toning because hypopigmented plaques occur in several places even though the laser is uniformly irradiated on the melasma. Also, the contrast between hypopigmented plaques and melasma makes them more visible and visually undesirable. Although rare (1.6%), it should be kept in mind that mottled hypopigmentation may occur when laser toning is performed. It may appear very quickly, even at the beginning of laser toning procedures (just after two times), so a careful observation is needed at every procedure.

Although there is no consensus on the course of mottled hypopigmentation, most are known to be long-lasting and difficult to recover. Therefore, the mechanism by which mottled hypopigmentation occurs and the prevention by that mechanism are important.

Mottled hypopigmentation is also called punctate leukoderma. Punctate leukoderma is a term

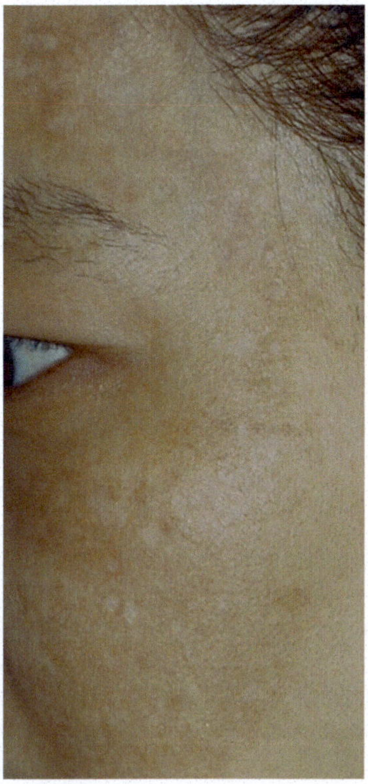

Fig. 12.17 Mottled hypopigmentation after ruby laser and laser toning in a 45-year-old female patient

that was used even before laser toning. Punctate leukoderma was first found after treatment of several skin diseases: 4-isopropylcatechol treatment of hypermelanosis, UV light treatment after taking psoralen for the treatment of vitiligo (solar ultraviolet exposure, PUVASOL, or PUVA) and UVB phototherapy treatment of psoriasis [50]. Falabella observed multiple hypopigmentations in 13 vitiligo patients who were treated with PUVASOL and described it as "leukoderma punctata" for the first time [51]. The pathogenesis of punctate leukoderma is thought to phototoxicity such as UV induced damage to the melanocyte [50].

The histological findings of mottled hypopigmentation are described in several papers. Wong et al. observed that in the hyperpigmentation sites melanin pigmentation was increased, the number of melanocytes was normal, and the dendritic process was developed, just like melasma sites [52]. On the other hand, the hypopigmentation site had a decreased amount of melanin pigmentations, the number of melanocytes and the dendritic process was both decreased (melanocytopenia). Ryu et al. reported otherwise [46]. The results of histological examination through H&E staining, MART staining, and S-100 staining showed that the number of melanocytes was normal and only melanin was reduced (i.e., melanopenic, not melanocytopenic). In one paper, the electron microscope was used to observe the hypopigmentation site. Melanin pigmentations were decreased. Melanocytes were observed, but they were malfunctioning melanocytes (Fig. 12.18) [44]. Jang et al. also observed that the hypopigmentation site showed higher gp100 expression than melasma or normal skin [53]. High gp100 expression means that the melanosome production activity of the melanocytes is impaired, which prevents the melanocytes from producing mature melanosomes.

The exact mechanism of mottled hypopigmentation by laser toning is not yet known. However, based on the mechanism of punctate

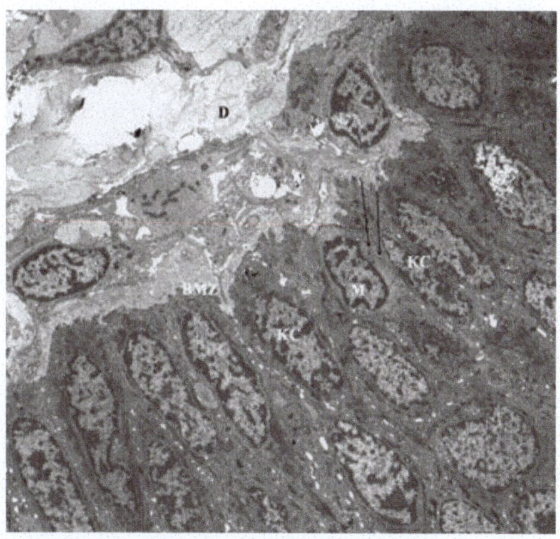

Fig. 12.18 Electron microscopy analysis of lesional hypopigmented skin after treatment with the Q-switched neodymium:yttrium-aluminium–garnet laser, showing surviving but malfunctioning melanocytes (M) and a relative decrease in or absence of melanin granules (arrows) in the melanocytes and surrounding keratinocytes (KC). The dermis (D) was unremarkable and the basement membrane zone (BMZ) appeared intact (Original magnification ×3000). (Reproduced from [44])

leukoderma induced by UV rays and the histological results of mottled hypopigmentation after laser toning, it can be estimated as follows. The main mechanism is thought to be the cumulative phototoxicity of melanocytes [51]. Specifically, the subcellular selective photothermolysis states that "there is an energy level that can only break melanosomes without damaging the cells," but in mottled hypopigmentation, melanocytes are damaged as well as melanosomes. I think if the damage is excessive, the number of melanocytes decreases, but if the damage is not excessive, the number of melanocytes is normal, but turns into malfunctioning melanocytes that are not able to produce melanin.

The reason why hypopigmentation occurs here and there is thought to be as follows. First, because melasma itself is not uniform, there is a high response to the same energy. Second, the Q-switched Nd:YAG laser beam is thought to be flat-top, top-hat mode, but they may not be entirely uniform [51]. I also think that due to many passes during laser toning, some parts accumulated more energy. (see Sect. 12.6.8).

The number of melanocytes should be noted. If the number of melanocytes is normal and only melanin is decreased (melanopenia), the function of the melanocytes will return, melanin will be produced and hypopigmentation will return to normal. But if the number of melanocytes is reduced (melanocytopenia) it is unlikely that hypopigmentation will return to normal. Therefore, the energy of laser toning should be "energy that breaks melanosomes only" and not "energy that reduces melanocytes."

Considering the mechanism "cumulative phototoxicity," the cumulative dose is considered to be a risk factor for mottled hypopigmentation. We will take the cumulative dose into account and review the parameters in papers of mottled hypopigmentation to find out which parameter is the problem.

Kim et al. observed mottled hypopigmentation after laser toning in a 42-year-old Korean woman. The fluence was 2.5 J/cm^2, which is higher compared to conventional laser toning parameters [50]. Kim et al. performed laser toning in 8 Korean women, and mottled hypopigmentation occurred in seven patients [44]. The parameters were 2000–3000 shots, 6–8 passes each time. The problem seems to be too many shots and too many passes. Tian et al. retrospectively analyzed 23 patients who underwent laser toning three times a week for 2 months [54]. All patients showed mottled hypopigmentation. Tian et al. concluded that 2 weeks is adequate for the interval between laser toning procedures.

When "cumulative phototoxicity" and the papers above are taken together, high energy, multipasses, multiple sessions, and too short intervals seem to be risk factors for mottled hypopigmentation [44]. Therefore, if mottled hypopigmentation is found, laser toning should be stopped immediately in order not to increase the amount of energy accumulated [46].

Other risk factors are also mentioned [44]. Periorbital areas in erythema-prone patients, history of allergic contact dermatitis, erythema and pruritis after laser, history of long-lasting erythema, thin skin such as the periorbital area, and Fitzpatrick skin type V are considered as risk factors.

Mottled hypopigmentation is not a common side effect, so most papers are case reports of a small number of patients. The treatment strategy for mottled hypopigmentation is as follows [51]. First, the hypopigmentation site should become darker, and second, the hyperpigmentation site should become lighter. Based on these two aspects of strategy, let's review papers regarding the treatment of mottled hypopigmentation.

Chang et al. applied sunscreen with SPF100 only on normal skin and melasma and applied narrow band UVB weekly on the hypopigmentation site [51]. All five patients showed clinical improvement. Wong et al. applied the topical immunomodulator 0.1% tacrolimus ointment to three patients, one patient showed a visual improvement, one patient had no improvement and one patient showed only slight improvement [52]. Kim et al. applied 578-nm copper bromide laser five times at 2-week intervals [48]. Melasma improved and the overall color difference was reduced, resulting in general improvement. Ryu et al. applied 50% GA peeling at weekly intervals and 0.025% tretinoin cream every evening for 3 months on a 49-year-old female patient, and significant improvement was observed [46]. Kim et al. performed a 308 nm excimer laser on hypopigmentation sites and a single pass of the 1064-nm Q-switched Nd:YAG laser at 0.7 J/cm^2 on hyperpigmentation sites [55]. After 15 trials at 2-week intervals, significant improvement was achieved.

Based on these papers and histological findings of mottled hypopigmentation, the treatment of mottled hypopigmentation is recommended as follows.

First, the hypopigmentation area shows histological findings similar to vitiligo. Therefore, as shown in the papers earlier, UV treatment (NB-UVB), 0.1% tacrolimus ointment, and 0.025% tretinoin cream, which are effective in treating vitiligo, can be used. But there is a technical limitation because it is not easy to selectively treat hypopigmentation that is only 2–3 mm in size. This is why excimer lasers with adjustable spot sizes are thought to be most suitable. Also, the most effective treatment for vitiligo is known as the excimer laser.

Second, the surrounding pigmentation area should be made brighter. But as seen in the papers above, although sunscreen, HQ-based topical medication, 50% GA peeling, 0.02 5% tretinoin cream can be used, selectively treating the pigmentation area is difficult. Since the pigmentation area is originally a melasma area, paradoxically, the most effective laser toning for melasma may be considered safe. However, because mottled hypopigmentation occurred with the energy that was initially used, the energy that is lower than the initial energy should be used. Therefore, the one-pass toning, without overlapping by Kim et al. is meaningful in this aspect. Vascular lasers such as a copper bromide laser could be tried. Fifty percent of GA peeling may increase the epidermal turnover, which may be helpful to the surrounding pigmentation area, and 0.025% tretinoin may have no definite effect but may be tried.

Finally, we could consider the pigmentation area as just pigmentation and use the laser for epidermal pigmentations according to the principle of laser. The hypopigmentation area has no pigmentations; thus, the laser cannot exert its effect on this area, i.e., the laser can selectively target the pigmentation area. But the safest laser must be used and the energy must be lowered as well. Although not published in the paper, I have attempted to treat mottled hypopigmentation with the 755-nm long-pulsed alexandrite laser, which is the safest laser for epidermal pigmentation.

12.6.6 Golden Parameter

There are several papers regarding the effects of laser toning, but as discussed earlier, there are also many side effects. Is there a golden parameter for laser toning that is effective without side effects? One laser book suggests 3.0 J/cm^2 in PTP mode and 1.5 J/cm^2 in conventional mode as golden parameters [56]. But I think this energy is still high.

Choi et al. performed laser toning with a 1064-nm Q-switched Nd:YAG laser on 30 patients with aggravated melasma after previous therapy such as laser toning, IPL, fractional lasers, and chemical peels [57]. The parameters were spot size of 6 mm, 10 Hz, 2.1–2.5 J/cm^2 on PTP mode, and the end point was slight erythema. After laser toning, the so-called genesis technique was performed by using a long-pulsed 1064-nm Nd:YAG laser at 15–17 J/cm^2 at a spot size of 7 mm, 5 Hz and 0.3 ms. Ten laser toning was performed at weekly intervals. The results showed that the modified Melasma Area and Severity Index (mMASI) decreased from 10.48 ± 3.64 to 3.22 ± 1.45 2 months after completing the ten treatment sessions ($p < 0.001$). Twenty-four patients (80%) had physician's global assessment (PGA) grade 4 (76–100% improvement) and six patients (20%) had PGA grade 3 (51–75% improvement). All 30 patients had no signs of worsening of melasma or mottled hypopigmentation. After 1–3 years of follow-up, all 30 patients had no recurrence.

In this study, 30 patients showed improvement without any side effects, although the patients had aggravated melasma after previous therapy such as laser toning. Twelve patients (40% of all patients) who had mottled hypopigmentation due to other treatments had visual improvement of the mottled hypopigmentation area because of the reduction of the pigmentation area, which reduced the color difference between the pigmented area and the mottled hypopigmentation area.

Earlier in the Sect. 12.6.2 we reviewed that the therapeutic range of laser toning is very narrow. We also reviewed that even if the appropriate energy is found, it is still very dangerous. So, it is safer to use less than adequate energy because it is better to be less effective than to have side effects. This is why I think that a fluence of 2.1–2.5 J/cm^2 in PTP mode and 1–1.25 J/cm^2 in conventional mode is the golden parameter of melasma treatment.

12.6.7 Dermal and Mixed Type Melasma

Among the side effects of laser toning, nonresponse is 10–20%. There are many possible causes, but I believe that dermal and mixed type melasma are one of the reasons. What happens to the melasma on the dermis after laser toning? I was unable to find any paper regarding this, but in one book Kim's electron micrograph photograph and description could be seen [25]. Kim observed the destruction of a large number of melanosomes in the dermis after laser toning, and then the melanin disappeared by melanophages.

In other words, the process of breaking and disappearing of melanosomes by laser toning is similar to tattoo treatment. The macrophage devours the melanosomes and then disappears by lymphatic drainage. It is the same process as pigments disappearing from the dermis.

Two results can be predicted. First, the time it takes for the pigmentation in the dermis to disappear will be at least 1–3 months, the time for lymphatic drainage, as is the same for tattoos. It is also known that the number of treatments needed for tattoo removals is five times for amateur tattoos and 10–15 times for expert tattoos. Melasma is not as dark as tattoos, but it can be estimated that quite a long time will be needed for its removal. Second, melanosomes in the dermis may be present as melanosomes alone, but most are present in melanocytes or melanophages. To destroy the melanosomes in these cells the energy should be "energy that only damages cells without affecting surrounding cells." But as we reviewed in the subcellular selective photothermolysis, the energy we use for laser toning is "energy that breaks melanosomes without cell damage." Also, because the laser travels inward from outside of the skin, the photons decrease gradually as they enter the skin. Therefore, the energy used for laser toning can break the melanosomes of the epidermal melasma inside the cell, but it will not be able to destroy melanocytes or melanophages of the dermal melasma. Therefore, in order to treat dermal melasma the energy needs to be increased. However, this will result in the breakage of the cells in the epidermis, and cause side effects. Then how can we treat dermal melasma?

There are two ways to treat dermal pigmentations, such as tattoos (see Sect. 7.2.4 in "Chap. 7"). First, the tattoo particles are exploded by the Q-switched Nd:YAG laser and then the fibroblast that phagocytized the tattoo particle, melanocytes with melanosomes and melanophages are destroyed. Second, by fractional laser or pinhole therapy, tattoo particles or melanin are directly coagulated or vaporized and then discharged out of the skin through the microscopic epidermal necrotic debris (MEND), also known as the melanin shuttle. As explained earlier, the first method is problematic and the second method is also not recommended because melasma is sensitive to stimuli and may worsen if coagulated or vaporized with Er:Glass laser or CO_2 laser. More will be explained in detail in Sect. 12.9.3.

Then is there another method? There is a strategy, not a method. The strategy is to first remove the epidermal pigmentations and later remove the dermal pigmentations, i.e., perform the sequential procedure. Specifically, the melanosomes of the epidermis are first treated with laser toning, and as the epidermal melasma significantly improves, the dermal melasma may be treated by raising the energy. However, it is not clear how many times laser toning is needed for epidermal melasma. Also, laser toning cannot completely eliminate epidermal melasma and it is difficult to distinguish dermal melasma by eye. This is the reason why I do not yet have a clear standard for this.

Based on the above, my treatment plans for dermal and mixed type melasma are as follows. The first ten laser tonings are performed 1–2 weeks apart with an "energy level that can break melanosomes only without damaging cells," treating only epidermal melasma. The next 10–20 laser tonings are performed 1–2 months apart with an "energy level that damages only the targeted cells without causing damage to the surrounding cells" treating dermal and mixed type melasma. This treatment plan may completely improve dermal and complex melasma, but the recurrence of melasma cannot be prevented 100% and it also takes a very long time, so I do not have many cases.

12.6.8 Laser Toning Parameter Suggestion

Next, let's see if the seven parameters of conventional laser toning performed at the private practice are correct according to the principles of the laser (Table 12.9).

First, I believe that the use of the 1064 nm wavelength for laser toning is correct because of the epidermal bypass effect (see "Chap. 5"). The safe wavelength for the epidermis is 755 nm due to the low absorption coefficient, but I think 1064 nm with a lower absorption coefficient is the safest for melasma.

Second, although conventional parameters used the energy of 1.6–3.5 J/cm^2, I believe that lower energy is appropriate because the therapeutic range of laser toning is narrow and the therapeutic range may differ for each patient; 2.0–2.5 J/cm^2 in PTP mode or 1.0–1.25 J/cm^2 in conventional mode or lower fluence is recommended. For one-shot toning, I use a fluence less than 4 J/cm^2, specifically 3.0–3.5 J/cm^2.

Table 12.9 Comparisons between conventional laser toning parameters and my laser toning parameters

Parameter	Conventional laser toning parameters	My laser toning parameters
Laser	1064-nm Q-switched Nd:YAG laser	1064-nm Q-switched Nd:YAG laser
Fluence	1.6–3.5 J/cm^2	≤2.0–2.5 J/cm^2 (PTP mode) ≤3.0–3.5 J/cm^2 (one shot toning)
Spot size	6–8 mm	Largest spot, 4 mm (one-shot toning)
Pass, shot	Multiple passes, >1000 shots	≤1000 shots, one shot toning
Interval	1–2 weeks	≥2 weeks
Sessions	5–10 sessions	5/10 sessions
Clinical end point	Immediate perilesional erythema	Delayed perilesional erythema

Third, the conventional parameter uses a spot size of 6–8 mm, but a larger spot size may be used for a faster procedure. I use the largest spot size possible in that energy. Why should large spot sizes be used for laser toning? One of the principles of laser is that the larger the spot size, the deeper the optical penetration depth (OPD). Then are we using large spot sizes in laser toning to treat melanosomes in the dermis by deepening OPD? There are three factors involved in OPD (Table 1.8), namely spot size, wavelength, and power density. The most important of these is the wavelength (see Sect. 6.4 in "Chap. 6"). Most laser toning uses the 1064-nm Q-switched Nd:YAG lasers, so there is no need to worry about the OPD. If so, then why use the large spot size? The advantages of large spot sizes are not only deeper OPD but also shorter procedure time. If smaller spot sizes are used for the entire face, many shots and longer time would be needed. Also, because laser toning requires only low energy, large spot sizes are possible. I also use the largest spot size possible, rather than the 6–7 mm spot size of conventional laser toning.

Then what are the disadvantages of large spot sizes? To irradiate the entire face without omission, overlapping is inevitable. When the spot size becomes larger, there is more overlapping

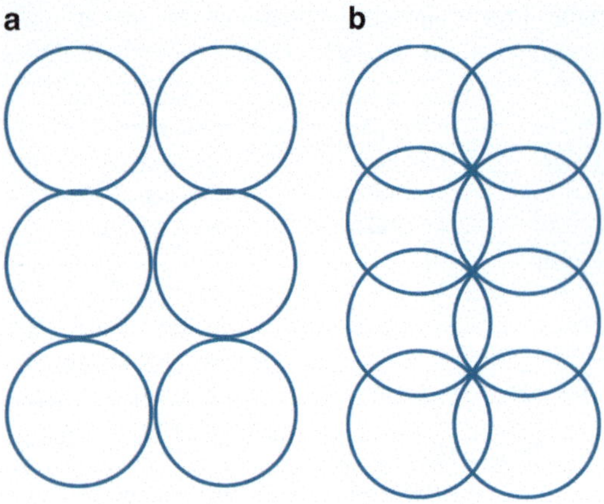

Fig. 12.19 (**a**) The spot is irradiated without overlapping. (**b**) The spot is overlapped to ensure that there is no missing area

area (Fig. 12.19). In the overlapping area, the energy may be accumulated. As multiple passes are performed, high energy can accumulate in certain areas, causing side effects, such as mottled hypopigmentation. So, when using a large spot size, multiple passes or shots should be avoided. Also, to irradiate only a small area, such as melasma or lentigo, smaller spot sizes should be used without overlapping. That is why during one shot toning, I use a smaller spot size of 4 mm without overlapping.

Fourth, the conventional parameter shoots more than 1000 shots by multiple passes at 10 Hz. But as we reviewed in the Sect. 12.6.5.3, many shots and multiple passes are not recommended. When performing conventional laser toning, I use less than 1000 shots and use one shot toning only on the lesion.

Fifth, the conventional parameter intervals are very short, usually 1–2 weeks. Also reviewed in the Sect. 12.6.5.3, a short interval is a risk factor, which is why I perform laser toning with an interval of more than 2 weeks.

Sixth, the conventional parameter treatment repetition is up to five to ten times. I recommend five times of laser toning per 10 treatment sessions, but after ten treatment sessions, I increase the interval of laser toning by 1–2 months.

Seventh, the conventional parameter considered the clinical end point as "perilesional erythema." But I think the clinical end point is "delayed perilesional erythema." As reviewed in subcellular selective photothermolysis, if it is an "energy level that can break melanosomes only without damaging cells," then why does erythema occur? There is no clear reason written in laser books as to why erythema occurs after laser. I consider the reason for erythema after laser as follows. First, in the case of millisecond long-pulsed lasers, residual heat remains and erythema occurs to compensate for this. In the case of nanosecond Q-switched lasers, erythema can occur because part of the energy is converted into heat. But most of the energy is used for photomechanical effect, so less erythema will occur. Second, erythema can occur because of inflammation. When the energy of the Q-switched laser is high and the cell wall is broken by the photomechanical effect, arachidonic acid is secreted and oxidized, and cytokines such as prostaglandin (PG) and leukotriene (LT) are secreted. These cytokines form erythema through capillary dilation and increased vascular permeability. Third, I think if the photomechanical effect breaks the cell wall and the basement membrane, and damages the vessel wall in the dermis, the vessel wall will expand in response. The second case is particularly problematic. Inflammation can lead to PIH, rather than ending with erythema and worsening melasma. Experience has shown that less PIH occurs if the erythema is not severe after laser treatment.

Based on the above, I think in an "energy level that can break melanosomes only without damaging cells" erythema should not occur. At least erythema that develops after some time, rather than immediately after the laser procedure, will be safer. This is why I regard the clinical end point of laser toning as "delayed perilesional erythema." On the contrary, "immediate perilesional erythema" is regarded as a "warning end point" meaning side effects.

Wattanakrai et al. enrolled 22 patients with melasma and performed laser toning and 2% HQ on one side of the face and 2% HQ only on the other side of the face. Fluence was 3.0–3.8 J/cm^2, and the clinical end point was either an immediate lightening of pigment or with mild erythema without petechiae [58]. The results showed that the side of the face treated with laser toning in combination with HQ had a higher improvement ($p < 0.001$), but three developed mottled hypopigmentation and four had rebound hyperpigmentation. After 12 weeks, all 22 patients had a recurrence of melasma. The clinical end point in this paper is worth noticing. Not only is the fluence of laser toning very high, but also the clinical end point is set incorrectly. In my personal experience, the immediate lightening of pigment or mild erythema suggests that the energy is too high.

12.7 Principle and Choice of Laser in Melasma Treatment

If we see melasma as a pigmentation, by the principle and strategy of the pigmentation lasers (see Sect. 7.8 in "Chap. 7"), I use the following treatment strategies for melasma.

Let's start by thinking about epidermal melasma treatment strategies. The competition tissue of the epidermal melasma is normal epidermal tissue. First, because of the horizontal relationship, selective photothermolysis is the main strategy. In the theory of selective photothermolysis, the wavelength is important. The epidermal bypass effect requires that the epidermal pigmentation laser use a laser of less than 800 nm. Lasers close to 800 nm are effective and safe. However, unlike the epidermal pigmentations, melasma is "active melanocytes" and have serious side effects. Therefore, a 1064-nm Nd:YAG laser with a much lower absorption coefficient is safer though not effective. This is why I first use a 1064-nm Q-switched Nd:YAG laser for laser toning. And for faster treatment of epidermal melasma, a 755-nm long-pulsed alexandrite laser is used. Long-pulsed lasers are used because the photothermal effect is safer than the photomechanical effect when considering the pulse duration. However, the fluence used in epidermal pigmentation may aggravate melasma, so the fluence should be lowered to 50% of the fluence used in epidermal pigmentation. Because the absorption coefficient changes with the concentration of the pigmentation, the energy should be adjusted so that the energy is "dark lesion weak, light lesion strong." The Q-switched laser has a fixed pulse duration, but when using the long-pulsed laser, longer pulse durations should be used first by thermal kinetic selectivity, and then the unresponsive lesions should be treated sequentially by using short pulse durations.

Second, epidermal cooling is not necessary. Since epidermal cooling lowers the temperature of both the normal tissue and the target tissue, the fluence must be increased for it to be effective. Therefore, cooling is meaningless when treating epidermal pigmentations.

Third, there is a fractional laser or pinhole method. However, CO_2 lasers or Er:YAG lasers should not be used because of the damage to the surrounding tissues due to vaporization. On the other hand, nonablative fractional lasers are considered safe because of their mechanism is coagulation. Nevertheless, I have concerns about the treatment of melasma with nonablative fractional lasers. This will be explained later in the Sect. 12.9.3.

Now let's think about dermal melasma treatment strategies. The competitive tissue of the dermis tissue is the normal epidermal tissue. Epidermal cooling may seem most important because it is a vertical relationship, but actually, epidermal cooling is of no use because of the use of Q-switched lasers in the treatment of dermal pigmentations.

According to the strategy, first, a laser of 800 nm or more should be used according to the theory of selective photothermolysis and the epidermal bypass effect. In order to target cells, a Q-switched laser using nanosecond should be used for the pulse duration. Thus, only the 1064-nm Q-switched Nd:YAG laser can be used. This is why I use Q-switched Nd:YAG lasers for dermal melasma. However, the energy should be increased because the dermal melanocytes or melanophages must be broken. For one-shot toning, the fluence is increased to 4–6 J/cm^2. Since ABNOM, the Nevus of Ota, and dermal melasma are present in separate cells, the "dark lesion weak, light lesion strong" energy theory is irrelevant.

Second, as mentioned earlier, epidermal cooling is meaningless.

Third, originally, dermal pigmentations require active use of fractional lasers or pinhole methods. But I do not recommend these treatment methods for ABNOM or dermal melasma. This will also be explained later in the Sect. 12.9.3.

Finally, lasers advance from the outside of the skin into the epidermis and the dermis, so it is advisable to first remove the epidermal lesions and then perform a stepwise procedure to treat the dermal lesions. Therefore, I first treat epidermal melasma and then increase the energy of 1064-nm Q-switched Nd:YAG laser to treat dermal melasma.

12.8 Issues in Recent Papers on Laser Treatment for Melasma

Many papers have been published that use lasers to treat melasma, but they have several problems. First, melasma occurs in various skin types and all races around the world, but most of the papers mainly contain studies on one or two skin types and one race. Second, various evaluation methods are used for each paper. For example, some papers use the melasma area severity index (MASI) and some papers use the modified melasma area severity index (mMASI). Therefore, a comparison between research papers is difficult. Also, there is no objective and accurate way of assessing melasma yet. Third, few papers are randomized controlled studies. Therefore, the objective result determination is difficult. Fourth, the biggest problem is that researchers do not know the principle of the laser and only use certain parameters, so even if the same laser is used, the results are different, i.e., it is effective in some papers but in some papers, only side effects occur. Therefore, we should look at papers on melasma treatment based on the principles of a laser.

A review paper summarized papers that used IPL to treat melasma [28]. Wang et al. (2004) compared 4% HQ (control group) and the combination of HQ and IPL (treatment group). Seventeen patients underwent IPL 4 times during 16 weeks. The results showed that the relative melanin index was decreased by 11.6% in the control group, while it decreased by 39.8% in the treatment group. The treatment group showed statistically significant improvement ($p < 0.05$). However, two patients developed PIH. Goldman et al. (2011) compared 56 patients, applied TCT including HQ and IPL on one side of the face (treatment side), and applied topical placebo and IPL on the other side (control side) of the face. After 10 weeks, 57% of the treatment side brightened or nearly brightened, but only 23% of the control side brightened. Figueiredo and Trancoso et al. (2012) compared 62 patients who received TCT with IPL and TCT only. After 6 months, the MASI score improved by 49.4% and remained at 44.9% at 12 months.

Based on the three studies above, we can conclude that "IPL has a moderate effect on melasma and may be an option in people who do not respond to topical medications. However, PIH can also occur, so caution must be taken." But there is no mention of parameters here. So, I searched all the papers for the specific parameters (Table 12.10).

Of the three papers, Wang et al. used the highest fluence. In general, a fluence of 15–20 J/cm^2 is used when treating epidermal pigmentations with a 560-nm filter. So although Wang et al. used the 570-nm filter, a fluence of 26–33 J/cm^2 is still very high. The clinical end point of IPL when treating epidermal pigmentations is usually "perilesional erythema," but in the paper by Wang et al. it was "graying of skin lesions," also implying that they used a higher power. Therefore, it can be estimated that this is the reason why PIH occurred, compared to the other two papers. If the fluence is not high and moderate, I believe that IPL can be used to treat melasma without any particular side effects. And even though IPL

Table 12.10 IPL parameters in three different studies

	Wang et al. [59]	Goldman et al. [60]	Figueiredo and Trancoso [61]
IPL	Vasculight, ESC/ Sharplan, Yokneam, Israel	Lumenis One, Lumenis, Santa Clara, CA	Limelight, Cutera, Brisbane, CA, USA
Cutoff filter	570 nm	560 nm	560 nm
Fluence	26–33 J/cm^2	14–18 J/cm^2	12–22 J
PD(delay) PD	3–4 (30–35) 4–5 (ms)	3–3.5 (10–30) 3–3.5 (ms)	
Second session	590–615 filters	Fluence 10% higher than the first IPL treatment	
End point	Mild perilesional erythema and graying of skin lesions	Mild darkening, without production of an erythematous footprint	Some mild, transient erythema, followed by a slight darkening
Treatment interval	4 sessions at 4-week intervals	At weeks 2 and 6	Single

may not be very effective it can still have moderate efficacy. However, I think it is safe to use less energy than the energy used to treat epidermal pigmentations because the problem of melasma is "active melanocytes."

12.9 Laser Treatment for Melasma

Next, we will review several papers about lasers that are known to be relatively effective in treating melasma.

12.9.1 Long-Pulsed Alexandrite Laser

Lee et al. used a long-pulsed 755-nm alexandrite laser to treat melasma [62]. The parameter of treatment was 60–80 J/cm^2 without a dynamic cooling device using a 15-mm spot size of the fractional handpiece, with a 0.5–1 ms pulse duration. One beam is 400 μm in size and 130 beams are irradiated. The fluence of 60 J/cm^2 in a 15-mm spot size of the fractional handpiece is equivalent to 9.5 J in energy. The clinical end point was "perilesional erythema and/or an ashy gray-colored microcrust formation." The results showed that the mean mMASI score improved 2 months after the final treatment and the patient self-assessment score was high. There was slight erythema, burning sensation, small microcrusts, but no special side effects. PIH developed in one patient but improved spontaneously after 2 months of follow-up.

This paper is about melasma treatment with a long-pulsed alexandrite laser. The results were relatively satisfactory. Since the epidermal pigmentation was treated, epidermal cooling was not performed, and the pulse duration was relatively short (0.5–1 ms). Since the thermal relaxation time (TRT) of the basal layer is known as 0.1–0.4 ms, I think it may be better to reduce it to 0.2 or 0.3 ms.

What is interesting about this paper is the use of fractional handpieces, I believe that using a fractional handpiece at the wavelength where the water is not a target and where scattering occurs is not suitable for fractional photothermolysis. Fractional photothermolysis does not irradiate the entire skin, but instead irradiates laser beams here and there and leaves normal tissue between the beams, reducing the side effects by quickly regenerating the necrotic tissues from normal surrounding tissues. However, in the wavelength at which scattering occurs, not only is the laser-irradiated where the beam is irradiated, but also absorption occur even in parts that are not irradiated due to scattering. This is why I believe that fractional handpiece at the wavelength at which scattering occurs is not suitable for fractional photothermolysis, but rather has the effect of only (1) lower energy, (2) smaller spot size and shallower penetration depth, and (3) strong energy may be irradiated where the laser is directly irradiated increasing the possibility of side effects.

In this paper, there is an interesting picture of a patient who had a history of mottled hypopigmentation due to laser toning in private practice, but the mottled hypopigmentation is improved as the skin pigmentations become uniform after the long-pulsed alexandrite laser. Hypopigmentation is still seen by Wood lamp, but after the pigmentation area improved, the overall improvement of the pigmentation of the face could be seen.

Cheng et al. performed a long-pulsed alexandrite laser four times at a monthly interval on 23 melasma patients [63]. The parameters were 0.2 5 ms, 8 mm spot size at 6–7 J/cm^2, and two to four passes were performed until mild erythema appeared. The mMASI scores decreased significantly and 10 patients (43.5%) described their improvement as marked and excellent (> 60% improvement). The treatments were well tolerated with only mild skin reaction with 83.7% complaining minor pain and two patients complaining severe pain. One patient had a blister that disappeared spontaneously within a week. One patient developed PIH after the first procedure and was excluded from the study.

This paper is also about melasma treatment with long-pulsed alexandrite laser. Similar to laser toning, the effect is relatively moderate, showing progressive improvement of melasma. The fluence was relatively low at 6–7 J/cm^2, but the energy is expected to be higher because of the overlap of two to four passes. The clinical end point is also mild erythema, suggesting that the energy that is used is similar to the energy used for epidermal pigmentation treatment. This paper, like the previous paper, also had one patient with PIH. Once again, I think it's better to irradiate only one shot for accuracy and lower the energy.

12.9.2 Nonablative Fractional Laser

The 1550-nm Er:Glass fractional laser was approved by the US FDA in 2005 for melasma treatment. However, in the case of lasers, US FDA approval does not always mean that the laser is safe and effective. There is a misconception about the US FDA approval: US FDA approval for drugs is very demanding, and US FDA approved drugs are safe, effective, and reliable. But US FDA approval for lasers is not as demanding as for drugs. The laser is approved by the FDA if it can prove its safety and its principles. Therefore, it should not be assumed that any laser that has been approved by the US FDA is always effective. Still, there are only two known lasers that are US FDA-approved lasers for melasma treatment: the 1550 nm-Er:Glass fractional laser (Fraxel. Solta medical) and the 1064-nm Q-switched Nd:YAG laser (Spectra, Lutronic Corp.) [28].

There are many papers about the 1550-nm nonablational fractional laser (NAFL) because it has been around for a long time [28]. Let's review some of these papers. Kroon et al. (2011) enrolled 20 patients and used TCT for 8 weeks (control group) and NAFL four times in an interval of 2 weeks (treatment group). Both groups showed similar improvement, but patient satisfaction was higher in the treatment group. Six months later, both groups had 50% recurrence, and there were no specific side effects except PIH. Therefore, the authors recommend the use of NAFL only in patients who are ineffective or cannot use topical whitening medications. Wind et al. (2010) compared the group treated with 1550-nm NAFL four to five times with the group using TCT. Both the evaluator and patient satisfaction were higher in the laser group, but PIH occurred in 31%. The authors of this paper presumed that the cause of PIH was higher than that of Kroon et al. (2011) because the fluence was increased from 10 to 15 mJ. Tourlaki et al. (2014) compared 1540-nm NAFL with TCT in 176 patients. After 1 month of treatment, 67.1% of patients showed improvement over 75%, and 21% of patients showed improvement of 51–75%. However, after 6 months only 21.1% of patients maintained an improvement of more than 75%.

Now we will review papers that used 1927-nm NAFL to treat melasma [28]. Polder and Bruce (2012) performed 1972-nm fractional laser three to four times at a monthly interval on 14 patients. The parameters were 10–20 mJ with a total density of 252–78 4MTZ/cm^2. Follow-up at 1, 3, and 6 months after treatment showed that the MASI scores improved 51%, 33%, and 34%, respectively. Lee et al. (2013) performed 1927-nm fractional laser on half of the face of 25 Oriental women, including eight melasma patients, three times at 3 weeks intervals. The parameters were 10 mJ with a density of level 3. The MASI score improved 5% for the half of the face that did not receive laser treatment, and 33% for the half of the face that received laser treatment, implying that laser treatment is effective for melasma treatment. Six months later, half of the face that did not receive laser treatment maintained the MASI score at 12%, while the half of the face that received laser treatment maintained at 28%. Niwa Massaki et al. (2013) retrospectively investigated 20 patients treated once with 1927-nm fractional laser. The parameters were 10–20 mJ/cm^2 with a 60–70% surface area coverage resulting in total energy of 1.72–4.42 kJ. One month after treatment, 4% HQ cream was used as maintenance therapy. The results showed more than 50% improvement in 60% of patients with just one treatment. The MASI score improved by 53.8%. But on an average of 10.2 months, 33.3% had a partial recurrence and 13% had a full recurrence. In addition, PIH occurred in two patients.

The overall evaluation of NAFL for the treatment of melasma is as follows [28].

First, the time of recurrence of melasma after NAFL is later than IPL or Q-switched lasers. IPL or Q-switched lasers recur within three months after the end of treatment, while NAFL recurs within 3–6 months. The reason for the late recurrence in NAFL may be related to the improvement of the dermis. Q-switched lasers and IPLs only treat epidermal pigmentations, but NAFL may also improve the dermis and result in rejuvenation, which may be helpful for melasma treatment. But even if we do not have NAFL, could we use another laser that helps rejuvenation in combination with IPL or Q-switched lasers? This is why after the laser toning, I use the Genesis technique with a 1064-nm long-pulsed Nd:YAG laser.

Second, similar to IPL, the number of treatments is about three to four times, less than that of Q-switched laser toning, which is performed about eight to ten times. In particular, the 1927-nm NAFL is more effective than other treatments with a single treatment.

Third, IPL or Q-switched lasers are recommended only for Fitzpatrick skin types I, II, and III, but NAFL may also be used for III and IV. I disagree with this, because IPL or Q-switched lasers may also be used on Fitzpatrick skin types III and IV if the energy is lowered. In fact, laser toning with Q-switched Nd:YAG lasers is used in skin types III, IV, and even V. So, this is only a general recommendation that has been used in the past. On the contrary, NAFL may also cause various side effects, including folliculitis, if the skin is sensitive regardless of the Fitzpatrick skin type.

12.9.3 Comments on Nonablative Fractional Laser

Because NAFL produces coagulation, and coagulation is a safe reaction, NAFLs have fewer side effects than other lasers. The occurrence of PIH with NAFL in the papers is probably due to high fluence. To reduce side effects and to be effective for rejuvenation, the parameters of NAFL should be "high fluence and low density." But in melasma, I think the fluence should also be lowered. Therefore, "low fluence and low density" should be used.

Nevertheless, I have some theoretical concerns about the treatment of melasma with NAFLs. First, a fractional laser with a wavelength of 1550 nm produces coagulation to the epidermis, basement membrane, and dermis, and the tissue is removed by microscopic epidermal necrotic debris (MEND). I am concerned that if the basement membrane coagulates and breaks, pigment incontinence may occur, resulting in the worsening of melasma [64].

Second, the fractional laser mechanism that improves melasma is to coagulate and discharge pigmentations, but if the parameter is set to low density for safety, melasma improvement will be insignificant and the number of treatments will increase. On the other hand, the advantage of the NAFL, which penetrates deep like 1550 nm is that it coagulates the deeper dermis, so the erythema that accompanies melasma is improved and dermal improvement effect can also be seen.

Third, in the case of 1927 nm, the absorption coefficient for water is high, so it is considered safer than 1550 nm because it does not penetrate deeply. But because the coagulation of the basement membrane is the same, I believe there is no difference in the outcome. Rather, because of the high absorption coefficient for water, a slight energy elevation may cause vaporization resulting in higher side effects. Therefore, lowering the fluence is more important in the 1927-nm laser than in the 1550-nm laser.

12.9.4 Vascular Laser

As there are vascular lesions in melasma, there is also a hypothesis that vascular treatment may be effective for melasma (Fig. 12.20). We will now review papers using a vascular laser to treat melasma.

Passeron et al. used TCT (Tri-Luma cream) once a day for 4 months in 18 white women with melasma [65]. The pulsed-dye laser treatment (PDL) treatment (V-beam; Candela Corporation) was started after 1 month of TCT applications. Three sessions of PDL were performed at 3-week interval on the half-face that was randomly assigned. The results showed that the efficacy was greater for the combination treatments. But only patients with Fitzpatrick skin type II and III were affected, and there was no difference in patients with skin type IV. Three patients who received PDL developed PIH, all of whom were Fitzpatrick skin type IV. Although this paper suggests that vascular lasers may be effective for melasma, PIH was developed in all patients with Fitzpatrick's skin type IV. This is why I think the use of PDL as a vascular laser seems inappropriate for melasma in Koreans. There are many Fitzpatrick skin types IV and V in Koreans. Other vascular lasers should be considered.

A 28-year-old woman, who was enrolled in the study above, visited 3 years later [66]. Examination showed that the left side treated only with TCT recurred, but the right side treated in combination with PDL did not recur (Fig. 12.21). RBX red subsurface analysis and

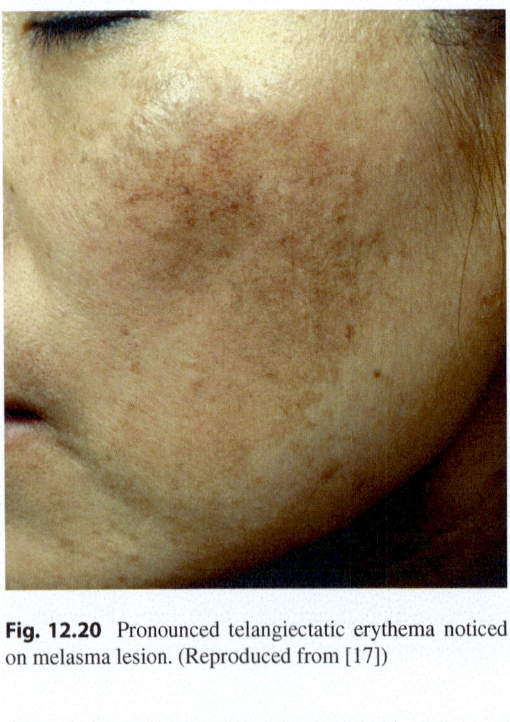

Fig. 12.20 Pronounced telangiectatic erythema noticed on melasma lesion. (Reproduced from [17])

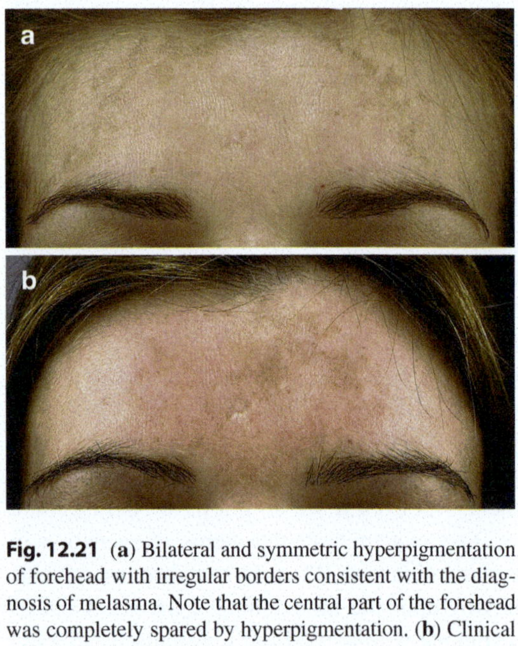

Fig. 12.21 (**a**) Bilateral and symmetric hyperpigmentation of forehead with irregular borders consistent with the diagnosis of melasma. Note that the central part of the forehead was completely spared by hyperpigmentation. (**b**) Clinical presentation of melasma for the same patient 3 years before treatment. Photograph was taken before any laser procedure, and a small scar in the middle of the forehead is not related to pulsed dye laser treatment. Present unaffected skin matched perfectly with localization of melasma observed before with a combination approach with Kligman's trio and PDL. (Reproduced from [66])

laser confocal microscopy revealed that blood vessels decreased in the right face treated with PDL. Thus, Passeron et al. thought that vascular treatment in melasma may prevent the recurrence of melasma.

Whether vascular lesions are the cause or effect of melasma is still controversial, but the paper above suggests that vascular therapy can help improve melasma and prevent a recurrence. However, due to the epidermal bypass effect, PDL, which is known as the best vascular laser, has a risk of PIH in Koreans due to its short wavelength. I think that the vascular laser with the longest wavelength, 1064-nm long-pulsed Nd:YAG laser is safer than PDL, and thus use the Genesis technique.

In addition to PDL, copper bromide laser is available as a vascular laser. Lee et al. performed copper bromide lasers on melasma patients [67]. The results showed that the mean MASI score decreased significantly after treatment. The values of L* reflecting the intensity of pigmentation increased, and the values of a* as the measurement of redness decreased after the treatments. Biopsy showed that Melan-A, which represents melanosomes, was decreased, and CD34 and endothelin-1, which represent vascular endothelial cells were decreased, and vascular endothelial growth factor (VEGF) was also decreased. However, there are studies contrary to the results of the paper above. Eimpunth et al. (2014) used copper bromide laser alone in melasma and Hammami Ghorbel et al. (2015) combined copper bromide laser and TCT in melasma, and both had no effect [28]. In other words, the effect of melasma treatment by copper bromide laser remains controversial.

12.9.5 Picolaser

With the recent release of picolasers (subnanosecond laser), interest in treating melasma using picolasers has increased. However, not many papers have been published yet.

Lee et al. performed picolaser in three patients, two patients with melasma, and one patient with PIH [68]. They were treated with a 755-nm alexandrite picolaser. All patients were Korean with skin type IV and no longer responding to Q-switched laser treatments. After the multiple treatment sessions, one patient reported fair improvement and two patients reported good improvement. Because this paper is a case report, it is difficult to conclude that picolasers are effective for melasma and PIH, but they do show the potential for melasma treatment. The biopsy results also show that picolasers treat pigmentations better and have fewer epidermal side effects than 532-nm Q-switched Nd:YAG lasers.

Lee et al. compared 755-nm picolasers and 1064-nm Q-switched Nd:YAG lasers for melasma treatment [69]. The right side of each patient's face received 755-nm picolaser, and the other side received 1064- nm Q-switched Nd:YAG laser. The clinical end point of both lasers was "mild erythema and swelling without petechiae." At the 3 months follow-up, greater clearance was observed at the 755-nm picolaser side compared to the 1064-nm Q-switched Nd:YAG side. This paper compares picolasers and Q-switched Nd:YAG lasers. However, it is not known whether the two lasers gave the same energy to the melanosomes. The clinical end points are the same, but the exact temperature is not known. Thus, it is too early to conclude that picolasers are more effective than Q-switched Nd:YAG lasers.

When considering laser-tissue reactions (see "Chap. 2"), I believe that the effects of both lasers are similar because both lasers break melanosomes. However, the side effects of the picolasers will be less than those of Q-switched Nd:YAG lasers. But this does not mean that picolasers do not have any side effects.

12.10 Combination Treatment

As mentioned earlier, there are various methods of treating melasma, but there is no effective single treatment. Therefore, several papers suggest that combination treatment is the best way to treat melasma, to which I also agree [5, 70].

But simply mixing all the effective methods may cause side effects due to overlapping procedures of the same mechanism. For example, peel-

Table 12.11 Strategy of treatment in melasma

Strategy of treatment in melasma
1. Decrease the activity of melanocyte
2. Inhibit melanosome formation
3. Promote melanosome degradation
A. Epidermal melanin removal
B. Dermal melanin removal

ing and long-pulsed alexandrite lasers both damage the epidermis and increase epidermal turnover, so side effects are more likely to occur when they are combined. Therefore, it would be ideal to classify treatments according to their mechanism and combine appropriate treatment methods without overlapping. The strategy of treatment in melasma may be divided into three types, considering the melanin production process. First, the activity of the melanocytes should be decreased. Second, melanosome formation should be inhibited. Third, melanosome degradation should be promoted (Table 12.11).

Most lasers do not inhibit melanin production like HQ, but they promote epidermal melanin removal similar to chemical peeling. Lasers used in pigmentation may selectively remove only the melasma pigmentation and not damage the surrounding tissues. In contrast, chemical peeling is nonspecific, damaging not only melasma but also surrounding tissue. I, therefore, believe that lasers are safer and more effective than chemical peeling in treating melasma.

12.11 Effective Therapy

Combining the above-mentioned presumed mechanisms of melasma, the principle of laser, and papers on the effects of melasma treatment, I believe that the following methods may be helpful in treating melasma (Table 12.12).

First, because we do not know 100% of the causes of melasma, we cannot treat melasma 100%. But if the patient takes birth control pills, switching them to low-dose estrogen contraceptives (e.g., Yaz®) may be helpful. Also, causative treatment such as avoiding chronic irritation (e.g., cosmetics) and thorough sun protection are most important for melasma treatment.

Table 12.12 Probable causes and effective therapy of melasma

Etiologies - genetics, hormone, UV, cosmetics, etc.
1. Epidermal barrier dysfunction—Moisturizer, iontophoresis
2. Basement membrane disruption—Superficial peeling (50% GA), genesis technique
3. Dermal inflammation—Nonablative rejuvenation, genesis technique, 'injectable glow'
4. Hyperpigmentation
1. Decrease the activity of melanocyte—Laser toning
2. Inhibit melanosome formation—Tranexamic acid, Vit C, glabridin
3. Promote melanosome degradation
I. Epidermal melanin removal—Laser toning, 755-nm long-pulsed laser
II. Dermal melanin removal—1064-nm Q-switched laser

Second, the damaged skin needs to be repaired. The epidermal layer will benefit from moisturizers and iontophoresis. The basement membrane will benefit from less irritating peeling such as 50% GA and genesis technique. To improve the dermal layer, nonablational lasers, Genesis technique, and intradermal injections of hyaluronic acid, also known as "injectable glow" may be helpful.

Third, to reduce the activity of melanocytes, laser toning is performed which has an effect of dendrectomy on melanocytes. Topical whitening medications to prevent melanin production may be helpful. Tranexamic acid, ascorbic acid (vitamin C), and glabridin are economical without side effects.

Finally, pigmentation that is already on the skin is regarded as the pigmentation itself and removed with a pigmentation laser. However, because the laser may worsen melasma, an appropriate laser with no side effects should be chosen, and the energy should be weak. I use laser toning and 755-nm long-pulsed alexandrite laser for epidermal melasma. Laser toning is performed on the whole face with a PTP mode of 2.1–2.5 J/cm^2, and then one-shot toning is performed at 4 J/cm^2 or less. In "Chap. 7" we reviewed that the safest laser for epidermal pigmentations is the long-pulsed alexandrite laser. The energy used for epidermal pigmentations in long-pulsed alexandrite lasers is usually 16–20 J/cm^2, but I use

8–10 J/cm^2, and I consider the clinical end point as delayed perilesional erythema which occurs usually when patients are finished with their face pack and ready to go home. Pigmentations that still persist even after prolonged epidermal melasma treatment or pigmentations that are gray or blue are considered dermal melasma and can be treated by 1064-nm Q-switched Nd:YAG laser by increasing the energy, similar to tattoo treatment.

12.12 Advices on Melasma Treatment

I have been treating melasma for more than a decade now and learned a lot through trial and error. The following is a list of advice that may be helpful to those who are new to melasma treatment.

First, when a melasma patient first visits, you should check what treatment has been attempted before. You should also ask if the treatment was effective or if there were any side effects. If there were no side effects and it was effective, and only the recurrence is the problem then the same procedure may be repeated. But if there were side effects, treatment changes should be considered. For example, if laser toning has been performed in the past and mottled hypopigmentation has occurred, then laser toning should not be attempted again, and it can be expected that it will not easily improve with conventional melasma treatment.

Second, you should not tell patients that melasma can be cured 100%. Despite all the melasma treatments, including behavioral therapy, medication, and laser treatment, melasma cannot be treated 100%. In addition, multiple repeated treatments are required. Recently I think that laser toning should be performed 20–30 times instead of 10 times when treating dermal melasma.

Third, the emphasis should not be on brightening the entire face, but on improving the dark pigmentation to match the overall face tone. This applies to all pigmentation treatments, including melasma. It is not easy to brighten the tone of the whole face. It is easier to make dark lentigines or melasma lighter, and this also has fewer side effects.

Fourth, combination treatments are needed. There are many causes and mechanisms of melasma, and there is no single treatment for melasma. However, as explained earlier, the underlying mechanism of each treatment should be considered so that the mechanism does not overlap.

Fifth, not everyone responds the same to each treatment. Some patients may develop side effects. Therefore, the patient should be carefully monitored whenever treatment is performed to see if there are any signs of improvement or side effects.

Sixth, melasma recur. Therefore, maintenance treatment should be prepared in advance. Prevention through behavioral therapy is also necessary, and sufficient consultation with the patient is needed in regard to dermal environment improvement and laser toning repetition.

References

1. Goldsmith LA, Katz SI, Gilchrest BA, Paller AS, Leffell DJ, Wolff K et al (2012) Fitzpatrick's dermatology in general medicine. McGraw-Hill Professional, New York
2. Jeong JY, Koo BS, Kim JH, Lee JD, Jang JM, Jung JW et al (2019) Melasma (Korean). MDworld, Seoul
3. Lee MH, Noh TK, Lee JH, Roh MR, Im Na J, Jung EC et al (2016) Clinicoepidemiological features of melasma in Korean patients at five university hospitals: a cross-sectional multicenter study. Korean J Dermatol 54(7):532–537
4. Kar HK, Gupta L, Chauhan A (2012) A comparative study on efficacy of high and low fluence Q-switched Nd:YAG laser and glycolic acid peel in melasma. Indian J Dermatol Venereol Leprol 78(2): 165–171
5. Rodrigues M, Pandya AG (2015) Melasma: clinical diagnosis and management options. Australas J Dermatol 56(3):151–163
6. Negishi K, Kushikata N, Tezuka Y, Takeuchi K, Miyamoto E, Wakamatsu S (2004) Study of the incidence and nature of "very subtle epidermal melasma" in relation to intense pulsed light treatment. Dermatol Surg 30(6):881–886. discussion 6
7. Lee WJ, Kim YJ, Noh TK, Chang SE (2013) Formation of new melasma lesions in the periorbital

area following high-fluence, 1064-nm, Q-switched Nd/YAG laser. J Cosmet Laser Ther 15(3):163–165
8. Kang S, Fitzpatrick TB (2019) Fitzpatrick's dermatology. McGraw-Hill Education, New York
9. Passeron T (2013) Melasma pathogenesis and influencing factors - an overview of the latest research. J Eur Acad Dermatol Venereol 27(Suppl 1):5–6
10. Kasai K (2007) Skin spots treatment clinics (Korean edition). Shinheung Med Science, Seoul
11. Grimes PE, Yamada N, Bhawan J (2005) Light microscopic, immunohistochemical, and ultrastructural alterations in patients with melasma. Am J Dermatopathol 27(2):96–101
12. Kang WH, Yoon KH, Lee ES, Kim J, Lee KB, Yim H et al (2002) Melasma: histopathological characteristics in 56 Korean patients. Br J Dermatol 146(2):228–237
13. Kang HY, Bahadoran P, Suzuki I, Zugaj D, Khemis A, Passeron T et al (2010) In vivo reflectance confocal microscopy detects pigmentary changes in melasma at a cellular level resolution. Exp Dermatol 19(8):e228–e233
14. Noh TK, Choi SJ, Chung BY, Kang JS, Lee JH, Lee MW et al (2014) Inflammatory features of melasma lesions in Asian skin. J Dermatol 41(9):788–794
15. Kang HY, Hwang JS, Lee JY, Ahn JH, Kim JY, Lee ES et al (2006) The dermal stem cell factor and c-kit are overexpressed in melasma. Br J Dermatol 154(6):1094–1099
16. Kim M, Kim SM, Kwon S, Park TJ, Kang HY (2019) Senescent fibroblasts in melasma pathophysiology. Exp Dermatol 28(6):719–722
17. Kim EH, Kim YC, Lee ES, Kang HY (2007) The vascular characteristics of melasma. J Dermatol Sci 46(2):111–116
18. Hernandez-Barrera R, Torres-Alvarez B, Castanedo-Cazares JP, Oros-Ovalle C, Moncada B (2008) Solar elastosis and presence of mast cells as key features in the pathogenesis of melasma. Clin Exp Dermatol 33(3):305–308
19. Kwon S, Park K (2014) Clues to the pathogenesis of melasma from its histologic findings. Pigment Disord 1(141):2
20. Kwon SH, Hwang YJ, Lee SK, Park KC (2016) Heterogeneous pathology of melasma and its clinical implications. Int J Mol Sci 17(6):824
21. Lee DJ, Lee J, Ha J, Park KC, Ortonne JP, Kang HY (2012) Defective barrier function in melasma skin. J Eur Acad Dermatol Venereol 26(12):1533–1537
22. Shin JH, Kang WH (2006) Two cases of melasma with unusual histopathologic findings. J Korean Med Sci 21(2):368–370
23. Torres-Alvarez B, Mesa-Garza IG, Castanedo-Cazares JP, Fuentes-Ahumada C, Oros-Ovalle C, Navarrete-Solis J et al (2011) Histochemical and immunohistochemical study in melasma: evidence of damage in the basal membrane. Am J Dermatopathol 33(3):291–295
24. Textbook compilation committee in Korean Dermatological Association (2014) Text book of dermatology, 6th edn. (Korean). Daehanuihak, Seoul
25. Committee C, SI C, Kim IH, Kang JS, Park SH, Chung KY et al (2016) Laser and light treatment in Asian skin. Koonja, Paju
26. Oluwatobi A, Ogbechie-Godec EN (2017) Melasma: an up-to-date comprehensive review. Dermatol Ther J 7(3):305–318
27. Ball Arefiev KL, Hantash BM (2012) Advances in the treatment of melasma: a review of the recent literature. Dermatol Surg 38(7 Pt 1):971–984
28. Trivedi MK, Yang FC, Cho BK (2017) A review of laser and light therapy in melasma. Int J Womens Dermatol 3(1):11–20
29. Rivas S, Pandya AG (2013) Treatment of melasma with topical agents, peels and lasers: an evidence-based review. Am J Clin Dermatol 14(5):359–376
30. Rendon M, Berneburg M, Arellano I, Picardo M (2006) Treatment of melasma. J Am Acad Dermatol 54(5 Suppl 2):S272–S281
31. Shankar K, Godse K, Aurangabadkar S, Lahiri K, Mysore V, Ganjoo A et al (2014) Evidence-based treatment for melasma: expert opinion and a review. Dermatol Ther (Heidelb) 4(2):165–186
32. Chan R, Park KC, Lee MH, Lee ES, Chang SE, Leow YH et al (2008) A randomized controlled trial of the efficacy and safety of a fixed triple combination (fluocinolone acetonide 0.01%, hydroquinone 4%, tretinoin 0.05%) compared with hydroquinone 4% cream in Asian patients with moderate to severe melasma. Br J Dermatol 159(3):697–703
33. Tse TW, Hui E (2013) Tranexamic acid: an important adjuvant in the treatment of melasma. J Cosmet Dermatol 12(1):57–66
34. Bala HR, Lee S, Wong C, Pandya AG, Rodrigues M (2018) Oral tranexamic acid for the treatment of melasma: a review. Dermatol Surg 44(6):814–825
35. Wu S, Shi H, Wu H, Yan S, Guo J, Sun Y et al (2012) Treatment of melasma with oral administration of tranexamic acid. Aesthet Plast Surg 36(4):964–970
36. Karn D, Kc S, Amatya A, Razouria EA, Timalsina M (2012) Oral tranexamic acid for the treatment of melasma. Kathmandu Univ Med J (KUMJ) 10(40):40–43
37. Tosti A, Grimes PE, Padova MP (2012) Color atlas of chemical peels. Springer-Verlag, Heidelberg: New York
38. Jeong JY (2010) Clinical skin care (Korean). Seoul, MDworld
39. Erbil H, Sezer E, Tastan B, Arca E, Kurumlu Z (2007) Efficacy and safety of serial glycolic acid peels and a topical regimen in the treatment of recalcitrant melasma. J Dermatol 34(1):25–30
40. Se YJ, Sung EC, Bak H, Choi JH, Kim I-H (2008) New melasma treatment by collimated low fluence Q-switched Nd: YAG laser. Korean J Dermatol 46(9):1163–1170

41. Kim JH, Kim H, Park HC, Kim IH (2010) Subcellular selective photothermolysis of melanosomes in adult zebrafish skin following 1064-nm Q-switched Nd:YAG laser irradiation. J Invest Dermatol 130(9):2333–2335
42. Kim JH, Jeong SY, Shin JB, Hc P, Kim IH (2008) Subcellular selective photothermolysis in zebrafish: an electron microscopic evidence after Q-switched Nd:YAG laser ablation. Korean J Dermatol 46(20):187
43. Mun JY, Jeong SY, Kim JH, Han SS, Kim IH (2011) A low fluence Q-switched Nd:YAG laser modifies the 3D structure of melanocyte and ultrastructure of melanosome by subcellular-selective photothermolysis. J Electron Microsc 60(1):11–18
44. Kim JE, Chang SE, Yeo UC, Haw S, Kim IH (2013) Histopathological study of the treatment of melasma lesions using a low-fluence Q-switched 1064-nm neodymium:yttrium-aluminium-garnet laser. Clin Exp Dermatol 38(2):167–171
45. Zhou X, Gold MH, Lu Z, Li Y (2011) Efficacy and safety of Q-switched 1,064-nm neodymium-doped yttrium aluminum garnet laser treatment of melasma. Dermatol Surg 37(7):962–970
46. Ryu HJ, Kim J (2013) A case of mottled hypopigmentation after low-fluence 1,064-nm Q-switched neodymium-doped yttrium aluminum garnet laser therapy. J Cosmet Laser Ther 15(5):290–292
47. Lee MC, Hu S, Chen MC, Shih YC, Huang YL, Lee SH (2009) Skin rejuvenation with 1,064-nm Q-switched Nd:YAG laser in Asian patients. Dermatol Surg 35(6):929–932
48. Kim MJ, Kim JS, Cho SB (2009) Punctate leucoderma after melasma treatment using 1064-nm Q-switched Nd:YAG laser with low pulse energy. J Eur Acad Dermatol Venereol 23(8):960–962
49. Gokalp H, Akkaya AD, Oram Y (2016) Long-term results in low-fluence 1064-nm Q-Switched Nd:YAG laser for melasma: is it effective? J Cosmet Dermatol 15(4):420–426
50. Kim T, Cho SB, Oh SH (2010) Punctate leucoderma after 1,064-nm Q-switched neodymium-doped yttrium aluminum garnet laser with low-fluence therapy: is it melanocytopenic or melanopenic? Dermatol Surg 36(11):1790–1791
51. Chan NP, Ho SG, Shek SY, Yeung CK, Chan HH (2010) A case series of facial depigmentation associated with low fluence Q-switched 1,064 nm Nd:YAG laser for skin rejuvenation and melasma. Lasers Surg Med 42(8):712–719
52. Wong Y, Lee SS, Goh CL (2015) Hypopigmentation induced by frequent low-fluence, large-spot-size QS Nd:YAG laser treatments. Ann Dermatol 27(6):751–755
53. Jang YH, Park JY, Park YJ, Kang HY (2015) Changes in melanin and melanocytes in mottled hypopigmentation after low-Fluence 1,064-nm Q-switched Nd:YAG laser treatment for melasma. Ann Dermatol 27(3):340–342
54. Tian B (2017) The Asian problem of frequent laser toning for melasma. J Clin Aesthet Dermatol 10(7):40–42
55. Kim HS, Jung HD, Kim HO, Lee JY, Park YM (2012) Punctate leucoderma after low-fluence 1,064-nm quality-switched neodymium-doped yttrium aluminum garnet laser therapy successfully managed using a 308-nm excimer laser. Dermatol Surg 38(5):821–823
56. Park SH, Yeo WC, Koh WS, Park JW, Noh NK, Yoon CS (2014) Laser dermatology plastic surgery, 2nd edn. (Korean). Koonja, Seoul
57. Choi CP, Yim SM, Seo SH, Ahn HH, Kye YC, Choi JE (2015) Retreatment using a dual mode of low-fluence Q-switched and long-pulse Nd:YAG laser in patients with melasma aggravation after previous therapy. J Cosmet Laser Ther 17(3):129–134
58. Wattanakrai P, Mornchan R, Eimpunth S (2010) Low-fluence Q-switched neodymium-doped yttrium aluminum garnet (1,064 nm) laser for the treatment of facial melasma in Asians. Dermatol Surg 36(1): 76–87
59. Wang CC, Hui CY, Sue YM, Wong WR, Hong HS (2004) Intense pulsed light for the treatment of refractory melasma in Asian persons. Dermatol Surg 30(9):1196–1200
60. Goldman MP, Gold MH, Palm MD, Colon LE, Preston N, Johnson LA et al (2011) Sequential treatment with triple combination cream and intense pulsed light is more efficacious than sequential treatment with an inactive (control) cream and intense pulsed light in patients with moderate to severe melasma. Dermatol Surg 37(2):224–233
61. Figueiredo Souza L, Trancoso SS (2012) Single-session intense pulsed light combined with stable fixed-dose triple combination topical therapy for the treatment of refractory melasma. Dermatol Ther 25(5):477–480
62. Lee MK, Min KS, Park EJ, Kim KH, Kim KJ (2016) A retrospective analysis of the treatment of melasma using a fractional long-pulsed alexandrite laser in Korean patients. Dermatol Surg 42(8):952–960
63. Cheng CY, Huang YL, Lee MC, Chang SL, Lin YF, Hu S (2017) Pulsed alexandrite laser for treatment of melasma in Asian patients. J Cosmet Laser Ther 19(4):210–214
64. Choi JR, Won CH, Oh ES, An J, Chang SE (2013) Does altered basement membrane of melasma lesion affect treatment outcome in Asian skin? Am J Dermatopathol 35(1):137–138
65. Passeron T, Fontas E, Kang HY, Bahadoran P, Lacour JP, Ortonne JP (2011) Melasma treatment with pulsed-dye laser and triple combination cream: a prospective, randomized, single-blind, split-face study. Arch Dermatol 147(9):1106–1108
66. Passeron T (2013) Long-lasting effect of vascular targeted therapy of melasma. J Am Acad Dermatol 69(3):e141–e142

67. Lee HI, Lim YY, Kim BJ, Kim MN, Min HJ, Hwang JH et al (2010) Clinicopathologic efficacy of copper bromide plus/yellow laser (578 nm with 511 nm) for treatment of melasma in Asian patients. Dermatol Surg 36(6):885–893
68. Lee YJ, Shin HJ, Noh TK, Choi KH, Chang SE (2017) Treatment of melasma and post-inflammatory hyperpigmentation by a picosecond 755-nm alexandrite laser in Asian patients. Ann Dermatol 29(6):779–781
69. Lee MC, Lin YF, Hu S, Huang YL, Chang SL, Cheng CY et al (2018) A split-face study: comparison of picosecond alexandrite laser and Q-switched Nd:YAG laser in the treatment of melasma in Asians. Lasers Med Sci 33(8):1733–1738
70. Li JY, Geddes ER, Robinson DM, Friedman PM (2016) A review of melasma treatment focusing on laser and light devices. Semin Cutan Med Surg 35(4):223–232

The manufacturer's authorised representative in the EU is Springer Nature Customer Service Centre GmbH, Europaplatz 3, 69115 Heidelberg, Germany. If you have any concerns regarding our products, please contact ProductSafety@springernature.com

Printed and bound by CPI Group (UK) Ltd, Croydon, CR0 4YY
30/09/2026
02225299-0014